D1553328

The American Way of Birth

Health, Society, and Policy

a series edited by Sheryl Ruzek

and Irving Kenneth Zola

The American Way of

B I R T H

Edited by Pamela S. Eakins

Temple University Press

Philadelphia

Temple University Press, Philadelphia 19122
Copyright © 1986 by Temple University. All rights reserved
Published 1986
Printed in the United States of America

The paper used in this publication meets the minimum requirements
of American National Standard for Information Sciences—
Permanence of Paper for Printed Library Materials, ANSI Z39.48-1984

Library of Congress Cataloging-in-Publication Data

The American way of birth.

(Health, society, and policy)
Includes bibliographies and index.
1. Childbirth—Social aspects.   2. Pregnancy—Social aspects.
3. Feminism.   4. Social change.   I. Eakins, Pamela S.   II. Series.
[DNLM: 1. Delivery.   2. Pregnancy. WQ 150 A5125]
RG652.A45   1986   304.6'3'0973   86-3803
ISBN 0-87722-432-3 (alk. paper)

To all our mothers, and all our daughters

Contents

PART II. The Conduct of Birth

PART III. Woman-Centered Birth

EPILOGUE

Acknowledgments

For the original impetus to compile this book, I would like to thank my children, Katherine and Taylor, because in giving birth to them, I first came to comprehend the importance of the subject.

I would like to thank my friends at The Birth Place whose insight helped bring this volume about especially Barbara Stern, Emmie Poling, Myra Gerson Gilfix, Cathy Sever, Susan Willis, Henci Goer, Suzanne Arms, Don Creevy, and Joe Hopkins.

For valuable comments, criticism, and support I thank my colleagues at the Center for Research on Women, especially Karen Skold, Wenda Brewster O'Reilly, Karen Offen, Marilyn Yalom, Edie Gelles, Harriet Blodgett, and Jane Novak.

For clarifying issues and turning my head in the right direction, I would like to thank Barbara Katz Rothman, Dorothy Wertz, and Nancy Stoller Shaw.

And finally, a thank-you to my editors, Sheryl Ruzek, Irving Zola, and Janet Francendese, for helping to focus the project, for keeping it on track, and for many words of encouragement.

Foreword

ANN OAKLEY

Over the past few decades, two social movements have contributed to a radical reappraisal of the ways in which different cultures stylize the conduct of birth. One movement is the new feminist scholarship, arising out of women's political protest against their oppression. This scholarship has taken childbearing out of its previous narrow institutional and intellectual enclosures and placed it instead in the more spacious setting of the dialectics of women's situation: production versus reproduction, personhood versus motherhood, individualism versus the altruism of love's losses and gains. The other social movement that has changed our awareness of what birth is, and can be, is the so-called consumer movement in health care.

Professionalized medicine, having had its undoubted successes in the preservation of human life, has entered a stage of crisis. In claiming exclusive jurisdiction over all matters pertaining to health and illness, the institution of professionalized medicine promised a paradise that cannot be created and at the same time threatened a hell that is, in some sense, already with us in the form of iatrogenic illness and mortality, and a disabling dependence on other people to remove from our lives, from the cradle to the grave, all disease and discomfort.

This therapeutic crisis of modern medicine is accompanied by the escalating costs of increasingly technologized forms of care. In countries with privately funded medical care systems, this cash crisis is in turn contributing to an escalation of inequalities between those who can buy medical care and those who cannot. In the case of childbirth, it is becoming doubtful whether the world can continue to afford the costs of professionalized medicine. Like other modes of radical awareness, this uncertainty is intrinsic to the very structure from which it escapes—in fighting spirit—from time to time. As socialism and feminism are ever-present possibilities created and maintained by patriarchal capitalism, so the critique of medicalized reproduction is perpetually generated and revitalized by the system itself.

Protest feeds off protest. Today's assertive health care consumers at times may be uneasy allies with the practitioners and theoreticians of feminism (and both may have their disagreements with the natural childbirth lobby); yet together they constitute a formidable mood of opposition against the obstetrical establishment. It is within this context that *The American Way of Birth* has emerged.

The two most salient questions of this book are:
1. How did we get where we are now? In other words, what is the origin of the (obstetrical) species?
2. Are the interests of all childbearing women the same? Or, what do women really want?

As far as the origin of the species is concerned, the rise of a birthing system in which (mostly male) obstetricians came to be "in charge" was clearly not a male conspiracy against women. It was not forced on women, nor did it happen by women's choice. It was not that women voluntarily chose to replace their untrained and supposedly dangerous "granny" midwives with more hygienic male manipulators. The new system did not replace a golden age of female-dominated childbirth management. That age was neither golden nor dark. In fact, in both United States and Great Britain, there is a good deal of evidence that the coming of man-midwives actually constituted a threat to the health of mothers and babies. This book presents the American data, the conclusions of which are supported by research in Great Britain as well. Margaret Versluysen (1981) has documented that while the dangers of eighteenth-century infant obstetric technology were many, the relocation of obstetric care to the hospital provided the degree of control over both reproduction and women that would-be obstetricians needed in their ascent to professionalized power.

But to talk of a coalition of interests between all doctors (or all midwives) is misleading. It is as unproductive as making the blanket statement that all women want the same thing, or that, conversely, women's real desires are a mystery (Riley, 1977). Yet within both feminist and consumer critiques of childbirth management the fallacy has crept in that, once medical mystifications have been peeled away, women will stand united on how they want childbirth to be. This is, of course, nonsense. In their capacity to become mothers women are theoretically—or symbolically—united. But in their social backgrounds and experiences they are as divided as anyone else. While it is debatable whether the classic sociological definition of social class is a variable in the debate over women's different and shared expectations of birth (Illsley, 1980), and while countless methodological traps lie in the path of those who seek to discover what patients want from medical care (Cartwright, 1983), it is nonetheless helpful to try to stratify by social group data on the attitudes and experiences of childbearing women. *The American Way of Birth*, in addressing these issues, begins to propel us out of the old unenlightening paradigms and into the illumination of new ones.

One paradigm of the first kind states that the target of study for medical sociologists, anthropologists, and others looking at birth is the officially provided services for maternity and infant care. A World Health Organization study group recently carried out a survey of perinatal care in Europe. During this exercise, the researchers discovered that many interesting and significant initiatives were happening outside the official services. In eight out of ten countries surveyed in Europe and North America, a well-developed network of alternative perinatal services was uncovered—ample evidence that the alternative developments charted in *The American Way of Birth* (from home births to lay midwives) are not at all exclusively American, but rather are part of an international mood of dissatisfaction with officially organized obstetric care (Houd and Oakley, 1983).

But any critique of the status quo in birth management is itself open to criticism unless it takes on the fundamental question of which factors shape good and bad pregnancy outcomes—however these are defined, which should naturally be as holistically as possible. The fact is that much of the twentieth-century improvement in obstetric mortality rates is the result of changes in the age and parity of the childbearing population, as well as long-term improvements in health affecting reproductive capacity (Macfarlane and Mugford, 1984). Even the final decline in the rate at which women died in childbirth that occurred in the mid-1930s is partly explained by such factors, and not wholly by the introduction of the sulfonamides in the treatment of puerperal fever (Oakley, 1984). Beyond these specifics, there is mounting evidence that social factors, especially stress, may profoundly affect a woman's chance of giving birth to a healthy baby. (Oakley, Macfarlane, and Chalmers, 1982). This kind of evidence is not overwhelmingly popular with obstetricians.

Perhaps being an obstetrician is like being a mother: it was Adrienne Rich (1980) who wondered whether the experience of motherhood was truly radicalizing or conservatizing. The answer is probably that it can go both ways. There are signs that the obstetrical establishment is changing. There are signs that women are becoming better able to recognize and articulate what they want. The most difficult task for both parties is to undo their reliance on what Thomas Szasz (1977) has called the theology of medicine.

Ultimately, there are no easy answers to the general problem of human suffering, especially with regard to the physical, psychological, social and metaphorical pangs of reproduction. This book systematically sorts through the issues surrounding the conduct of American birth, first through tracing the origin of modern obstetrics, second through describing the social relationships inherent in the American birth process, and third, through examining various avenues toward social change. It is only through a careful examination of the past and an analytical look at the present that we can begin to construct a future in which the pain of birthing, in all senses, is understood, acted on, and diminished.

REFERENCES

Cartwright, A. *Health Surveys: In Practice and in Potential.* London: King Edward's Hospital Fund, 1983.

Houd, S., and Oakley, Ann. *Alternative Perinatal Services in the European Region and North America: A Pilot Survey.* Copenhagen: World Health Organizations, 1983.

Illsley, Raymond. *Professional or Public Health? Sociology in Health and Medicine.* London: The Nuffield Provincial Hospitals Trust, 1980.

Macfarlane, A. J., and Mugford, M. *Birth Counts.* London: HMSO, 1984.

Oakley, Ann. *The Captured Womb: A History of Medical Care for Pregnant Women.* Oxford: Blackwells, 1984.

Oakley, Ann; Macfarlane, A.; and Chalmers, I. "Social Class, Stress and Reproduction." In *Disease and the Environment,* edited by A. R. Rees and H. Purcell. Chichester: John Wiley, 1982.

Rich, Adrienne. "Motherhood: The Contemporary Emergency and the Quantum Leap." In *On Lies, Secrets and Silence.* London: Virago, 1980.

Riley, E. D. M. " 'What Do Women Want?'—The Question of Choice in the Conduct of Labour." In *Benefits and Hazards of the New Obstetrics,* edited by T. Chard and M. Richards. London: Spastics International Medical Publications, 1977.

Szasz, Thomas. *The Theology of Medicine.* Baton Rouge: Louisiana State University Press, 1977.

Versluysen, Margaret. "Lying In Hospitals in Eighteenth Century London." In *Women, Health and Reproduction,* edited by H. Roberts. London: Routledge and Kegan Paul, 1981.

INTRODUCTION

The American Way of Birth

PAMELA S. EAKINS

Giving birth constitutes what anthropologists call a rite of passage: it is the point at which a critical and deeply personal life transition occurs from one stage to another, a transition that occurs when a life boundary—the moment that divides two stages of life—is crossed. In many cultures and for many women, giving birth becomes the bridge from childhood to adulthood.

But, as the poet Adrienne Rich points out, how women have given birth, who has helped them and for what reasons, are not simple questions of the history of midwifery and obstetrics. These are, rather, political questions. One does not give birth in a void, but rather in a cultural and political context. Laws, professional codes, religious sanctions, and ethnic traditions all affect women's choices in childbirth (Rich, 1976:117). Thus, the conduct of birth is culturally produced.

THE CULTURAL PRODUCTION OF CHILDBIRTH

How childbirth is culturally produced depends on the location in which the event is carried out, the suggested or mandated protocol or theory governing the action, the accepted instruments or tools, and the attitudes and behaviors of the participants in the birth setting.

For example, the act of giving birth necessarily takes place on someone's territory, and, from culture to culture, the territory on which childbirth takes place varies. It may be marked and separate from the women's normal sphere, and highly specialized—as it is in the United States—or it may occur within the realm of women's everyday life (Jordan, 1980). Whether specialized or ordinary, that territory is a sphere of control.

Robert Ardrey defines territory as an arena of space that "a group of animals defends as an exclusive preserve" (1966:3). In the animal kingdom, the challenger to territory is at a disadvantage and is nearly always defeated or expelled. The defender, states Ardrey, becomes imbued with a "mysterious flow of energy and resolve" to protect his home ground, while the intruder, eternally marked by inhibition, is handicapped by some innate deference to the other's right to the territory. Thus, not only is there a compulsion to defend territory, but there also seems to be an almost universal respect for concomitant rights to territory. So profound are these dynamics among territorial animals that it seems to be the case that all territorial species, including human beings, experience a universal recognition of such territorial rights (Ardrey, 1966).

This issue is central to women's experience of birth in America. Ninety percent of all American women will give birth, and 95 percent of them will do it within the hospital system. A woman giving birth in the United States enters hospital territory typically unfamiliar with its sights, sounds, and structures. She is only partially familiar with the medical world view, and therefore the very rules under which she is laboring. Conversely, her doctor, who understands, and even develops and changes the rules, is on home ground.

The rules of the game play a major role in the management of birth. In the United States, protocols for managing birth are highly specific. Conveyed in medical texts and hospital procedures manuals, they tell doctors how to screen pregnant women for risk factors and how to handle complications that arise during pregnancy, childbirth, and the postpartum period. Yet how does the medical establishment impose these protocols on the general public?

First, the importance of following medical protocol is communicated to the laity through advice columns, media interviews, professional-lay interactions, folktales, and so on. A popular household medical text states:

> Even during a normal, uneventful, and uncomplicated pregnancy, a doctor's advice is invaluable to the mother. He supervises her diet, the amount and kind of activity she can engage in, and many other aspects of her day-to-day life. . . . I feel that the best advice I can give you is this: as soon as you are fairly sure that you are pregnant, put yourself in the care of a well-trained obstetrician, and do what he, not your grandmother or a neighbor, says you should do (Miller, 1978:237).

Once a woman puts herself in the care of a medical professional, she will follow a standardized medical protocol. She will be treated primarily as a medical problem throughout pregnancy, birth, and the postpartum. She will be seen at standardized intervals throughout pregnancy wherein she will be processed routinely: blood pressure check, urine check, weight gain check, fetal growth check, fetal heart rate check, and so on. At birth, she will usually labor and deliver in a hospital obstetric ward that has been designed for organizational efficiency and the central availability of medical technology. Her labor, which will take place in bed in a standard-issue hospital gown, may be induced or augmented with pitocin, a drug that stimulates uterine contractions by means of intravenous infusion. The labor may be speeded further by amniotomy: artificially breaking the bag of waters. She will be without food or drink but will be kept hydrated intravenously. Her movements will be restricted by the intravenous needle and an electronic fetal heart monitor. She will often receive epidural analgesia: pain relief through a needle and catheter inserted into the lower back near the spine. She will probably receive an enema and may have her pubic area shaved more often than not, for delivery, she will be taken to a room with sterile surgical equipment, transferred to a narrow table, where she will lie supine with her legs secured in stirrups. She will be given an episiotomy: a surgical incision in the wall of the vagina to allow more room for the descent of the baby and to obviate uncontrolled tears. She will run a four out of ten chance that her baby will be delivered by instruments, either by forceps or a Cesarean section (Romalis, 1981; Jordan, 1980). An estimated 95 percent of American births follow this routine. Some researchers have stated that many women experience a deep-seated sense of loss and failure associated with the hospital birth experience (Seiden, 1978; Bromberg, 1981; Peterson and Mehl, 1977) but are unable to explain their feelings of alienation.

ALIENATION IN AMERICAN BIRTH

In 1957 the *Ladies Home Journal* ran a letter from a maternity nurse concerning "cruel" conditions in maternity wards. In response, the magazine received hundreds of letters testifying to "dehumanization and unconcern for mother and baby." Of the respondents, 93 percent reported negative experiences. One woman wrote:

> I have had three children and three different doctors who delivered my children at three different hospitals ... Women are herded like sheep through an obstetrical assembly line, are drugged and strapped on tables while their babies are forceps-delivered. Obstetricians today are businessmen who run baby factories. Modern painkillers and methods are used for the convenience of the doctor, not to spare the mother (as quoted in Wertz and Wertz, 1977:170).

Despite two decades of innovation in the management of hospital birth, a 1982 *Parents' Magazine* poll showed that 65 percent of its readers would "do it [their birth] differently next time." Of 64,000 respondents, 32 percent said that they wanted to use more prepared childbirth techniques; 30 percent wanted more discussion of their wishes with their doctor before the birth; 16 percent wanted a different doctor; 14 percent wanted no medication; and 8 percent wanted a different hospital (Yarrow, 1982).

Did the women who wrote to the *Ladies Home Journal* in 1957 and the women who completed the *Parents Magazine* survey in 1982 represent only those who were dissatisfied? What about the millions of satisfied American women who did not respond?

Unfortunately, those women who may be satisfied with their birth experiences are not speaking out. In fact, we hear few women speak in defense of the roles, rules, and rituals surrounding medicalized birth. Why? What does it mean to women to give birth in the contemporary American medical system?

MEDICALIZING CHILDBIRTH

An aspect of life that comes to be viewed as a medical event—that is, when it comes under the jurisdiction of medical professionals who are charged by society to prevent disease, relieve pain, and improve and preserve health—is said to have been "medicalized."

Medicalization implies that disease has been discovered. In every culture, the medical structure determines how signs and symptoms come to be labeled as disease and diagnoses and treats what comes to be defined as disease. In every culture, the medical structure establishes: (1) a definition of disease; (2) prescribed roles for "professionals" and "patients"; (3) where the diagnosis and treatment of disease will occur; (4) a particular set of methods and tools by which diagnoses are made and treatments rendered.

By accepting common definitions and a common style of practice, medical professionals can arrive at a consistent view of reality that fosters the development of consistent conclusions—in short, an "expert" definition of the situation. An expert definition of the situation requires that baselines be established. An "ideal" type of physiological behavior is articulated, and deviations from that course are described.

In American culture, disease is viewed as any deviation, obvious or latent, from what is believed to be the normal or average condition in appearance, structure, or function of an organ, a group of organs, or the body as a whole. It follows that pregnancy, defined as a *potentially* pathological deviation from the normal or average condition of the female body, comes logically under the jurisdiction of obstetrics, that branch of medicine dealing with the care of the mother from the time of conception until the maternal organs of reproduction have returned to their pregravid (prepregnant) state.

The American medical profession has defined an ideal course of pregnancy and birth in great detail and has developed increasingly technical—and thus increasingly "professionalized"—methods by which to keep pregnancies and births on this "ideal" track. When medical professionals specify what constitutes deviation from the ideal course and offer remedies—just as they have been socially charged to do—the laity is relieved of responsibility. The locus of decision making passes from the layperson to the expert.

Within the framework of this system, the public accords medical professionals the power both to define and to take action. As a special interest group, medical professionals define normality and pathology in childbirth through the cumulative representation of medical "facts," which, taken together, constitute the medical standard of the day. The birth event is consequently structured according to the definition of normality and pathology that has thus been arrived at: standards for treatment are instituted.

Regarding the medical standard of the day, it becomes apparent that undergirding medical definitions and medical treatments is a medical world view, a commonly accepted set of assumptions about the way things work. Even though the set of assumptions changes from time to time,[1] this world view is commonly accepted, and so it must be if we are to entrust our health to experts. The medical world view is so pervasive that it is invisible and generally taken for granted. Unless it is challenged, its presence goes unseen. "A worldview is like air. We don't notice it unless there is something wrong with it—if we breathe it and it seems polluted."

Medical professionals are thus invested with the right, and therefore the power, to make decisions; the laity maintains the right to expect that decisions will be made responsibly. It becomes, in fact, the duty of the medical profession to render decisions responsibly, and should this obligation be defaulted through negligence or some other deficiency, severe social sanctions, in the form of claims and lawsuits, are invoked.

We thus give medical professionals—those with the narrowest, most circumscribed, and most specialized definition of childbirth, one that places the preservation of physical health

---

[1]For an excellent discussion of the current controversy surrounding the electronic fetal heart monitor, for example, see Myra Gerson Gilfix, "Electronic Fetal Monitoring: Physician Liability and Informed Consent," *American Journal of Law and Medicine* 10(1984):31-90.

as the single most important measure of the outcome—*the sole right to err*.[2] Our judgment concerning whether or not a mistake has been made in the management of a childbirth case depends on the medical standard of the day. We ask: was everything within our (medical) power done for the baby/mother? Was anything (medical) that might have been done, not done? In asking whether a doctor acted responsibly, we are essentially asking: Did the doctor make decisions and act according to the dominant beliefs of the medical profession? Did the doctor act responsibly in accordance with the medical standard of care?

In American hospitals, the procedures of operation are devised and controlled to such an extent that "natural birth"—uncomplicated childbirth taking place with little medical intervention in accordance with the mother's wishes—is seen as anomalous. Even the idea of natural birth has been standardized. For example, in the 1978 volume *Psychological Aspects of Gynecology and Obstetrics*, Dr. Heinz Luschinsky recommends the following procedures for attending natural birth:

If the patient, in early labor, arrives at the hospital late in the evening and lives too far away to be sent home, she should be kept in the hospital. Since she will be in a strange environment, heavy sedation should be given. "At this point," says Dr. Luschinsky, "I like to give 12.5 mg. morphine, 50 mg. Librium, and possibly 100 mg. Nembutal, with instructions not to disturb her if she is asleep."

As the labor progresses, he recommends that "the patient should be emotionally supported...with staff encouragement." If drugs are needed, they should be no more than 100 milligrams of Demerol and 25 milligrams of Librium at approximately 4 centimeters' diliation. And he advises that when the labor gets "stormy," an epidural may be administered. If an epidural is not given, and the patient becomes "angry, uncooperative and combative...50 mg. Demerol may be given intravenously, but the physician should be prepared to counteract its influence at birth by administering Narcan, [a drug that reverses respiratory depression in newborns]."

[2]Sociologist Barbara Katz Rothman gave an excellent presentation on this subject at the conference on "Technological Approaches to Obstetrics: Benefits, Risks, Alternatives IV," October 18–19, 1984, San Francisco, CA.

In other words, the act of keeping the mother subdued—controlling her behavior—may actually inhibit the baby's ability to breathe at birth. And it raises a fundamental question: Who defines what constitutes appropriate birthing behavior?

ROLES IN THE BIRTH PROCESS

When an aspect of life, such as pregnancy and birth, becomes medicalized, medical professionals acquire the power to officially "excuse" the pregnant/birthing woman from her typical social obligations (such as work or school) by giving her the official label of patient. In the role of patient, she must behave in a socially acceptable way *for a sick person* if she is to be exempted from her normal responsibilities. She must be seen as unable to pull herself together; she must come across as incapacitated (Parsons, 1951). (In fact, if she desires to be legitimately and officially excused—as recognized by Medicaid, employment benefits, insurance carriers, and so on—she must report to a doctor and voluntarily commit herself to treatment.)

In this culture, pregnancy is defined as a "transitional" sickness, a status that temporarily excuses a sick person from social obligations (Mechanic, 1968). However, pregnant women typically are expected to fulfill as many of their social obligations as they can because pregnancy and birth are only deviations from a woman's "normal" condition and are, after all, "normal" physiological functions. Our culture has difficulty defining how pregnant women ought to behave as patients because we have not yet come to terms with what women's most important social obligations ought to be vis-à-vis bearing children. Are such women sick, or not? Are they incapacitated, or not? Should pregnant women be excused from work? With what benefits? For how long?

As a patient, the pregnant woman turns the management of her pregnancy over to medical professionals, and decision making passes from her private sphere into the sphere of medical jurisdiction. This shift in the nature of the interaction and in the relative power of the pregnant woman occurs along with the *shift in the allocation of responsibility for the outcome.* The physician acts on his or her territory according to medical protocols, accepting the responsibility for the health and welfare of the patient, while the woman, as patient, relinquishes relative decision-making power to the professional in exchange for relative freedom from responsibility. The pregnant woman, concerned first and foremost with her baby's life and health, places decision-making power in the hands of those believed to be most qualified to render opinions: those who have been professionally trained and socially sanctioned to handle such matters.

As knowledge becomes power for a physician, the pregnant woman experiences a concomitant loss of power. As one woman stated:

> The doctor talked to me in terms of its being *his* birth. I was going to go in and he was going to take care of everything. The doctor said "Sweetheart, you just have to have the baby, that's all you have to do. I'm going to do the rest."

The patient, as an "alien," has little command over resources on the medical site because such access comes with command of domain. This lack of power affects both the way she is viewed by the medical system and the society at large, and the way she views herself.

Becoming a patient involves a change in social and moral status. Socially, the patient, particularly the hospitalized patient, holds a position in the hierarchy of the medical system, and that place is most likely in the lower rungs. Further, the patient's status in the medical setting will, in part, be determined by her location within the larger social structure. What race is she? How old is she? Is she married? Is she wealthy?

All of these factors affect how the patient will be judged and ultimately treated by the medical system, and if the behavior of a laboring woman does not conform to hospital routine, there will be repercussions (Danziger, 1978). One study has shown, for example, that when private obstetrical patients (those with more money or those with insurance) lose control, they are reassured by their doctors, but when institutional obstetrical patients (those who rely on "charity") lose control, they are reprimanded, they may even be strapped down (Scully, 1980).

Turning control over to medical professionals constitutes

socially acceptable behavior (Rothman, 1982:18). It is a simple case of "doctor knows best." If I do not follow "doctor's orders," I have only myself to blame for a negative outcome. If the doctor makes a mistake, I may, in good conscience, sue, in which case the responsibility for compensation moves into the hands of insurance companies, and, as a last resort, into the judicial system.[3] Our social structures—that is to say, the medical and legal systems—dictate our socially appropriate roles. How we ought to behave, and where the responsibility lies, is no mystery, although in some cases it may take a court proceeding to clear up clouded details. In this way, the formal definition of what is considered to be socially appropriate behavior becomes ever more refined.

The power relationship is clear. Medical professionals, through ownership and exclusive control over highly specialized knowledge—knowledge that is highly valued—acquire the ability both to define and to manage the situation. If the woman is not at a disadvantage on the basis of her sex, class, or race, she will be at a disadvantage territorially. She will be at a disadvantage because of her lack of knowledge. She will experience a loss of rights as a patient because she will be considered incapable of assessing her own physical status and incapable of making decisions regarding her own care.

SATISFACTION WITH THE BIRTH EXPERIENCE

Recent studies in medicine and social science suggest that women's satisfaction with the birth experience significantly affects their level of self-esteem as well as the character of their relationships with their children. The research suggests that the three most important factors determining the quality of the birth experience for the mother are control, awareness, and support (Entwisle and Doering, 1981). If these three factors are present in a hospital environment, it is likely that the hospital has allowed the woman to control her circumstances, that the hospital has allowed her to remain unanesthetized, that the hospital has allowed her to surround herself with

---

[3]Lawsuits are also brought in cases of "maloccurrence," that is, when there is a negative medical outcome (e.g., a damaged baby) and an award by the court may constitute the only possibility for paying costly medical bills.

support people. And, to quote psychiatrist R. D. Laing, *"To allow is to exercise as much, if not more power, than to forbid"* (italics added, Laing, n.d.).

The way we "do" birth in America affects women's self image, the way identity, ability and worth are conceptualized. The individual woman, after giving birth, stands in judgement of herself, of her attitudes and behavior. She judges herself as she is judged by others.

Does this mean that women are, or should be, at war with their doctors? It does not have to. With the increasing centralization of the medical model has come an increase in the mechanized/technological approach to birth. The promise of technology has been followed by rising expectations, on the part of parents, for a perfect outcome. Expectations for a perfect outcome in turn have led to the practice of "defensive" medicine; when the outcome of birth is not perfect, doctors and hospitals realistically face the threat of being sued.

Combining high expectations with defensive medicine can lead to a breakdown in communication, along with a sense of distrust, between doctor and patient. Legal experts maintain that lawsuits are more likely to occur when a communication breakdown occurs, especially when the patient feels her own needs or desires have not been taken into account or respected. These needs and desires, may, on a deep level, include the woman's longing for the acknowledgment that she is moving through a profound psychological, social, and spiritual transformation.

The medical profession asks women: "What do you want: a healthy baby or a good experience?" Women of all races, creeds, colors, classes, and nationalities want both. Furthermore, having a healthy baby does not preclude the possibility of giving birth in a setting in which the profundity of bringing forth a new generation is recognized and honored as central to women's experience. In fact, juxtaposing "healthy baby" with "good experience" is like juxtaposing apples and oranges. The two are not mutually exclusive, nor are they even comparable.

How can we break the negative cycle in which women feel alienated from their birth experience? One radical approach would be to move the doctor-patient relationship to a new level of trust and caring in which the world view of each party is understood and respected. For the short term, however, we can expect American childbirth to become increasingly technical and that, concurrently, there will be a growing movement toward "humanization." What is needed to solve the incongruities in these apparently divergent trends is a new vision: one that combines excellent outcomes with a truly woman-centered experience.

Feminist scholars, by examining how the structural relations of birth have emerged and how they are maintained, have begun to illuminate some pathways to positive change.

THE FEMINIST STUDY OF CHILDBIRTH

The study of childbirth is a relatively new endeavor in the social sciences, emerging in the past decade largely because of feminist scholarship that places women at the center of their own experience. Beginning with women's experience, rather than taking gender as an isolated variable, has dramatic analytical consequences. It has the potential, for example, to challenge the basic assumptions and conceptual frameworks of social science. In understanding stages of the life cycle, for example, feminist research starts with women's experience rather than looking at the male life cycle and then fitting women in as a subset.

In this context of feminist thought, *The American Way of Birth* was born. Every contributor to this volume writes in the spirit of Adrienne Rich's words:

> We need to imagine a world in which every woman is the presiding genius of her own body. In such a world women will truly create new life, bringing forth not only children (if and as we choose) but the visions, and the thinking, necessary to sustain, console, and alter human existence—a new relationship to the universe (1976:292).

REFERENCES

Ardrey, Robert. *The Territorial Imperative.* New York: Atheneum, 1966.
Bromberg, Joann. "Having a Baby: A Story Essay." In *Childbirth: Alternatives to Medical Control,* edited by Shelly Romalis. Austin: University of Texas Press, 1981.

Danziger, Sandra K. "The Uses of Expertise in Doctor-Patient Encounters During Pregnancy." *Social Science and Medicine* 12 (1978):359-367.

Entwisle, Doris R., and Doering, Susan G. *The First Birth: A Family Turning Point.* Baltimore: The Johns Hopkins University Press, 1981.

Jordan, Brigitte. *Birth in Four Cultures.* Montreal: Eden Press, Women's Publications, 1980.

Laing, R. D. "The Politics of Birth." In *Active Birth.* Epson, England, n.d.

Luschinsky, Heinz. "Natural Childbirth." In *Psychological Aspects of Gynecology and Obstetrics,* edited by Benjamin B. Woman. Oradell, N.J.: Medical Economics Company, Book Division, 1978.

Mechanic, David. *Medical Sociology: A Selective View.* New York: Free Press, 1968.

Miller, Benjamin E. *The Complete Medical Guide.* New York: Simon and Schuster, 1978.

Parsons, Talcott. *The Social System.* Glencoe, Ill.: The Free Press, 1951.

Peterson, Gail H., and Mehl, Lewis E. "Studies of Psychological Outcome for Various Childbirth Alternatives." In *21st Century Obstetrics Now:* Vol. 1, edited by Lee Stewart and David Stewart. Marble Hill, Mo.: NAPSAC, 1977.

Rich, Adrienne. *Of Woman Born.* New York: W. W. Norton, 1976.

Romalis, Shelly, ed. *Childbirth: Alternatives to Medical Control.* Austin: University of Texas Press, 1981.

Rothman, Barbara Katz. *In Labor: Women and Power in the Birthplace.* New York and London: W. W. Norton, 1982.

Scully, Diana. "How Residents Learn to Talk Women into Unnecessary Surgery." *MS Magazine* 8 (May 1980):89-93.

Seiden, Anne M. "The Sense of Mastery in the Childbirth Experience." In *The Woman Patient,* edited by M. T. Notman and C. C. Nadelson. New York: Plenum Press, 1978.

Wertz, Richard W., and Wertz, Dorothy C. *Lying-In: A History of Childbirth in America.* New York: The Free Press, 1977.

Yarrow, Leah. "When My Baby Was Born." *Parents' Magazine* (August 1982).

PART I
The Medicalization of Birth

The development of American obstetrics is generally seen as part of a rational trend toward more scientific and safer medical practices that began during the Age of Enlightenment. The eighteenth century, a period characterized by surging technology and a new faith in science, witnessed great advances in the understanding of the human body and, not coincidentally, a decline in the predominant religious viewpoint held by the American Puritans in the seventeenth century. In the Age of Enlightenment, says historian Eugen Weber, "The general laws of nature of the seventeenth century were brought to bear not only on the world as it was, but as it could be made to be: man could manipulate them for his benefit. He need not only admire his world—he could master and remake it" (1972:221). Similarly, women no longer had to perceive the outcome of birth as solely in the hands of God. Eighteenth century Americans were ready to experiment with new medical techniques (Wertz and Wertz, 1977) and welcomed doctors freshly trained in Europe into the American birthplace.

Nevertheless, the "scientific" birth did not arise entirely from a dispassionate interest in improving maternal and child health outcomes; medicalization was as much a political and economic as a scientific process. In Chapter 1, Nancy Schrom Dye shows that medicalized birth was carefully differentiated from the traditions of "social childbirth," in which all women had community responsibilities for attending friends and neighbors in birth; doctors had to claim superior knowledge of anatomy and physiology and a superior method of practice. These claims were then systematically marketed to the public. The doctors had to convince the public that the knowledge they possessed was not only important but also necessary, and they had to eliminate rival practitioners. Midwives presented an obstacle to both establishing professional status and attracting practitioners. The role of midwives had to be undermined so that attending at birth could be seen as necessitating specialized knowledge and skill, and so that the doctors would have access to the low-income women (traditionally attended by midwives) for teaching obstetric techniques to new practitioners.

In short, obstetrics had to become a profession. A professional must have a full-time occupation, a commitment to a calling, a formalized organization, an education of exceptional duration, a service orientation, and autonomy. Becoming part of a profession involved becoming set apart from the laity through the establishment of rules of competence, conscientious performance, and loyalty. Further, it had to recognize common occupational interests, maintain control over standards of performance, and control access to the occupation (Moore, 1970). During the nineteenth century, doctors were engaged in all these areas, and redefining birth as a pathological event (one requiring the intervention of an expert) helped set obstetrics apart as a medical profession. Male midwives and the new doctors, focusing on birth complications, experimented with a variety of instruments: "perforators" to evacuate the contents of the fetal skull to reduce head size to allow passage through the pelvis; hooks and cutting instruments to dissect and extract fetal pieces; obstetrical forceps, and other "mechanical improvements." And, as Diana Scully points out in Chapter 2, the more surgery and instruments were used, the more necessary they became. As attending at birth became increasingly specialized, and as more doctors became available, every woman's labor came to be defined as potentially pathogenic—that is, every labor carried within it the possibility of surgery. Eventually, in fact, *not* having surgical capability in American childbirth would come to be seen as virtually criminal, both figuratively and literally.

Redefining childbirth in this way was decidedly controversial. Scully details the debate that arose over increased intervention in childbirth. Although some observers said that the new male birth attendants were actually increasing, rather than alleviating, suffering and dangers to childbearing women, increased intervention became the norm within a few decades. Scully shows how Dr. J. Marion Sims and the New York Women's Hospital, which Sims founded in 1856, introduced aggressive surgery as the first, rather than the last, measure in solving reproductive problems. Solving the "midwife problem" and solidifying the practice of aggressive obstetrics were accomplished, in part, by establishing large hospital-medical school complexes and formal professional organizations. By the second half of the nineteenth century, obstetrics had solidified into a true profession.

The intervention of scientists and physicians was supposed to decrease maternal mortality, along with death rates in general, but, as Janet Carlisle Bogdan informs us in Chapter 3, the rates remained artificially high as a direct result of septic death associated with aggressive intervention and hospital birth. (The problems created by medical intervention in childbirth, such as an increased risk of infection, would not be alleviated until the late 1930s, when antibiotics were introduced.) Doctors had created a new form of practice that "scientifically" diagnosed and treated the problems of childbirth. Whether or not this practice reduced mortality in the nineteenth century was not as important as the belief that it did.

In less than a century, the conduct of birth had been completely revised. Childbirth, which for many centuries had been the exclusive domain of women, now took place on medical territory. To give birth to their babies, women entered a hospital bureaucracy, complete with institutionalized routines and protocols, in which all aspects of labor and delivery were now under the management of a medical (and male-dominated) professional.

REFERENCES

Moore, Wilbert E. *The Professions: Roles and Rules.* New York: Russell Sage Foundation, 1970.

Weber, Eugen. *Europe Since 1715: A Modern History.* New York: W. W. Norton, 1972.

Wertz, Richard W., and Wertz, Dorothy C. *Lying-In: A History of Childbirth in America.* New York: The Free Press, 1977.

1

The Medicalization of Birth

NANCY SCHROM DYE

Giving birth has always fascinated us. No other experience involves the intersection of biology and culture and the union of nature and art that birth entails. At once a biological process and a cultural event, childbirth has been shaped and defined by attitudes toward women, toward medical knowledge and authority, and toward nature itself. We live in a society in which giving birth is defined as a medical event, requiring the supervision and expertise of a physician. But birth has not always been so defined. Indeed, the central question of childbirth history in America has become: How did the management of birth, for centuries indisputably the province of women, become a medical event, controlled and managed by physicians?

Scholars (Leavitt, 1983; Wertz and Wertz, 1977) have identified three distinct periods in the history of American childbirth. The years from the early seventeenth century through the mid-eighteenth centuries marked an era characterized by what Dorothy and Richard Wertz have aptly called "social childbirth," during which all women had community responsibilities for attending friends and neighbors in birth. The second era in American childbirth history began in the mid-eighteenth century, as a generation of American physicians became aware of the revolution in obstetrical knowledge and practice taking place in Britain and France. This period, spanning from the 1750s through most of the nineteenth century, was a transitional stage, during which physicians staked their claim to the management of birth. The third era covered the years from the 1870s to the 1940s. These decades witnessed the consolidation of medical authority over birth.

In each of these three periods, developments in the professionalization of medicine, the state of knowledge concerning parturition, technology, and cultural attitudes toward birth help explain how and why birth ultimately became the medical experience it now is in contemporary America.

CHILDBIRTH IN EARLY AMERICA

This morning was very Cloudy, Not only abroad as to the weather but in the house with respect to my wife who for about Three hours was in great Extremity. I thought I had not been earnest enough with God yet. . . . Then again Engaged in a Short but fervent Devotion and Ten Minutes past Eight my wife was delivered of a Daughter. I cryed unto God most high, unto God who is a very present Help in time of Trouble . . . and He brought Salvation. He put joy and gladness into our Hearts; and O that we may never forget his Benefits! —"The Diary of Ebenezer Parkman," September 14, 1725.

A great number of unpleasant and stormy Sabbaths have happened this winter and have prevented my attending meeting for a long time—and now *my situation* incapacitates me for it—how long it may be before I again visit the Courts of my God I know not—my hour of Difficulty and danger is not far distant—'tis a dreaded event—and nothing but a firm reliance of the supporting aid of my Maker and Sovereign could make the expectation supportable—O may I be prepared for whatever awaits me—may I be resigned to life or Death. —Diary of Elizabeth Cranch Norton, January 27, 1799.

For early Americans, death—particularly the death of infants and young children—was an everyday reality. Throughout the seventeenth and eighteenth centuries, Americans perceived birth as a time of sickness and danger and often described birthing as a terrible ordeal. Although American women probably died less frequently in childbirth than did their English counterparts (Wertz and Wertz, 1977:19-20), virtually every woman in the small communities that constituted colonial America must have known friends and relatives who died or were invalided in birth. Whatever the statistical probabilities, death in childbirth seemed close at hand, and birth itself was viewed as an unpredictable and potentially calamitous event, very much part of the daily precariousness of human existence.

Diaries testify to the frequency with which birth and death were closely related experiences in colonial America. Mary Vial Holyoke, of Salem, Massachusetts, bore twelve children between 1760 and 1782; eight died in infancy or early childhood. Like many colonial diaries, hers is a sparely written chronicle of birth and infant death. From September through December of 1767, for instance, Mary Holyoke (Dow, 1911:67) recorded the following:

September 5. I was brought to bed about 2 o'Clock A.M. of a daughter.

September 6. The Child Baptized Mary.

September 7. The Baby very well till ten o'Clock in the evening and then taken with fits.

September 8. The Baby remained very ill all day.

September 9. It Died about 8 o'Clock in the morning.

September 10. Was buried.

September 11. Mrs. Woodbridge brought to bed.

September 17. Mrs. Van and Mrs. Cranch brought to bed.

October 2. Mrs. Mackay's baby Buried.

October 8. Mrs. Van's Baby Buried.

October 11. I first got to meeting. Mrs. Oliver brought to bed. Child named Peter.

November 13. Mrs. Walter brought to bed.

November 15. Mr. Walter's Child Christen'd Lynd.
December 15. Mrs. Webster brought to bed.

It is in this context of frequent birth and frequent death that early American childbirth must be placed. Colonial Americans dealt with the omnipresent possibility of death by committing their welfare to an omnipotent divine Providence. God, and God alone, could control the outcome of pregnancy. When the eighteenth-century Massachusetts clergyman Ebenezer Parkman attributed his wife's difficult labor to his not being "earnest enough with God," he was giving voice to the sentiments typically held in the first centuries of American history.

Colonial Americans surrounded birth with well-defined rituals and traditions, perhaps in an attempt to lend some order and security to a process that seemed beyond human control. Parkman's diary provides a particularly revealing picture of the social context of birth. Parkman married his second wife, Hannah, in 1737. In the first three years of their marriage, Hannah Parkman experienced three pregnancies. Her first child, born late in 1738, lived sixteen days. Almost exactly a year after her first labor, Hannah Parkman delivered a premature stillborn son. And late in 1740, after suffering from eclampsia, she gave birth to a daughter.

Hannah Parkman's births, like those of all colonial women, were community events. When she began labor, her husband rode through the countryside to summon his wife's friends and relatives to her side:

> My Wife had been Somewhat ill all night but in the morning was so full of Pain that I rode away to fetch Granny Forbush [a midwife] to her. The Snow which fell last night added to the former . . . made it extraordinarily difficult passing. I was overmatch'd with it at old Mr. Maynards. Ebenezer Maynard and Neighbor Pratt took their horses and rode before me, by which means I succeeded. Brother Hicks carry'd up his wife, and fetch'd Mrs. How and Ensign Forbush's wife. Ensign Maynard brought his wife and fetch'd Mrs. Whipple. Mr. Williams also brought over his (Parkman, December 27, 1740).

As various historians have noted (Wertz and Wertz, 1977:2–10; Scholten, 1977:429–434; Leavitt, 1984), this "gathering together of women" served several social functions: the presence of friends and relatives at birth ensured women that they would have support during labor and the first weeks of mothering. But the particular ways in which Parkman and other diarists described this custom suggest that the tradition met psychological needs as well. Like other colonial husbands, Parkman made extraordinary efforts to ensure that his wife was surrounded by friends when she gave birth; they, in turn, made extraordinary efforts to be present. Parkman made careful note of each woman who attended his wife, and how long she stayed. Women's attendance at birth seems to have been an important responsibility, as Parkman had occasion to learn in 1747: "Mrs Chamberlin (wife of John) here," he noted. "Had talk with her about her being disgusted at my desiring my wife might be excused from being at her last groaning—it being sabbath Day, and when I was not very well" (Walett, 1963:59).

Until the 1760s, midwives were the only practitioners to attend women in labor. Although a physician attended Hannah Parkman in each of her first three pregnancies, bleeding her in an attempt to control her eclamptic convulsions, and prescribing blistering and various anodynes for the phlegmasia alba dolens she suffered after her first pregnancy, he did not attend her in childbirth. Labor and delivery were clearly the midwife's province.

Unfortunately we know very little about the identity or practices of colonial midwives. Most seem to have lacked formal training. Many probably practiced medicine or "physic," for the line between midwifery and "doctoring" was not firmly drawn in a society in which medical knowledge was neither monopolized nor mystified. The journal of an eighteenth-century Maine midwife, Martha Ballard (Nash, 1904), the most complete account we have of early American midwifery practice, indicates that in addition to attending some thirty to forty births each year, she gathered medicinal plants; prescribed salves, elixirs, and syrups; applied poultices and plasters; cut the tongues of "tongue-tied" infants; and treated burns, fevers, injuries, and all manner of diseases. When remedies failed, she washed and laid out the dead.

Only a few colonies regulated midwifery, and at best such regulation was sporadic. Nevertheless, community standards did exist. Competent midwives enjoyed respect and high status (Wertz and Wertz, 1977:10-15; Thoms, 1933:1-20). Those whose competence was questioned could find themselves in serious trouble. In 1648, a Boston midwife named Elizabeth Tilley stood accused of "the miscarrying of many women and children under her hand," of treating her patients cruelly by "using threatening words," and of interfering too much in the birth process. Mrs. Tilley was arrested and jailed pending trial, and her case generated considerable controversy. In all, Bostonians submitted six petitions to the governor and the magistrates. One, signed by six women and three men, reiterated the charges against her. Five others, signed by more than 100 women, testified to her "ability and kindness" (Tilley, 1648).

Because birth was viewed as a perilous event, women midwives and attendants managed birth but did not believe that they exercised significant control over the experience. Indeed, birth, for early Americans, was out of the realm of human control altogether.

THE REVOLUTION IN OBSTETRICAL KNOWLEDGE, 1762-1870

In our present highly artificial state there are numerous causes at work, and numerous difficulties experienced, unknown to more primitive times and conditions, and we therefore require greater skill and more extensive resources. Females have in fact become more in want of help and less able to assist. Many new discoveries have been made lately, which enable us to facilitate delivery and ease its pains, so that it is now robbed of many of its former terrors and dangers. —Frederick Hollick, *The Matron's Manual of Midwifery and the Diseases of Women During Pregnancy and Childbed*, 1848.

I was amused by a doctor telling me, lately, some women refused to take ether for extracting teeth or anything, thinking it wicked so to evade the discipline of life of which physical pain is a part. As if, with all the etherial relief, there is not suffering enough left in the world, not to speak

of the kind no gas can reach. —Fanny Appleton Longfellow
to a friend, July 11, 1847.

In 1758 William Shippen, Jr., like a growing number of
affluent young gentlemen interested in a medical career, left
for Europe to round off his medical education in Britain and
France. His most important training took place in London.
There he studied under the anatomist William Hunter from
whom he learned the anatomy and physiology of pregnancy.
He also sat in on the lectures offered by William Smellie, the
most famous of English "men-midwives," who instructed him
in practical midwifery, including how and when to use the
still-novel obstetrical forceps. Shippen returned to America in
1762 with a full set of Hunter's anatomical engravings and a
conviction that midwifery was a proper branch of medical
science, to be investigated, taught, and practiced. By 1765 he
was offering instruction to physicians and those midwives
"who have the virtue enough to own their own ignorance"
(Donegan, 1978:115–120).

As Shippen's educational biography suggests, the eighteenth
century witnessed the laying of the foundation of modern
obstetrical knowledge and practice. One cornerstone was new
knowledge of the anatomy and physiology of gestation. The
anatomical dissections and painstaking engravings of Hunter
and others enabled physicians to visualize the pregnant
uterus and how the fetus positioned itself in the womb. At the
same time, French physicians charted the mechanical
processes of labor and pioneered the science of pelvic measure-
ments, thus establishing a basis for predicting whether labors
would be normal or difficult (Wertz and Wertz, 1977:29–76).

The second cornerstone of modern obstetrics consisted of
developments in birth technology, most importantly the
obstetrical forceps. The forceps revolutionized obstetrical practice because they gave practitioners an alternative to the
mutilating operations of craniotomy and embryotomy that
killed infants and often mothers as well. In fact, forceps were
invented early in the seventeenth century by one Peter Chamberlen the Elder, but, because four generations of Chamberlen
physicians managed to keep the reason for their astounding
success with difficult labors a family secret, a published
description of the forceps and their use did not appear until

1734. Thereafter, however, knowledge of the instruments and their use became widespread (Donegan, 1978:38-83; Radcliffe, 1947:5-37).

By the time of the Revolution, American physicians were well aware of these obstetrical advances. Some, like Shippen, studied abroad. Others circulated copies of William Smellie's *Treatise on the Theory and Practice of Midwifery* and other English works. New medical schools established professorships of midwifery, and physicians began to present papers on obstetrical cases to fledgling medical societies. Once Amercians began to publish their own medical journals early in the nineteenth century, obstetrics was the subject of numerous articles.

Physicians who served as accoucheurs found much demand for their services. As Catherine Scholten (1977:430-436) has documented, affluent women in coastal cities readily turned to physicians for care in childbirth. Although midwives continued to practice throughout the nineteenth century in the countryside and among the urban poor, by the early 1900s physician attendance had become the norm for urban women of means.

Why did many American women turn so readily to physicians? How were doctors successful in establishing themselves as childbirth attendants? Why did midwives, so long preeminent in the management of birth, virtually disappear during the first half of the nineteenth century?

The alacrity with which women turned to doctors indicates that they believed that medical practitioners could make birth safer and easier. Then, too, as Scholten (1977:430-432) has argued, doctors' newfound interest in obstetrics indicated their belief in the power of human agency. By the early nineteenth century, both women and their doctors shared a growing faith in the power of human beings to master the natural world. Although many nineteenth-century women continued to dread childbirth, they had come to believe that pain and death were not necessarily God-given outcomes.

The new faith in human agency was particularly evident in the history of obstetrical anesthesia. Although social conservatives opposed its use, arguing that God intended women to suffer in childbirth, many physicians and their patients eagerly adopted ether and chloroform when they were introduced in the 1840s (Duffy, 1964:32–44; Leavitt, 1983). Fanny Longfellow, the first American woman to experience an etherized birth, was ecstatic, concluding that the anesthesia was "certainly the greatest blessing of the age" (July 1847). The success of physicians in gaining acceptance as accoucheurs was the result not only of innovations in birth technology but also, equally important, of their access to knowledge. Throughout the late eighteenth and nineteenth centuries, physicians developed ways to transmit clinical findings and medical discoveries. The widespread availability of medical books (including English translations of continental writers), the new medical societies and schools, and the appearance of medical journals all provided a growing network for medical communication.

The obstetrical history of ergot is an excellent example of the early nineteenth-century communication revolution in medicine. Traditional histories credit John Stearns, an early nineteenth-century New York physician, with the discovery that ergot induces powerful uterine contractions. But Stearns, who published his *Observations on the Secale Cornutum, or Ergot, With Directions for Its Use in Parturition* in 1822, candidly acknowledged that he had learned about ergot from "an ignorant Scotch woman" (quoted in Thoms, 1933:40). Midwives like Stearns's "ignorant Scotch woman" may well have known of ergot's uses for centuries. Unlike doctors, however, they had no effective way to communicate their findings and experiences. Given the fact that a significant percentage of American women was illiterate in 1800, it is quite probable that even personal correspondence was not an option for many (Lockridge, 1974).

The lack of a communications network for midwives helps explain their rapid decline. Doctors criticized midwives but seem to have made little concerted effort to curtail their practice. Indeed, as Dorothy and Richard Wertz have suggested (1977:44), American physicians apparently envisioned an alliance between themselves and educated midwives. The acrimonious midwife debate that raged among English practitioners had no counterpart in the United States. Denied access to the new knowledge and technology of birth, however, midwives faded into obscurity. Their closest nineteenth-century counterpart in middle-class America was the "monthly nurse"—a woman hired to assist at birth and with the first weeks of baby care. The monthly nurse, unlike the traditional midwife, was a servant and clearly subordinate to the physician.

Nevertheless, physicians were not without their critics in the first half of the nineteenth century. Social conservatives condemned the presence of men in the lying-in chamber as indecent and called for either a return to midwives or for the training of female physicians (e.g., Gregory, 1848; Skinner, 1850; Donegan, 1978:164-228). Sectarian practitioners such as botanics and homeopaths also criticized regular practitioners' management of birth, arguing that birth was a process that could be more easily understood and managed by intelligent women themselves. Giving birth, they maintained, was a natural physiological process that rarely, if ever, warranted the heroic measures they accused physicians of being all too willing to employ: bloodletting, ergot, opium, and the use of instruments (e.g., Hersey, 1836:xii–xiii, 136-148; Skinner, 1850:3-5).

Nineteenth-century physicians agreed that childbirth was fundamentally a natural and healthy process. As a group, they may not have been as prone to intervene in the birthing process as their critics suggested. One young practitioner described his management of an 1828 case in the following manner: "Encouraged my patient with assurances of her safe delivery, and telling her that nature should never be meddled with, when she has the power to accomplish her purposes alone, I lay down" (Metcalf, February 21, 1828).

Yet, if doctors believed that childbirth was fundamentally a normal, healthy process, how did they justify their presence at birth? Many argued that modern urban life was in itself unnatural and rendered women unfit to give birth without medical assistance. As Harvard professor Walter Channing explained, labor

> ordinarily terminated with but little agency on the part of the practitioner, and it was obviously intended that labor should always be thus easily terminated. The circumstances, however, in which women have been placed in the progress of civilization have tended so far to interfere with the original design as to render delivery almost always a painful, frequently a formidable, and sometimes even a dangerous process.

Nineteenth-century obstetrical literature is full of references to the supposed ease with which Native American and black women gave birth. These women, doctors argued, were less "civilized," and therefore closer to nature, than the middle-class urban women who made up their practices.

Doctors also based their claim to childbirth attendance on their superior knowledge of anatomy and physiology. As E. Augustus Holyoke, a late eighteenth-century physician, concluded after describing a disastrous midwife-managed delivery that ended in the complete inversion of the patient's uterus, "what better can be expected from an Operator utterly destitute of all knowledge of the figure, situation, and anatomy of the parts" (1783). More than fifty years later, Maria Meservey, a physician practicing in Delaware, agreed that lay practitioners' ignorance caused untold amounts of mischief. As she wrote to a friend, "The old midwife has her patients go through a strange sort of gymnastics and in every case there is an inverted or a prolapsed uterus (the result of her haste in removing the afterbirth). . . . I do not believe there is any need of a woman being left so broken down—I always intend to have my patients get up as well and strong as before marriage" (February 19, 1867).

As early as the 1820s, obstetrical practitioners began to insist that a medical education be a requirement for managing birth. "No one can thoroughly understand the nature and treatment of labour who does not understand thoroughly the profession of medicine as a whole," insisted John Ware (1820:7), and Channing concurred. Midwifery, he stressed, could not be understood without a thorough study of physiology and anatomy.

By the mid-nineteenth century, doctors had become American's primary birth attendants. In many respects, the transition from social childbirth to medically managed childbirth was remarkably smooth. But it is easy to overestimate the authority of doctors at the time. Their control of birth was limited in good part by the relatively low status and divided nature of the medical profession. When J. Marion Sims's father reacted to his decision to study medicine by declaring, "to think that my son should be going around from house to house through this county, with a box of pills in one hand and a squirt in the other, to ameliorate human suffering, is a thought I never supposed I should have to contemplate"

(Sims, 1884:116), he probably reflected the sentiments of many Americans. And although nineteenth-century doctors did not face serious competition from midwives, "regular" practitioners did contend with sectarians, who challenged their legitimacy.

Although doctors made much of their knowledge, the obstetrical learning of even the most conscientious of physicians was sadly deficient. Nowhere were such limitations more evident than in the confusion over the etiology and prevention of puerperal fever, the main cause of maternal death throughout the nineteenth century. Puerperal fever was so widespread that some degree of postpartum infection seems to have been commonplace, even expected. Theories purporting to explain this bewildering affliction that affected only parturient women abounded; the disease was caused by miasma, by climatic conditions, or by infected women themselves. That scrupulous cleanliness could dramatically reduce the incidence of puerperal fever had been documented since the 1770s (White, 1773; Gordon, 1795). And in the 1840s, Oliver Wendell Holmes, in Boston, and Ignaz Semmelweis, in Vienna, independently came to the conclusion that doctors themselves spread the disease from woman to woman by carrying infectious matter on their persons, especially on their hands (Holmes, 1843, 1855). Holmes's essay "The Contagiousness of Puerperal Fever" was widely read and discussed, and many physicians put into practice his recommendation that practitioners with a patient who developed puerperal fever stop attending midwifery cases for a considerable length of time. But at a time when doctors were unaware of the existence of bacteria and unimpressed with statistics, Holmes's explanation seemed to many no more convincing than others. Moreover, without a technique for effective antisepsis, no practitioner, however careful, could protect his patients.

Equally important, as Leavitt (1983:294-296) has documented, was the fact that women themselves limited doctors' authority. Although childbirth lost the public aspects that had characterized birth in early America, women continued to give birth at home with friends as well as a doctor in attendance. Nineteenth-century standards of decorum circumscribed physicians' practices (Donegan, 1978:141-157). For example, obtaining permission to conduct a vaginal examination during labor involved delicate negotiations between the physician and an intermediary—a friend or nurse—who would convey the request to the patient. Finally, nineteenth-century women knew a great deal about birth. Giving birth and attending birth remained frequent and familiar experiences throughout the century. Because knowledge of the birthing process was not yet the exclusive property of physicians, patients and their friends felt free to challenge or contradict their doctors' authority. Doctors often deferred to the wishes and sensibilities of their patients. One doctor recorded that a case he had just attended involved a "very severe labor without the aid of forceps. I urged the use of instruments but she objected so strongly that I yielded to her wishes" (Snow, 1865). Then, too, women maintained folk beliefs that conflicted with medical knowledge. One practitioner reported his patient's reaction when he informed her that her baby had been born with a caul. "The woman was sorry I had destroyed it," he wrote, "as it would tell when the child was going to be sick. [I] told her I was sorry but could not help it, as I was ignorant of its use." (Metcalf) In day-to-day practice, then, obstetrics was not based entirely on the systematic application of anatomical and physiological knowledge. Instead, obstetrics was often haphazard, determined in good part by the clinical experience of the doctor and by the social values and customs of his patient (Leavitt, 1983:294-295).

THE MEDICALIZATION OF BIRTH, 1870-1940

The old idea that childbirth is limited to a process of expulsion or extraction of a child from a uterus in a woman's abdomen by way of the narrow tortuous canal of the human pelvis; by the forces of nature alone, or with the aid of man stretching or tearing or cutting the soft parts or even severing the pelvis itself, has passed away in the light of aseptic abdominal surgery. Today no man is a competent obstetrical specialist who is not a trained abdominal surgeon as well as a qualified pelvic operator.... Normal women come to us demanding a cesarean delivery to avoid the agonies of childbirth. While none would grant this request, it is well to remember that what is a fantasy today may be a fact tomorrow. A cesarean section is the easiest way for any primaparous woman to have her baby, and it is the surest way of having a live baby. It is the only painless childbirth that occurs today.—O. Paul Humpstone, "Cesarean Section versus Spontaneous Delivery," *American Journal of Obstetrics and Gynecology* 1 (June 1921).

We cannot sit back and say, "One woman in 150 dies in childbirth. It is a chance all women have to take. Let nature take its course." All women should not have to take that chance. —R. F. Wadsworth, "Mothers in Danger," *Collier's* 86 (July 5, 1930).

In the early twentieth century, childbirth came to be defined entirely in medical terms. Several developments hastened the full medicialization of birth. The professionalization of medicine in the years around the turn of the century was accompanied by the specific efforts by obstetricians to win prestige and recognition for their own specialty. This they did by upgrading standards of training and practice, by eliminating midwifery as a feasible alternative in maternity care, and by linking forces with the surgical specialty of gynecology. The development of antiseptic and aseptic techniques made possible another development essential to the medicalization of birth: the move from home to hospital as the primary birthplace. Finally, the early twentieth-century maternal and child welfare movement, fueled by new, urgent concern about the high death rates of American mothers and babies, encouraged women to think of childbirth as a medical process that demanded specialized care.

Late nineteenth-century obstetricians were uncomfortably aware of their field's limitations. Obstetrics, so exciting and full of promise a century earlier, had become a medical backwater that attracted too few talented young practitioners. The key to improving obstetrics, doctors came to believe, lay in better instruction (Williams, 1912; Kobrin, 1966). Most students' training consisted solely of entirely didactic lectures, with no opportunities for observing, let alone managing, actual labor. Poor training encouraged careless, incompetent practice and a lack of respect toward obstetrics. But how could clinical training be improved? Given nineteenth-century standards of modesty and decorum, a practitioner could hardly parade students into his patients' bedchambers to view their labors. Obstetricians, in short, lacked clinical material.

Ambitious, scientifically oriented practitioners made their way to the *Frauenkliniks* of Austria and Germany, the centers of late nineteenth-century research and practice. In European teaching hospitals, where destitute women served as clinical material in exchange for free medical care, doctors worked without the cultural constraints imposed on physicians in America (Morton, 1937:50–70). When American practitioners came home, they too began to look to poor women for instructional purposes. As Virginia Drachman (1979:80) has suggested, "in the post Civil War period, doctors evolved a working agreement with the growing population of poor urban women.... They gave them medical attention and, in return, used them as a resource for clinical instruction." Poor and working-class women were thus essential to the medicalization of birth (Dye, 1983).

To reach working-class women, doctors established outpatient obstetrical clinics in impoverished urban neighborhoods. They also took a new interest in lying-in hospitals. Founded early in the nineteenth century, lying-ins existed primarily as charitable institutions for the refuge of homeless women and the reclamation of "fallen" women with illegitimate children. For decades, physicians had little to do with the lying-ins. Late in the century, however, many doctors took on hospital practices to take advantage of the opportunities for clinical observation and experimentation (Vogel, 1980).

Doctors enjoyed far more authority and autonomy in the lying-ins than they did in private practice. In the hospital, a doctor did not have to worry about pleasing the patient and her family by accommodating himself to cultural standards of decorum or popular birthing customs. Instead, hospitals and dispensaries enabled practitioners to restructure the doctor-patient relationship along new lines. In hospital birth, there was no room for negotiation between doctor and patient: the physician expected to be acknowledged as the expert and to control the management of labor. Doctors came to expect patients to be passive and to accept their medical authority. The full medicalization of birth rested in no small part on this restructuring of the social relationship between doctors and their patients (Dye, 1983:2–3).

Nevertheless, very few women used hospitals. In 1900 only 5 percent of American women gave birth in them, for hospitals were associated with depravity and were exceedingly dangerous. It was, of course, the high incidence of puerperal sepsis that rendered hospital birth so perilous. From 1872 to 1873, for example, 56 percent of the patients at the New England Hospital for Women and Children showed evidence of sepsis, and fully 9 percent suffered severe systemic infections (Call, 1908:396–397).

As doctors gradually became convinced that puerperal fever was a bacterial infection and not a specific disease, they adapted surgical antiseptic technique to obstetrics. The popularization of obstetrical antisepsis in the early 1880s was the result in good part of the work of Henry Garrigues, the attending obstetrician at New York's Charity Hospital. One of the first physicians to insist that hospital birth could be made safe, Garrigues introduced stringent standards of cleanliness in the obstetrical wards, kept maternity patients in isolation, and made liberal use of bichloride of mercury to disinfect women before, during, and after labor. By 1883 Garrigues could demonstrate that his methods had dramatically reduced sepsis (Garrigues, 1877:592–643; 1886:19–31). Other hospitals adopted antisepsis with similar results. In the 1890s, asepsis supplemented antisepsis, as hospitals began to sterilize instruments and dressings. Puerperal fever rates again dropped dramatically. By 1907, for instance, more than 92 percent of New England Hospital patients remained free from infection (Call, 1908:392–404).

Antisepsis, though far from perfect in its application in late nineteenth-century hospitals, ushered in a new era of operative obstetrics, as lower sepsis rates gave doctors more confidence about performing surgical procedures. From the 1890s through the 1920s, the incidence of Cesarean section, internal version, forceps deliveries, and labor induction, or accouchement force, rose dramatically. New operations such as pubiotomy and symphysiotomy, both of which involved fracturing and separating pelvic bones to widen the birth passage, also found acceptance. By the early twentieth century, many physicians employed forceps in more than 20 percent of their hospital cases (Danforth, 1922:610–611). The career of Irving Potter, an early twentieth-century obstetrician in Buffalo, New York, illustrates the extent to which the new operative obstetrics could reach. Potter attended more than 1,100 births a year. The great majority he delivered by podalic version, a technique that involved reaching into the uterus, turning the infant to a feet-first position, and pulling on the baby's feet to effect rapid delivery, thus eliminating the second stage of labor (Potter, 1918:215-220). The technique of podalic version had been used for centuries in complicated labors, but never before had it been advocated as a routine procedure. Many obstetricians denounced such trends in no uncertain terms, and the differences between radicals and conservatives became an ongoing theme in obstetrical literature from the 1890s through the 1930s (e.g., Bedford, 1888:897-903; Smith, 1898:785-791; Williams, 1912:493-499; Anspach, 1923:566-574). This new emphasis on operative treatment, however, linked obstetrics closely with gynecology, and professional organizations began to formalize this connection. Obstetrics thus became defined as a surgical specialty.

In their efforts to improve the status of obstetrics, doctors also moved to eliminate rival practitioners. Chief among these, of course, was the midwife. By 1900 far more midwives were practicing in the United States than there had been in 1850, largely because of the great influx of European immigrants. Urban midwives, most of them new immigrants, and "granny" midwives in the rural South attended between 40 and 50 percent of American births in 1900 (Kobrin, 1966:351; Litoff, 1978). Although midwives did not pose an economic threat to obstetricians (their clienteles rarely overlapped), obstetricians insisted on eliminating these midwives for two reasons. First, as Frances Kobrin (1966:354-357) has argued, midwives served poor immigrant urban women—precisely the women doctors wanted as clinical material in lying-in hospitals. Second, obstetrics could hardly command prestige and attract talented young practitioners if midwives continued to practice. As Joseph DeLee explained, "If an uneducated woman of the lowest classes may practice obstetrics . . . it certainly must require very little knowledge and skill—surely it cannot belong to the science and art of medicine" (1916: 407-408). By the 1920s, through a combination of regulatory and licensing requirements in some states, outright prohibition of midwifery practice in others, and the expansion of free hospital care for the urban poor, midwives had once again been rendered insignificant as birth attendants in all but the most rural areas of the United States (Litoff, 1978).

Obstetricians received help in their campaign against midwifery from early-twentieth-century social reformers concerned about maternal and child welfare. A coalition of clubwomen, settlement residents, public health officials, and social workers founded such organizations as the American Association for the Study and Prevention of Infant Mortality and lobbied successfully for the establishment of the federal Children's Bureau in 1912—the first federal agency empowered to investigate the causes of maternal and infant mortality. These social reformers did much to collect and publicize statistics concerning maternal and infant mortality in the United States and emphasized that the American mortality rates were among the highest in the Western world. In 1915, for example, out of every 10,000 births, 60 mothers died. Only tuberculosis killed more women of childbearing age. In the same year, about one in ten babies born did not live until their first birthdays. The majority of those deaths were in the first month of life (Meigs, 1917; Adair, 1935:389). Although some reformers defended midwives, pointing out that the mortality rates with general practitioners were often higher (Williams, 1912:1–5; Levy, 1923:88–95), most argued that the death rates were so high because many women did not have access to skilled medical care. Persuade women to go to obstetrical dispensaries and hospitals for birth, reformers believed, and the death rates would drop (Women's Municipal League of Boston).

Social reformers introduced prenatal care. As instituted by such organizations as the Women's Municipal League of Boston, prenatal care programs had both medical and educational purposes. Nurses monitored the general health of their impoverished patients to watch for toxemia and other complications. Prenatal workers also served as educators, providing women with information about nutrition, stressing the importance of breast-feeding, and insisting on the necessity of medical attendance at birth, preferably in a hospital. In time, prenatal programs developed formal ties with lying-in hospitals, thus serving outreach and referral functions (Women's Municipal League of Boston). In short, the maternal and infant welfare movement of the early twentieth century linked the concerns of the lay public with those of the medical profession. It was through the efforts of reformers that the medical profession developed serious concern for the poor mortality rates in America. At the same time, reformers worked to medicalize birth in America by adopting medical approaches to childbirth and by communicating the importance of skilled medical attention and hospitalization to women.

Finally, the medicalization of birth depended on redefining the nature of the birth process. Throughout much of the nineteenth century, as we have seen, most physicians defined parturition as fundamentally natural. But many early twentieth-century obstetricians were not content with the largely passive role of "watchful expectancy" that their predecessors had advocated. Chief among those who worked to redefine birth as a pathologic process that demanded active management was Joseph DeLee, a Chicago obstetrician. A perfectionist in his own work, DeLee made no secret of his impatience with what he believed to be the generally low standards of obstetrical practice and with those who believed that childbirth was a simple physiologic process. By no means the most radical of obstetricians in terms of the techniques he advocated (indeed, he regarded himself as conservative compared with doctors like Irving Potter, the advocate of routine podalic version), he nonetheless emphasized the essential pathologic character of labor. "Labor has been called, and still is believed by many to be, a normal function," he stated in 1920:

Everything, of course, depends on what we define as normal. If a woman falls on a pitchfork and drives the handle through her perineum, we call that pathologic—abnormal, but if a large baby is driven through the pelvic floor, we say that is natural, and therefore normal. If a baby were to have his head caught in a door very lightly, but enough to cause a cerebral hemorrhage, we would say that is decidedly pathogenic, but were a baby's head crushed against a tight pelvic floor, and a hemorrhage in the brain kills it, we call this normal, at least we say that the function is natural, not pathogenic.... In fact only a small minority of women escape damage during labor, while 4 percent of the babies are killed and a large indeterminable number are more or less injured by the direct action of the natural process itself. So frequent are these bad effects that I have often wondered whether Nature did not deliberately intend women should be used up in the process of reproduction, in a manner analogous to that of the salmon, which dies after spawning?

DeLee proposed his "prophylactic forceps operation" as a way to minimize birth's natural dangers. By reducing the pain of the first stage of labor with narcotics and scopalomine, DeLee reasoned that he lessened psychic trauma and physical exhaustion. By performing routine episiotomy, he argued that he preserved the perineum from injury. By eliminating the second stage of labor with the routine use of low forceps, DeLee stressed that he spared both mother and child from injury. And by administering pituitrin and manually extracting the placenta, DeLee stated that he reduced hemorrhage and infection. In all, the new technique, down to the last detail, was carefully planned to maximize human control of labor.

Although DeLee's prophylactic forceps operation met with strenuous opposition when he presented the technique to the American Society of Gynecologists in 1920, many of his techniques and attitudes soon became the norm in American obstetrics. In particular, his approach embodied a new view of nature. Whereas nineteenth-century physicians had generally seen nature as a fundamentally benign force that sometimes went awry or that was perverted by the artificial habits and fashions of modern urban civilization, DeLee saw nature itself as much too capricious and cruel to be left to its own devices. Then, too, he reflected the growing concern in the early twentieth century for the well-being of the child as well as the mother. Throughout the history of obstetrics, the mother had been the sole focus of all obstetrical measures. DeLee's emphasis on the destructive aspects of normal labor for the infant provided an additional rationale for interventionist obstetrics—while a mother might be expected to survive a difficult labor without permanent damage, the dangers to infants were far graver and more difficult to predict. Hence, DeLee and others reasoned, it was better to rely on carefully managed and predictable surgical intervention to counteract what was in essence a destructive natural process.

DeLee's new definition of childbirth as inherently pathologic found ready adherents not only among obstetricians but also among middle-class women. The highly publicized American maternal and infant death rates created new and urgent concern over how to ensure safety in childbirth. Throughout the first decades of the twentieth century, popular periodicals and women's magazines reflected women's fears and urged them to "abandon the moth-eaten tradition that bringing little children into the world is a 'natural process' and therefore in the hands of God" (Richardson, 1915:24). In particular, child-birth reformers cautioned women to "avoid the smiling family practitioner of old who says that there is nothing to worry about—that childbirth is merely a physiological function" (Boyd, 1931:293-295).

One consequence of the heightened anxiety and the new attitudes toward birth was the fact that middle-class women began to enter hospitals to have their babies. Before the 1920s, few doctors and even fewer middle-class women looked to the hospital for private maternity care. By the mid-1920s, however, about 50 percent of births in large cities took place in hospitals. On the eve of World War II, more than 75 percent of urban births were hospitalized. And by 1960, nearly 100 percent of all births—urban and rural—took place in hospital maternity wards (Devitt, 1977:48-49). In the nineteenth century, hospitals had symbolized disease and poverty; by the 1920s, they had come to symbolize absolute cleanliness and safety.

Tragically, hospitalization and operative intervention did not make childbirth safer in the 1920s and 1930s. Maternal mortality remained high throughout these decades, and sepsis remained the major cause of maternal death (Adair, 1935:384-394; Antler and Fox, 1976:581). The maternal death rate in that period never dropped below the 1915 level of 60 maternal deaths per 10,000 live births. In 1932 the national maternal death rate stood at 63 maternal deaths per 10,000 births, and the urban rate, where hospital birth had become common, was considerably higher: 74 maternal deaths per 10,000 live births (Adair, 1935:389). Maternal mortality did not decline significantly until the late 1930s. Its decline then had nothing to do with hospitalization or surgical intervention. Rather, it was the result primarily of new, more stringent efforts on the part of obstetricians to oversee obstetrical practice (Antler and Fox, 1976) and, perhaps more important, the

introduction in the late 1930s and 1940s of sulfa and antibiotics to treat puerperal sepsis.

With the virtually universal hospitalization of birth, the
medicalization of childbirth was complete. Hospital birth, as
various scholars have emphasized, was by definition physician-
controlled birth (Leavitt, 1983:297-304; Wertz and Wertz,
1977:132-177). The birth rituals specific to the hospital, many
of them originating in the late nineteenth-century regimens to
control sepsis, were strikingly different from the rituals and
traditions that had surrounded birth at home. Equally important was the fact that once birth took place in institutions, it
was isolated from society as a whole. As a result, by the
middle of the twentieth century, women knew very little about
the process of birth and had no alternative but to accept
physicians' authority. Women throughout American history
may well have dreaded parturition, but childbirth was a frequent, familiar event about which women knew a great deal.
Indeed, as we have seen, nineteenth-century women frequently
regarded their own knowledge of birth as equal or even superior to that of physicians. Once birth routinely took place in
hospitals, however, few women had the opportunity to participate in births other than their own, and, given the
widespread adoption of general anesthesia, often did not experience even their own births. As knowledge of birth became
monopolized, birth itself became mystified.

Several factors, then, help explain how birth became a
medical event in the United States. Women's fear of pain and
death in childbirth, coupled with a new faith in the human
power to understand and master nature, help explain why
Americans turned to physicians in the late eighteenth century. Technological developments—forceps, anesthesia, antisepsis—help explain Americans' growing willingness to put their
faith in doctors to make birth safer and less painful. The
extraordinarily successful efforts to professionalize medicine
in the late nineteenth and early twentieth centuries, coupled
with the relative political weakness and disorganization of
alternative practitioners such as midwives, help explain how
physicians achieved an unprecedented degree of social and
scientific authority in the United States (Starr, 1982:3-29).
Technological and professional developments in and of themselves, however, are not sufficient to explain the medicaliza-

tion of childbirth. Doctors' access to and ultimate control of knowledge concerning birth are, in the final analysis, the most potent factors in explaining why birth became a medical event. In the nineteenth century, as we have seen, doctors developed an extensive and effective communications network—a network from which women were largely excluded. Nevertheless, doctors' ideas about birth and its management competed with those of other practitioners and with the experiential knowledge and traditions of women. As alternative practitioners were eliminated and alternative models of birth management discredited, however, and as birth moved out of the home and into the hospital, American women came to depend on medicine as the only source of knowledge about a central female experience.

REFERENCES

Adair, Fred L. "Maternal, Fetal, and Neonatal Morbidity and Mortality." *American Journal of Obstetrics and Gynecology* 29(1935): 384–394.

Anspach, Brooke M. "The Trend of Modern Obstetrics—What Is the Danger? How Can It Be Changed?" *American Journal of Obstetrics and Gynecology* 6(1923):566–574.

Antler, Joyce, and Fox, Daniel M. "The Movement Toward a Safe Maternity: Physician Accountability in New York City, 1915–1940." *Bulletin of the History of Medicine* 50(1976):569–595.

Bedford, Henry. "The So-Called Physiological Argument in Obstetrics." *American Journal of Obstetrics and the Diseases of Women and Children* 21(1888):897–903.

Boyd, Mary. "Why Mothers Die." *The Nation* 132(1931):293–295.

Call, Emma. "The Evolution of Modern Maternity Technic." *American Journal of Obstetrics and the Diseases of Women and Children* 58(1908):392–404.

Channing, Walter. Lecture notes. *Walter Channing Papers*. Boston: Massachusetts Historical Society, 1822.

Danforth, W. C. "Is Conservative Obstetrics to Be Abandoned?" *American Journal of Obstetrics and Gynecology* 3(1922):609–616.

DeLee, Joseph B. "Progress Toward Heal Obstetrics." *American Journal of Obstetrics and Gynecology* 73(1916):407–415.

_____. "The Prophylactic Forceps Operation." *American Journal of Obstetrics and Gynecology* 1(1920):34–44.

Devitt, Neal. "The Transition from Home to Hospital Birth in the United States, 1930–1960." *Birth and the Family Journal* 4(1977): 47–58.

Donegan, Jane. *Women and Men Midwives: Medicine, Morality, and Misogyny in Early America.* Westport, Conn.: Greenwood Press, 1978.

Dow, George Francis, ed. "Diary of Mary Vial Holyoke." In *The Holyoke Diaries, 1709–1856.* Salem, Massachusetts, 1911.

Drachman, Virginia. "The Loomis Trial: Social Mores and Obstetrics in the Mid-Nineteenth Century." In *Health Care in America: Essays in the Social History of Medicine,* edited by Susan Reverby and David Rosner. Philadelphia: Temple University Press, 1979.

Duffy, John. "Anglo-American Reaction to Obstetrical Anesthesia." *Bulletin of the History of Medicine* 38(1964):32–44.

Dye, Nancy Schrom. "Scientific Obstetrics and Working-Class Women: The New York Midwifery Dispensary." Paper presented at meeting of American Historical Association, San Francisco, December 1983.

Garrigues, Henry J. "On Lying-In Institutions, Especially Those in New York." *Transactions of the American Gynecological Society* 2(1877):592–643.

_____. *Practical Guide in Antiseptic Midwifery in Hospitals and Private Practice.* Detroit: George D. Davis, 1886.

Gordon, Alexander. *Treatise on the Epidemic Puerperal Fervor of Aberdeen.* London, 1795.

Gregory, Samuel. *Man-Midwifery Exposed and Corrected; or, The Employment of Men to Attend Women in Childbirth, and in Other Delicate Circumstances Shown to Be a Modern Innovation.* Boston: G. Gregory, 1848.

Hersey, Thomas. *The Midwife's Practical Directory; or, Woman's Confidential Friend . . . The Whole Designed for the Special Use of the Botanic Friends in the United States.* Baltimore: privately printed, 1836.

Hollock, Frederick. *The Matron's Manual of Midwifery and the Diseases of Women During Pregnancy and Childbirth.* New York: T. W. Strong, 1848.

Holmes, Oliver Wendell. "The Contagiousness of Puerperal Fever." *U.S. Quarterly Journal of Medicine and Surgery* 1(1843):503.

_____. *Puerperal Fever as a Private Pestilence.* Boston, 1855.

Holyoke, E. Augustus. "On Uterine Inversion." *Proceedings of the Massachusetts Medical Society.* Boston: Harvard University, Countway Library of Medicine, 1783.

Humpstone, O. Paul. "Cesarean Section versus Spontaneous Delivery." *American Journal of Obstetrics and Gynecology* 1(1921): 987–989.

Kobrin, Frances. "The American Midwife Controversy: A Crisis in Professionalization." *Bulletin of the History of Medicine* 40(1966): 350–363.

Leavitt, Judith. "'Science' Enters the Birthing Room: Obstetrics in America since the Eighteenth Century." *Journal of American History* 70(1983):281–304.

———. "Shadow of Maternity: Childbirth and Death Fears." Paper presented at the Sixth Berkshire Conference on the History of Women, June 3, 1984.

Levy, Julius. "Maternal Mortality and Morbidity in the First Month of Life in Relation to Attendant at Birth." *American Journal of Public Health* 13(1923):88–95.

Litoff, Judy Barrett. *American Midwives: 1860 to the Present.* Westport, Conn.: Greenwood Press, 1978.

Lockridge, Kenneth A. *Literacy in Colonial New England. An Inquiry into the Social Context of Literacy in the Early Modern West.* New York: W. W. Norton, 1974.

Longfellow, Fanny Appleton. Manuscript Collection. Cambridge, Massachusetts: Longfellow Historical Site, 1847.

Meigs, Grace L. *Maternal Mortality—From All Conditions Connected with Childbirth in the United States and Certain Other Countries.* U.S. Children's Bureau Bulletin #19. Washington: Government Printing Office, 1917.

Meservey, Maria. Correspondence, Shaw-Webb Papers. Worcester, Mass.: American Antiquarian Society, 1867.

Metcalf, John George. *Obstetrical Notebook, 1824–1832.* Boston: Harvard University, Countway Library of Medicine.

Morton, Rosalie Slaughter. *A Woman Surgeon; The Life and Work of Rosalie Slaughter Morton.* New York: Frederick A. Stokes, 1937.

Nash, Charles Elventon, ed. *The History of Augusta; First Settlements and Early Days as a Town, Including the Diary of Mrs. Martha Moore Ballard (1785 to 1812).* Augusta, Maine: Charles F. Nash and Son, 1904.

Norton, Elizabeth Cranch. *Diary of Elizabeth Cranch Norton.* Boston: Massachusetts Historical Society, 1799.

Potter, Irving W. "Version, with a Report of Two Hundred Additional Cases Since September, 1916." *American Journal of Obstetrics and the Diseases of Women and Children* 77(1918):215–220.

Radcliffe, Walter. *The Secret Instrument (The Birth of the Midwifery Forceps).* London: William Heinemann, 1947.

Richardson, Anna Steese. "Safety First for Mother." *McClure's* 45(1915):24.

Scholten, Catherine. "'On the Importance of the Obstetrick Art': Changing Customs of Childbirth in America, 1760 to 1825." *William and Mary Quarterly* 34(1977):426–445.

Sims, J. Marion. *The Story of My Life.* New York: D. Appleton, 1884.

Skinner, George W. *Nature Defended, and the Abuses of Custom Exposed: Being an Argument Advocating the Claims of Female*

Midwifery. Newburyport, Mass., 1850.

Smith, Thomas C. "What Have You To Offer That Is Better? A Question for Critics." *American Journal of Obstetrics and the Diseases of Women and Children* 38(1898):785-791.

Snow, George. *Obstetrical Casebook, 1865-1875.* Boston: Harvard University, Countway Library of Medicine.

Starr, Paul. *The Social Transformation of American Medicine.* New York: Basic Books, 1982.

Thoms, Herbert. *Chapters in American Obstetrics.* Springfield, Ill.: Charles C. Thomas, 1933.

Tilley, Elizabeth. Petitions in the Case of Elizabeth Tilley. Boston: Massachusetts Historical Society, 1648.

Vogel, Morris. *The Invention of the Modern Hospital, Boston, 1870-1930.* Chicago: University of Chicago Press, 1980.

Wadsworth, R. F. "Mothers in Danger." *Collier's* 86 (July 5, 1930).

Walett, Francis G., ed. "The Diary of Ebenezer Parkman, 1719-1747." *Proceedings of the American Antiquarian Society,* 71-76. Worcester, Mass.: American Antiquarian Society.

Ware, John. *Remarks on the Employment of Females as Practitioners in Midwifery. By a Physician.* Boston: Cummings and Hilliard, 1820.

Wertz, Richard W., and Wertz, Dorothy C. *Lying-In: A History of Childbirth in America.* New York: The Free Press, 1977.

White, Charles C. *A Treatise on the Management of Pregnant and Lying-In Women.* London, 1773.

Williams, J. Whitridge. "Medical Education and the Midwife Problem in the United States." *The Journal of the American Medical Association* 58(1912):1-7.

Women's Municipal League of Boston. *Bulletin of the Women's Municipal League of Boston,* 1910-1920.

2

From Natural to Surgical Event

DIANA SCULLY

Medical customs differ from society to society because they are affected by the cultural context in which they develop. All societies have customs that guide labor and childbirth and that reflect, to some degree, the culturally patterned beliefs of the birth attendants.

In contrast to many societies where birth is regarded as a natural process and attended by woman-midwives, in the United States today, birth is defined as a medical-surgical event. As such, it most frequently takes place in hospital surgical suites with surgically trained male obstetricians in attendance. To understand how male physicians gained control of childbirth from women-midwives and redefined childbirth from a natural state to a pathological condition requiring the intervention of surgeons and their instruments, it is necessary to examine the history of obstetrics in the

Portions of this chapter are adapted from the book *Men Who Control Women's Health* by Diana Scully. Copyright © 1980 by Diana Scully. Reprinted by permission of Houghton Mifflin Company.

United States.[1] This chapter places male-dominated medicine within the context of nineteenth-century United States values and examines the significant trends and controversies in pre-anesthesia midwifery and childbirth. This period in childbirth set the pattern for twentieth-century obstetrical practices and determined what the role of the modern woman's doctor would be.

NINETEENTH-CENTURY CHILDBIRTH

In the early nineteenth-century United States, the average woman gave birth at home attended by a woman-midwife. Medicine had little control over childbirth, although general practitioners, with little specific training, did conduct some home deliveries. Early in the century, the encroachment of medicine into midwifery met with some resistance from medical professionals. Objections took two forms. The first obstacle to the medicalization of childbirth can be traced to the remnants of Victorian morality that made physical contact with the female genitalia an odious task for physicians and an indiscretion on the part of women who permitted it. The second obstacle was the belief that medical intervention in childbirth was unnecessary and often harmful.

Writing around 1848, Dr. Samuel Gregory noted that the first use of a man-midwife was in 1663 by the Duchess of Villiers, "a favorite mistress of Louis XIV of France." Gregory asserted that modern women, by following a precedent set two centuries before, were inviting a "violent attack against chastity." But even the duchess, he asserted, had had "some modest scruples": She wore a hood over her head whenever a man attended her (Gregory, 1974:9).

Other types of modesty-preserving devices protected the delicate sensibility of man-midwife and patient (Wertz and Wertz, 1977). A delivery position was used in which the woman was placed on her side so that the man-midwife, working from behind, could avoid eye contact. Some men-midwives covered themselves and the patient with a sheet, their work apparently not hindered by the dark, and one man-midwife is

---

[1]Male-midwifery (which became obstetrics) and pelvic surgery (which became gynecology) had relatively separate professional histories until 1920 when the American Board of Obstetrics and Gynecology incorporated and formally united the two specialties (Mengert, 1971).

reported to have disguised himself as a woman by wearing a ruffled nightcap and gown (Wertz and Wertz, 1977).

Richard Wertz and Dorothy Wertz point out that the prohibition against exposure of the female body clearly retarded clinical training in obstetrics. They relate the incidents surrounding the first use of a woman for instructional purposes. Before this, students were not allowed to observe deliveries; their training came entirely from reading books. In 1850 Dr. James White of Buffalo, apparently believing that he had found a solution to this problem, demonstrated a live birth with a poor Irish immigrant woman pregnant with her second illegitimate child, because "doctors could classify such women as not needing or deserving the same symptomatic treatment given to respectable women," Twenty male medical students observed for five minutes, long enough to prompt a local physician to write in the town paper that the students had become sexually aroused. The case came to the attention of the American Medical Association, which "deprecated the exposure of a patient during delivery as unnecessary since a physician had to learn to conduct labor by touch alone or he was unfit to practice" (Wertz and Wertz, 1977:86). Although some physicians favored the improved medical training that such exposure to women would permit, others feared that if men could not perform obstetrical operations without seeing what they were doing, women would be so offended that they would choose female midwives over male physicians.

Regarding the belief that medical intervention in childbirth was unnecessary and often harmful, many physicians felt that unless the fetus was in an unnatural position, female midwives were competent to oversee childbirth, and such doctors even ridiculed the idea of employing physicians. A professor at the University of Edinburgh likened men-midwives to a species of frog in which the male draws the ova from the female. If this is a fact, he proclaimed, "this frog practice is doubtless the only precedent, in the whole animal kingdom, in favor of accoucheurs and male-midwifery" (Gregory, 1974:12).

In "The Married Woman's Private Medical Companion," published in 1847, Dr. A. M. Mauriceau alerted his readers:

I have long labored under the conviction, that the office of attending women in their confinement should be entrusted

to prudent females. There is not, according to my experience, and the reports of the most eminent surgeons,
more than one case in three thousand that required the least
assistance. I am aware, however, that there are crafty
physicians who attempt, and often succeed, in causing the
distressed and alarmed female to believe that it would be
altogether impossible for her to get over her troubles without
their assistance; and, for the purpose of making it appear
that their services are absolutely necessary, they will be
continually interfering, sometimes with their instruments,
when there is not the least occasion for it. There is no doubt
in my mind that one half of the women attended by these
men are delivered before their proper period; and this is the
reason why we see so many deformed children, and meet
with so many females who have incurable complaints
(Mauriceau, 1974:188–189).

Echoing the sentiments of many physicians of the period,
Samuel Gregory, a prominent physician who founded the New
England Female Medical College in 1848, petitioned physicians
to give up midwifery "whatever might be the pecuniary
sacrifice" because he believed that the

> introduction of men into the lying-in chamber, in place of
> female attendants, has increased the suffering and dangers
> of childbearing women, and brought multiplied injuries and
> fatalities upon mothers and children; it violates the sensi-
> tive feelings of husbands and wives, and causes an untold
> amount of domestic misery; the unlimited intimacy between
> a numerous profession and the female population silently
> and effectually wears away female delicacy and profes-
> sional morality, and tends, probably more than any other
> cause in existence, to undermine the foundation of public
> virtue (Gregory, 1974:1).

Women midwives also perceived the danger to both their
clients and their profession and fought against instrument-
aided childbirth or, as it was sometimes called, "meddlesome
midwifery." English-born Elizabeth Nihell, a famous eighteenth-century midwife, led such an attack. In a paper entitled,
"A treatise on the Art of Midwifery, Setting Forth various
Abuses therein, especially as to the Practice with Instruments,
the whole serving to put all Rational Inquirers in a fair way of

very safely forming their Own Judgement upon the Question which is best to employ in Cases of Pregnancy and Lying-In, a Man-Midwife or a Midwife," she wrote:

My very natural and strong attachment to the profession which I have long exercised, created in me an insuppressible indignation at the errors and pernicious innovations introduced into it, and every day gaining ground, under the protection of Fashion, sillily fostering a preference of men to women in the practice of midwifery (Graham and Flack, 1960:158).

Nevertheless, the small percentage of complicated deliveries (e.g., if the fetus lay in an abnormal position, obstructing birth, or if the pelvis was too narrow to permit passage of the fetus), childbirth meant excruciating labor pain and often death for the woman and the fetus, no matter who was in attendance.

Before about 1860, the time that anesthesia came into general use, women could obtain little relief for normal birth pain. And the Cesarean section was certainly no solution for birth complications, because the operation was fatal for women and therefore had been used for centuries as a method of delivering a child only after the death of the mother (Speert, 1973).

Thus, seeking answers to such problems and focusing on the complications of childbirth, men-midwives invented and experimented with an array of instruments. Craniotomies were performed with an instrument called a perforator, which was used to perforate the fetal skull and evacuate the contents, thus reducing the size of the head and allowing the fetus to pass through the pelvis. There were also hooks and breaking-and-cutting instruments used to perform and embryotomy, in which the fetus was dissected and extracted in pieces (Gregory, 1974:29). Obstetrical forceps, also used by men-midwives, had the potential for averting some of the deaths in childbirth.[2]

The more surgery and instruments were used, the more necessary they seemed to become. Nevertheless, men-mid-

[2]See Chapter 1 for a discussion of the history of forceps.

wives' claim of improved care and better outcomes in complicated births did not go unchallenged. First, men-midwives possessed only crude skill with the newly developed obstetrical instruments, which frequently led to internal injuries or death for the mother or fetus. Forceps, as used in the nineteenth century, were particularly damaging. Wertz and Wertz (1977) point out that current obstetrical technique favors the application of "low" forceps in which the fetus's head is low in the birth canal and already visible. Two hundred years ago, men-midwives used "high" forceps, applied before the fetal head was engaged in the mother's pelvis, and "mid" forceps, in which the head was engaged but not visible. "These latter operations presented extreme danger to both mother and child, the possibilities of physical damage, infection in damaged tissue, hemorrhage, and a crushed fetal head" (Wertz and Wertz, 1977:37).

In addition, according to eighteenth- and nineteenth-century reports, instruments were often used unnecessarily for the sake of experimentation. Gregory, the prominent nineteenth-century physician, wrote: "There is a great propensity in many accoucheurs [men-midwives] to try their dexterity in the use of these mechanical 'improvements'" (1974:29). It was Gregory's belief that men-midwives were sometimes guilty of malpractice, performing the more complicated craniotomy and embryotomy on the poor for experimental purposes and on the middle class and wealthy because a higher fee could be charged. He wrote, "What is most unaccountable ... is, that when they have wounded the mother, killed the infant, and with violent torture and inexpressible pain, extracted it by piecemeal, they think no reward sufficient for such an extraordinary piece of mangled work" (Gregory, 1974:32).

As a result of the sometimes inept and needless use of these instruments, women often suffered not only extremely painful childbirth but damage to their internal organs as well. Among the worst of these injuries was the vesicovaginal fistula, which can be caused by obstetrical instruments or by prolonged labor. This injury, which is a tear in the wall between the vagina and bladder, resulting in a continuous seepage of urine, causes severe discomfort and unpleasant odors—and often ended in social isolation for the victim.

J. MARION SIMS:
A PROTOTYPE OF THE MODERN WOMEN'S DOCTOR

Largely because of the efforts of the nineteenth-century pelvic surgeon J. Marion Sims, a surgical technique for closing vesicovaginal fistula was discovered. Sims is so important in the history of childbirth that an examination of his career is warranted. Perhaps more than any other physician, Sims was the prototype for the twentieth-century women's doctor.

Within medical literature, Sims is among the most famous and celebrated of early surgeons. His major achievements, in addition to closure of vesicovaginal fistula, include work on female infertility, the invention of the Sims speculum and numerous other instruments, and the founding of the New York Women's Hospital—from which he was ironically fired for his aggressive surgical experimentation on immigrant women by the "Board of Lady Managers" appointed by him.

Statues of Sims currently stand in New York's Central Park opposite the New York Academy of Medicine and on the capitol grounds of South Carolina and Alabama. At the time of Sims's death, a noted colleague said, "If I were called upon to name the three men who in the history of all times had done the most for their fellow men, I would say George Washington, William Jenner, and Marion Sims" (Harris, 1950:373).

Sims's obituary in the *Journal of the American Medical Association* concluded, "His memory the whole profession loves to honor, for by his genius and devotion to medical science and art he advanced it [gynecology] in its resources to relieve human suffering as much, if not more, than any man who has lived within this century" (Harris, 1950). The opposing view, however, held that his "greatest general influence was to encourage an extremely active, adventurous policy of surgical interference with women's sexual organs" (Barker-Benfield, 1976:91).

Sims, a Southerner, began his career in 1835 as a general practitioner, avoiding female problems because "if there was anything I hated, it was investigating the organs of the female pelvis" (Sims, 1889:231). His attitude was, of course, shared by other physicians of this period. Sims's dislike of the female pelvis, however, turned into fascination as he became interested in the case of Anarcha, a local slave who had developed a vesicovaginal fistula as the result of a prolonged labor and instrument damage sustained when he delivered her. Realizing that slave women with this condition were viewed by many owners as economic burdens because they were good for neither breeding nor work, Sims discovered that slaves provided a readily available source of material for surgical experimentation. He guessed that other slaves in rural Alabama had the same condition and soon found that "plantation owners were delighted to hand over to him such unprofitable incurables and he soon had seven young negro women who were otherwise quite healthy collected in a little [backwoods] hospital he had specifically built" (Graham and Flack, 1960:237).

Slaves had no rights. When surgery was to be performed, the owner, not the slave, gave permission. It is reported that when Sims once could not obtain permission to operate, he actually purchased the woman from her owner (Shryack, 1966:167).

Interestingly, in his autobiography Sims referred to his work on vesicovaginal fistula as experimentation, not surgery. From 1845 to 1849 he kept the seven women in his hospital. Without anesthesia, which was not in general use as yet, he performed repeated experiments on them in an attempt to find a way to close a fistula permanently. The operations were, in his own words, so painful that "none but a woman could have borne them" (Graham and Flack, 1960:237). He operated on one woman, Anarcha, thirty times without anesthesia and the others with "comparable frequency." As each experiment failed, the women's conditions worsened and became more painful, though his attention to cleanliness kept them from dying of sepsis.

His pursuit of a surgical solution for the vesicovaginal fistula has been described as a monomania and Sims called a surgical zealot. Colleagues praised his "courage" and "endurance," but the local community became critical. Rumors began to circulate "that it was a terrible thing for Sims to be allowed to keep on using human beings as experimental animals for his unproven surgical theories" (Harris, 1950:99). Reflecting on his lack of success, Sims stated:

My repeated failures brought about a degree of anguish that I cannot now depict even if it were desirable. All my spare time was given to developing a single idea, the seemingly visionary one of curing this sad affliction, which not infrequently follows the law pronounced by an offended God when he said of women: "In sorrow and suffering shalt thou bring forth children" (Graham and Flack, 1960:237).

Sims also speculated on the degree of anguish endured by his patients and puzzled over their apparent willingness to submit to his experiments. White women, he stated, "seemed unable to bear the operation's pain and discomfort," and he theorized that stoicism was part of the "negro racial endowment."

The explanation was simple: In addition to the fact that it would have done a slave little good to resist a white man's orders, during the four years they were contained in his hospital Sims fed and sheltered the women and gave them "tremendous quantities of opium." Opium was used as a buffer against pain and "to prevent any activity of the bowels which might endanger the success of an operation." As a result of the administration of opium, the women had "severe constipation," lasting up to five weeks; the tactic "nowadays ... would be considered little short of murderous" (Harris, 1950:100). Apparently, the women became addicted to opium and were able to ensure themselves a supply of the drug only by submitting to Sims's continued experiments.

In his thirtieth experiment on Anarcha, Sims perfected the long-sought technique for closing vesicovaginal fistula, which, for him, resulted in fame and professional prominence and, for women, relief from this obstetrical injury. But history tends to record success, not failure. There is no record of the number of slaves like Anarcha, who, because they were unprofitable for owners to keep, were used in medical and surgical experiments.

It was later, however, during his tenure at the New York Women's Hospital, that Sims was credited with introducing the idea of aggressive surgery.

At the Women's Hospital this conception of surgery as nothing but a last-resort measure was radically revised.

Insofar as gynecology was concerned, Marion Sims tended to look upon the knife not as the last weapon, but as the first. In espousing this viewpoint he sometimes brought himself into conflict with the distinguished members of his Consulting Medical Board, several of whom considered unduly reckless his suggestion for operating not only on cases of vesicovaginal fistula but also on diverse other diseases and malformations of the female reproductive system (Harris, 1950:160).

By the time of his death in 1883, Sims's reputation and influence as the "evangelist of healing to women" spanned the world. His book *Clinical Notes on Uterine Surgery* influenced other surgeons to take an active policy on surgical interference. "It's vivid recitals of success along unconventional lines had emboldened them to try surgical experiments which otherwise they would not have had the courage to undertake" (Harris, 1950:268). Marion Sims was, as Barker-Benfield noted, an "architect of the vagina" (1976:91). Welcome or not, the mold had been cast.

THE ELIMINATION OF THE WOMAN-MIDWIFE

Aggressive surgical techniques became more acceptable. By the turn of the twentieth century, medical journals had begun to carry numerous articles charging that midwives were "hopelessly dirty, ignorant, and incompetent" (Edgar, 1911:882) and were responsible for the high rates of maternal death from puerperal sepsis (Korbin, 1966:351).[3] Furthermore, many medical men were convinced that women were incapable of medical training. In his 1820 "Remarks on the Employment of Females as Practitioners in Midwifery," the physician Walter Channing had argued:

They [female midwives] have not that power of action, or that active power of mind, which is essential to the practice of the surgeon. They have less power of restraining and governing the natural tendency to sympathy, and are more

[3]Puerperal fever, however, was related more to the use of hospitals than the use of midwives. See Chapter 3 for an in-depth discussion of its encroachment and alleviation.

disposed to yield to the expression of acute sensibility. Where the responsibility in scenes of distress and danger does not fall upon them, when there is someone on whom they can lean, in whose skill and judgement they have confidence, they retain their collection and presence of mind; but there they become the principal agents, the feelings of sympathy are too powerful for the cool exercise of judgement. The profession of medicine does not afford a field for the display and indulgence of those finer feelings, which would be naturally called into operation by the circumstances in which a practitioner is placed (Channing, 1974:5).

Many believed, as Channing did, that the accoucheur must be a fully trained physician and surgeon. As for female physicians, "It is needless to go on to prove this; it is obvious that we cannot instruct women as we do men, in the science of medicine" (Channing, 1974:7).

By the turn of the twentieth century, most of the resistance within the medical community to men in childbirth had disappeared. However, the emerging profession had not yet demonstrated its ability to reduce maternal death. In fact, research revealed that the medical profession still lost at least as many women in childbirth as did women-midwives (Williams, 1912).

It is ironic that physicians who were, at the time, incapable of reducing the mortality rate claimed that the elimination of women-midwives and the expansion of obstetrics constituted the solution to high infant mortality rates. Only a small faction believed that the problem would be better handled by training and licensing women-midwives. One spokesperson for the American Association for the Study and Prevention of Infant Mortality argued, "If the [female] midwife does better work untrained than the general practitioner, what type of work would she do after six months or one year of careful training?" (Noyes, 1912:1056).

The major impetus for the elimination of women-midwives, while couched in terms of better care, may actually have been economic. As another spokesperson put it:

Some 30,000 women have taken enough practice away from the physician to obtain a livelihood. Unquestionably the field of the physician has been invaded and the community is the loser because this form of practitioner is a make-shift, admittedly incapable of coping with the abnormalities of pregnancy, labor and the puerperium. The more midwives there are and the more successful they are, just so much the worse for the community at large which is thereby being supplied by second-class service (Emmons and Huntingdon, 1912:394).

Not only was the volume of business for obstetricians decreased by women-midwives, but, since midwives' clients were mostly poor and working-class women, the "material" with which to train new generations of obstetricians was diminished as well.

Part of the solution to the "midwife problem" was the establishment of large hospital–medical school complexes with obstetrics clinics and lying-in facilities. Early twentieth-century hospitals were often overcrowded and dirty and intended largely for the poor and homeless. Although humanitarian concerns motivated some physicians, it was also true that hospitals for the poor provided a constant supply of clients who could be used for clinical observation, experimentation, and instruction. Then, as now, people unable to afford private physician fees received care that was free or at reduced cost in return for providing medicine with "training material." Thus, with one stroke, two objectives could be achieved. The need for women-midwives among the poor would be eliminated, and students would be provided with ample "material" on which to train (Korbin, 1966:357).

Thus, as women-midwives were being systematically eliminated from the business of birth, childbirth was entering the machine age and the sterile, technologically oriented environment of American hospitals. Presaged by the Chamberlen forceps,[4] birth came under the domination of new experts who not only perceived the process as problematic rather than natural but who were also surgeons trained to intervene. Consistent with the traditions established by J. Marion Sims, aggressive intervention became the norm in twentieth-century obstetrics.

[4]For a discussion of the development of the Chamberlen forceps, see Wertz, Richard W., and Wertz, Dorothy C., *Lying-In: A History of Childbirth in America.* New York: The Free Press, 1977.

REFERENCES

Barker-Benfield, G. J. *The Horrors of the Half-Known Life.* New York: Harper and Row, 1976.

Channing, Walter. "Remarks on the Employment of Females as Practitioners in Midwifery" (1820). In *The Male Mid-Wife and the Female Doctor: The Gynecology Controversy in Nineteenth-Century America,* edited by Charles Rosenberg and Carroll Smith-Rosenberg. New York: Arno Press, 1974.

Edgar, J. Clifton. "The Remedy for the Midwife Problem." *American Journal of Obstetrics* 63(1911):882.

Emmons, Arthur, and Huntingdon, James. "The Midwife. Her Future in the United States." *American Journal of Obstetrics* 65(1912): 393–403.

Graham, Harvey, and Flack, Isaac. *Eternal Eve: The Mysteries of Birth and the Customs That Surround It.* London: Hulctinson Press, 1960.

Gregory, Samuel. "Man-midwifery Exposed and Corrected" (1848). In *The Male Mid-Wife and the Female Doctor: The Gynecology Controversy in Nineteenth Century America,* edited by Charles Rosenberg and Carroll Smith-Rosenberg. New York: Arno Press, 1974.

Harris, Seale. *Woman's Surgeon.* New York: Macmillan, 1950.

Kobrin, Frances. "The American Midwife Controversy: A Crisis in Professionalization." *Bulletin of the History of Medicine* 40(1966): 350–363.

Mauriceau, A. M. "The Married Woman's Private Medical Companion" (1847). In *The Male Mid-Wife and the Female Doctor: The Gynecology Controversy in Nineteenth Century America,* edited by Charles Rosenberg and Carroll Smith-Rosenberg. New York: Arno Press, 1974.

Mengert, William. *History of the American College of Obstetricians and Gynecologists, 1950–1970.* Chicago: American College of Obstetricians and Gynecologists, 1971.

Noyes, Clara. "Training of Midwives in Relation to the Prevention of Infant Mortality. *American Journal of Obstetrics* 66(1912):1056.

Shryock, Richard. *Medicine in America.* Baltimore: Johns Hopkins University Press, 1966.

Sims, J. Marion. *The Story of My Life.* New York: Appleton, 1889.

Speert, Harold. *Iconographic Gyneatrica: A Pictorial History of Gynecology and Obstetrics.* Philadelphia: F. A. Davis, 1973.

Wertz, Richard W., and Wertz, Dorothy C. *Lying-In: A History of Childbirth in America.* New York: The Free Press, 1977.

Williams, J. Whitridge. "Medical Education and the Midwife Problem in the United States." *The Journal of the American Medical Association* 58(1912):1–7.

3

Aggressive Intervention and Mortality

JANET CARLISLE BOGDAN

Demographic transition theory describes changes in fertility and mortality as nations industrialize and move through the stages of technological modernization. According to transition theory, premodern or preindustrial populations such as seventeenth-century France or Sweden are characterized by high mortality as well as high fertility rates. In general, one balances out the other, and such populations remain fairly stable. Then mortality begins to decline, but births remain high, and thus, population grows rapidly. Soon the birth rate declines, birth and death rates once again come into balance, rapid growth ceases, and the mortality or demographic transition is complete (Wrong, 1977:21–27). Western European and North American countries followed this pattern of mortality decline and population stabilization in the eighteenth and nineteenth centuries. Contemporary developing nations are at some point along its path today.

This chapter focuses on one aspect of mortality: maternal deaths. How important are they in premodern or traditional mortality patterns? What part did they play in the mortality transition and how did they change from the colonial period to the nineteenth century? Given what we know about the changing pattern of deaths as a society moves from a premodern to a modern mortality situation, what would we expect the pattern of maternal death decline to be as overall mortality declines? Using New York City as a case study, this chapter will look at whether it fits the pattern of expected decline, and if it does not, why?

PREMODERN MORTALITY PATTERNS

Under traditional mortality conditions, overall life expectancy is low (forty-five or less) for both sexes. Females may have lower life expectancy at birth and in several age groups. Death comes most often to the youngest and oldest in the population and typically is the result of infectious, parasitic, and diarrheal diseases. Moreover, mortality fluctuates markedly over short periods, and at any particular time may vary widely from one area to another and from one subgroup to another within a population. By and large, premodern people are at the mercy of environmental and sociopolitical conditions beyond their control: when epidemics strike or disease is rife, mortality rises. When war erupts or the vicissitudes of climate disrupt the seasonal cycles of everyday life, wrecking harvests or destroying crops, food is scarce and people die in great numbers (Wrigley, 1969:passim).

A modern mortality pattern, however, implies control over numerous environmental forces and includes higher female than male life expectancies at every age and a high overall life expectancy (sixty and above). The major causes of death are chronic and degenerative diseases, not communicable ones, since a much larger proportion of the population lives to older ages and communicable diseases have been brought under control. Death rates are still highest among the youngest and oldest members of a population (Wrigley, 1969).

THE LITERATURE ON MATERNAL DEATHS AND THE MORTALITY TRANSITION

Only two studies examine the path of maternal deaths during the transition from overall low to high life expectancies in a society, and their findings are contradictory. Consequently, we do not have a clear model with which to compare what happened to maternal deaths in America generally and New York City specifically as overall mortality declined. Samuel Preston's analysis of 165 populations representing forty-eight nations in the period 1861 to 1964 shows maternal deaths to be only the fourth or fifth largest contributor to deaths among women of childbearing ages and only the third or fourth largest contributor to the mortality *decline* at ages fifteen to thirty-nine (Preston, 1976:90–99). Sigismund Peller, though, found that among the ruling families of Sweden, Norway, and England, mortality among women in their childbearing years declined considerably from the sixteenth to the nineteenth centuries. However, maternal mortality declined only slightly (see Table 3.1). Moreover, in the mid-nineteenth century, puerperal deaths increased to 42 1/2 percent of the total deaths for women in their fertile years. In other words, as health in general improved, health among fertile-age group women also improved, but *deaths in childbirth remained high.* Why? Peller suggests simply that the danger accompanying deliveries did not decrease along with the danger to general health (Peller, 1943:447).

MORTALITY IN EARLY AMERICA

Recent scholarship on mortality in colonial America suggests the varying pattern typical among premodern populations: a wide range of death rates from one area to another that

TABLE 3.1. Deaths of European Women Ages 15–50, Sixteenth through Nineteenth Centuries

Years	% Reaching 15 Who Died by 50	Deaths per 1,000 Deliveries	% Marrying Who Died in Childbed	% of Deaths Attributable to Childbirth
1500–1599	48.5	1.90	11.2	23.0
1600–1699	42.3	1.94	11.4	27.0
1700–1799	36.2	2.02	10.1	27.0
1800–1899	29.1	1.88	8.5	25.4
1850–1899	17.4	1.49	6.5	42.5

Source: Calculated from Sigismund Peller, "Studies on Mortality Since the Renaissance," *Bulletin of the History of Medicine* 23(1943):429, 443, 446.

TABLE 3.2. Seventeenth- and Eighteenth-Century American Life
Expectancies at Birth by Sex for Those Living to Age 20

	17th Century		18th Century	
Location	*Men*	*Women*	*Men*	*Women*
Andover	64.6	62.1	58.9	60.3
Ipswich	66.0	67.3	61.0	58.0
Plymouth	69.2	62.4	—	—
Salem	57.1	42.4	56.0	57.0
Virginia	48.8	39.8	—	—
N. Carolina	50.0	—	48.0	—
Maryland	46.0	—	—	—

Sources: Maris Vinovskis, "Mortality Rates and Trends in Massachusetts
Before 1860," *Journal of Economic History* 32(1972):198–199; Philip Greven,
*Four Generations: Population, Land and Family in Colonial Andover,
Massachusetts* (Ithaca, N.Y.: Cornell University Press, 1970), 192; Susan L.
Norton, "Population Growth in Colonial America: A Study of Ipswich,
Massachusetts," *Population Studies* 25(1971):440–441; John Demos, *A Little
Commonwealth: Family Life in Plymouth Colony* (New York: Oxford, 1970),
192; Darrett B. Rutman and Anita H. Rutman, "Now-Wives and Sons-in-Law:
Parental Death in a Seventeenth Century Virginia County," in *The
Chesapeake in the Seventeenth Century: Essays on Anglo-American Society,*
edited by Thad W. Tate and David L. Ammerman (Chapel Hill: University of
North Carolina Press, 1979); James M. Gallman, "Mortality Among White
Males: Colonial North Carolina," *Social Science History* 4(1980):300; and
Lorena Walsh and Russell B. Menard, "Death in the Chesapeake: Two Life
Tables on Early Colonial Maryland," *Maryland Historical Magazine*
69(1974):224.

fluctuate over short periods of time and that are essentially
dependent on local conditions. As one can see in Table 3.2,
seventeenth-century Northern colonies fared better than did
Southern ones. In fact, the populations of Andover, Ipswich,
and Plymouth enjoyed higher life expectancies than did U.S.
white populations until the 1930s and higher than U.S. black
populations until the 1950s (U.S. Bureau of the Census, Part
I, 1975:56).

Although eighteenth-century mortality pattern in America
was similar to the seventeenth century's in its geographic and
temporal variation, mortality and life expectancy in the
eighteenth century varied over a narrower range than it had
in the seventeenth. Whereas in the seventeenth century, life
expectation could vary from one place to another by almost

thirty years, in eighteenth-century America, the variation was not larger than thirteen years and typically was close to four. In the eighteenth century, mortality improved in some areas and declined in others. From town to town in Massachusetts, life expectations converged. Town death rates, which had been low in the early eighteenth century, increased, becoming comparable with cities like Boston (Blake, 1959:247-51). What were the underlying factors?

Not only had the numbers and size of communities increased from the seventeenth to the eighteenth century, but trade and communication had grown as well. Smallpox, diptheria, and other scourges that arrived with ships bound from both Europe and the West Indies made their way in from the coast, and even small and inland towns began suffering the epidemic and endemic diseases initially typical only in seaport communities (Greven, 1970:107; Shryock, 1966:2-3). As trade and travel ended the isolation of rural communities, the relative immunity from communicable diseases that such communities had enjoyed also ended.

SEX DIFFERENCES IN MORTALITY

Puzzling sex differences in mortality occurred in both centuries. Preston's and others' research suggests that a sex mortality differential favoring women is typically well established—especially in a Western population—long before life expectancy at age twenty reaches sixty years (Preston, 1976:91-95; Coale and Demeny, 1966:2-11). Thus, we would expect women to enjoy higher life expectancy than men in places where life expectation at birth is fifty years or more. That was not uniformly the case in either seventeenth- or eighteenth-century Northern colonies (see Table 3.2).

Because we have no information that might explain such variation, investigators surmise various reasons for particular mortality patterns. For the differences between men and women from ages fifteen to forty-five, childbirth is usually indicated as the likely cause for excess female mortality (Demos, 1970:66, 193; Vinovskis, 1972:201).

Whether childbirth is the major cause elevating women's death rates above men's is far from certain. In fact, at all ranges of life expectancy, factors other than childbirth typically present greater risk to women in the fertile years. According to Preston's (1976) data, respiratory tuberculosis can be expected to kill women during their fertile years more than twice as often as childbirth except when life expectancy at birth is more than seventy years. A study of cause of death in some early New Hampshire towns suggests the same conclusion (Estes, 1981:308–310).

Mortality information for seventeenth- and eighteenth-century America, then, shows the varied death experience usually found in a premodern society. Seventeenth-century life expectation at age twenty varied from a high of sixty-nine to a low of forty (see Table 3.2). At older ages, life expectancies for men and women were more equal (see Table 3.3). In the eighteenth century, a convergence appears to have occurred. Life expectancies still varied, but over a narrower range. Very little cause-of-death information is available for these centuries, but the age pattern of sex differences in life expectancies has led researchers to assert that death in childbirth is the cause of women's lower life expectancy when life expectancies during women's fertile years fall below men's (Demos, 1970:66, 193; Vinovskis, 1972:201). We cannot know at this time whether this assertion is true: sufficient information to study the problem simply is not available.

Although Preston's work does not deal with changes in specific cause of death according to age and sex, and so does not describe how maternal mortality falls among fertile-age women in relation to other causes of death as a population moves from one level of life expectancy to another, his findings urge us to consider a decline in maternal mortality as part of a larger or more extensive decline, rather than as an isolated occurrence. Peller, however, finds mortality among fertile-age women decreasing substantially while maternal mortality remains high. His study cautions us against assuming that a mortality decline among women of childbearing age necessarily means a decline in maternal mortality.

NINETEENTH-CENTURY NEW YORK CITY

With these cautions in mind, let us turn to the nineteenth century and especially to New York City. Nineteenth-century urban areas suffered higher death rates and lower life expec-

TABLE 3.3. Seventeenth-Century Massachusetts Life Expectancies at Ages 20 to 90

	Expected Age									
	Andover				Ipswich		Salem		Plymouth	
	1640–1669		1670–1699							
Present Age	Men	Women	Men	Women	Men	Women	Men	Women	Men	Women
20	64.3	62.1	64.8	62.1	66.0	67.1	57.1	42.4	69.2	62.4
30	70.8	66.8	68.7	65.9	—	—	60.2	51.0	70.0	64.7
40	72.7	67.7	71.4	69.0	70.0	72.9	65.1	61.9	71.2	69.7
50	73.5	71.3	73.5	72.4	73.1	72.9	70.1	65.4	73.7	73.4
60	76.4	77.6	75.2	75.9	76.1	75.8	75.5	77.2	76.3	76.8
70	80.3	82.1	80.2	81.9	79.5	82.7	81.0	81.0	79.9	80.7
80	86.4	90.0	86.7	89.5	86.2	86.3	—	—	85.1	86.7
90+	95.0	95.0	95.0	96.2	95.0	95.0	—	—	—	—

Source: Maris Vinovskis, "Mortality Rates and Trends in Massachusetts Before 1860," *Journal of Economic History* 32(1972): 198–199.

tations than did rural areas. More populous areas generally were less healthy places in which to live in times before it was commonly understood how disease was spread and how it could be prevented. A large mass of people, inadequately fed, housed, and clothed, and living in close quarters in an environment lacking sufficient sanitary safeguards, led to high death rates from rapidly spreading epidemic sicknesses like cholera and smallpox, and endemic sicknesses such as tuberculosis, diphtheria, and scarlet fever (Weber, 1899:343–367). New York City's death rates were usually higher than those in other Northern cities, but the pattern was similar: during an epidemic visitation, the city death rate jumped; afterward, since death had eliminated the most vulnerable among the population, the rate fell quickly, only to climb gradually again before taking another precipitous jump (see Figure 3.1). At every age, New York City male death rates exceeded females', a pattern that may have been usual in urban areas at this time (Downing, 1853). In Figure 3.1, the peaks in death rate were the result of cholera, which struck New York City in 1832, 1834, 1849, and 1854. In 1866 the disease struck again, but with far less impact on the death rate. In addition, crowding was at its worst during the mid-century years when the death rate soared (Ernst, 1949:52–53).

Death rates of New York City men and women between ages twenty and forty were lower than those of the city's general population (see Table 3.4 and Figure 3.2), although peak death rates occurred in the same years. New York's crude death rate (CDR: annual number of deaths in a population per 1,000) averaged twenty-six during the first quarter of the nineteenth century; it rose to thirty-one-and-a-half during the second quarter, rose again in the third quarter of the century to thirty-three, and then fell to first-quarter levels in the century's final quarter.

Among all women between ages twenty and forty, the CDR before 1850 remained around fourteen. In 1854, a cholera year, it climbed to twenty-two, dropping back down to stay near fourteen until 1865, when it rose to sixteen and then began to inch down. Men's CDRs followed a path similar to women's but were higher at each point except 1842, when they dropped and women's rose slightly.

Only women, of course, die in childbirth, and as we have

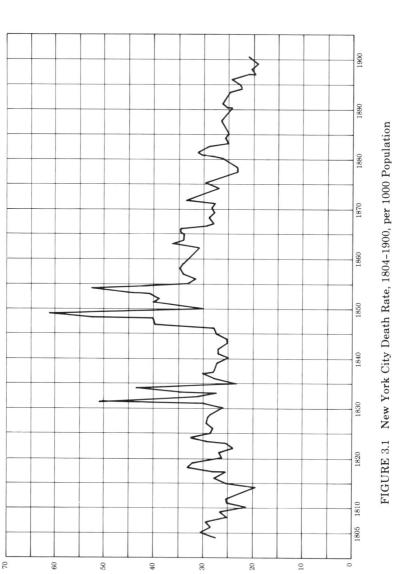

FIGURE 3.1 New York City Death Rate, 1804–1900, per 1000 Population

Sources: For 1804–1865: John Duffy, *A History of Public Health in New York City, 1625–1866* (New York, 1968), App. I, pp. 575–577. For 1866–1900: Ira Rosenwaike, *Population History of New York City* (Syracuse, N.Y.: Syracuse University Press, 1972), App. A, p. 177.

TABLE 3.4. Average Death Rates in New York City, 1804-1900, Per 1000 Population

Years	Death Rate	Years	Death Rate
1804-1809	28.1	1854-1859	34.0
1810-1814	22.9	1860-1865	29.7
1815-1819	29.0	1866-1869	31.0*
1820-1824	27.1	1870-1874	29.6
1825-1829	28.8	1875-1879	25.6
1830-1834	35.6*	1880-1884	27.7
1835-1839	27.6	1885-1889	25.9
1840-1844	26.2	1890-1894	25.1
1845-1849	39.3*	1895-1900	21.7
1850-1854	40.7*		

*Includes years of cholera outbreaks (1832, 1849, 1854) or civil war (1866).
Sources: For years 1804-1865: John Duffy, *A History of Public Health in New York City, 1625-1866* (New York, 1968), App. I, pp. 575-577. For years 1866-1900: Ira Rosenwaike, *Population History of New York City* (Syracuse, N.Y.: Syracuse University Press, 1972), App. A, p. 177.

seen, these deaths are usually assumed to explain women's high death rates. In his study of the life cycles of cohorts of nineteenth-century Massachusetts women, Peter Uhlenberg remarks that women between ages twenty-five and thirty-five were more likely to die than men in that age range before 1890—which, he maintains, shows that "the influence of deaths related to pregnancy may have been significantly large" (1969:410). As discussed earlier, both Vinovskis (1972) and Demos (1970) assumed the same relationship in accounting for sex differences in life expectations in their studies of seventeenth- and eighteenth-century Salem and Plymouth.

Unfortunately, the data needed to study the question of the cause of death are often missing. Determining when women died in seventeenth-century Salem, for example, is already difficult without the added complication of establishing what they died of. Women's lives are rarely chronicled in the usual public places—in wills and probate records, for example—and when women do appear in such records, they are often difficult to trace because of name changes on marriage. Because information is scarce, indirect measures of childbed mortality are often used: the number of women dying during their fertile

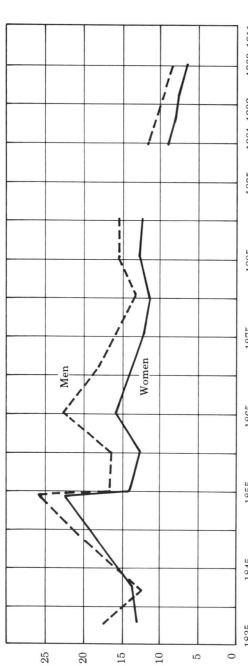

FIGURE 3.2.   Death Rates per 1,000 for Selected Years, 1838–1911, in New York City, for Ages 20–40 By Sex*

*Rates from 1838 to 1890 are for Manhattan; after consolidation in 1898, New York City included the five present boroughs. The rates recorded here after 1890 are based upon the present geographical New York City.

Sources: Rates were calculated from population and death statistics in the following: Charles A. Lee, "Medical Statistics Comprising New York, and Its Immediate Causes during a Period of Sixteen Years," *American Journal of Medical Science* 19(1836): 50; H. G. Dunnel, City Inspector, "Annual Report of Interments in the City and County of New York for 1838," *New York Journal of Medical Sciences* n.s. 1(1839): 233; Review of John Griscom, "Mortality of the City of New York, 1842," *American Journal of Medical Science* n.s. 6(1843): 437; New York City Inspector, "Annual Report of the City Inspector," 1854, 1855; Federal and State Censuses, 1830–1865, recorded in: Franklin B. Hough, *Statistics of Population of the City and County of New York as Shown by the State Census of 1985, with the Comparative Results of This and Previous Enumerations, and Other Statistics Given by the State and Federal, from the Earliest Period* (New York, n.p., 1866), pp. 44–46, 48–50, 78–79, 99–102; U.S. Secretary of the Interior, *A Compendium of the Ninth Census, 1870* (Washington, D.C.: Government Printing Office, 1872); U.S. Department of the Interior, *United States Tenth Census, 1880* (Washington, D.C.: Government Printing Office, 1883); U.S. Census Office, *Eleventh Census, 1890* (Washington, D.C.: Government Printing Office, 1893). Interpolation was used where necessary to estimate population in intercensal years. Death rates from 1901 through 1911 are from the New York City Department of Health, *Summary of Vital Statistics,* 1965.

years, for instance, or how frequently maternal death is recorded in diaries of the period.

For nineteenth-century New York City, however, direct data on female deaths are available. For some years, counts of deaths by sex and cause were reported, along with population information by sex and age (Bogdan, 1986). These data suggest, contrary to Uhlenberg's findings, that men between twenty and forty years of age were more likely to die than women of the same age. Moreover, childbirth did not seem to be the major factor in changes in the female death rate.

Nevertheless, it is not possible to comment directly on maternal mortality throughout the nineteenth century. To do so would require information on both maternal deaths and live births, the numerator and the denominator, respectively, of a maternal mortality formula. Although data on maternal deaths do exist, data on live births are not available until 1866 (Bolduan, 1916:6, 11). Only from that year forward can we trace maternal mortality in New York City. For earlier years, available age-, cause-, and sex-specific death rate data can be used to examine the path of New York City maternal death rates (number of childbed deaths divided by number of fertile-age women in population times 1,000), as well as to examine women's mortality in relation to overall mortality and to same-age male mortality. We can analyze some major components of female mortality and comment of the effects, if any, of changes in childbed mortality on overall female mortality.

The similar shapes of the death rate curves in Figure 3.3 suggest that young adults of both sexes were dying at different but parallel rates. Men and women did diverge on rates from some causes of death: for every 100 women dying from alcoholism in 1860, for example, 527 men died; for every 100 suicides among women, there were 405 among men (U.S. Department of the Interior, 1883:xxiv). But men and women shared high death rates from the century's principal killer of young adults, respiratory tuberculosis (see Table 3.5). Respiratory tuberculosis accounted for between 32 and 43 percent of deaths among New York City's young adults from at least 1870 until after 1890 (Columbia University, 1941:n.p.). Tuberculosis was the largest killer of the period. It was responsible for a greater percentage of deaths among fertile-age

TABLE 3.5. New York City Tuberculosis Death Rates per 1000 for Men and Women Ages 15-44

Years	Rates		
	Men	Women	All
1866–1870	5.85	5.35	4.53
1871–1875	5.62	5.00	4.17
1876–1880	5.04	4.63	3.81
1881–1885	5.56	4.65	4.02
1886–1890	5.38	3.97	3.63
1891–1895	4.62	3.24	3.00
1896–1900	4.00	2.73	2.50

Source: Calculated from figures at Columbia University, DeLeMar Institute of Public Health, *Population, Births, Notifiable Diseases, and Deaths Assembled for New York City, 1866-1938* (New York: Columbia University Press, 1941), Vol. 2.

women, almost 40 percent, than among men in the same age range (see Table 3.6). Childbed deaths, on the other hand, averaged less than 10 percent of fertile age women's deaths (see Table 3.7). Childbirth posed a lesser threat to fertile age women than did tuberculosis (see Figure 3.3). From at least 1842, a woman between the ages of fifteen and forty-five was less likely to die than a

TABLE 3.6. New York City Respiratory Tuberculosis Deaths as a Percentage of Total Deaths Among Men and Women Ages 15-44, for 1866-1900

Years	Women	Men
1866–1870	37.7	34.7
1871–1875	38.5	36.4
1876–1880	42.9	41.0
1881–1885	39.0	38.6
1886–1890	35.8	36.0
1891–1895	31.7	36.0
1896–1900	31.8	37.0

Source: Calculated from figures at Columbia University, DeLeMar Institute of Public Health, *Population, Births, Notifiable Diseases, and Deaths Assembled for New York City, 1866-1938* (New York: Columbia University Press, 1941), Vol. 2.

TABLE 3.7. New York City Puerperal Deaths as a Percentage of Total Deaths, 1838-1900

Years	Percent
1838-1842	5.3
1853-1855	8.4
1856-1860	8.9
1861-1865	7.2
1866-1870	7.5
1871-1875	11.5
1876-1880	10.1
1881-1885	9.5
1886-1890	8.4
1891-1895	7.9
1896-1900	8.0

Sources: Thomas K. Downing, New York City Inspector, "Table of Semi-Centennial Mortality of the City of New York, 1804-1853," and New York City Inspector's reports, 1836-1865, continued as annual reports of New York City Board of Health from 1866 to 1893. Figures from 1893 to 1900 from Columbia University, DeLeMar Institute of Public Health, *Population, Births, Notifiable Disease, and Deaths Assembled for New York City, 1866-1938* (New York: Columbia University Press, 1941), Vol. 2.

man in that age group. Moreover, when she did die, she was about four times likelier to succumb from tuberculosis than she was to die from causes connected with childbirth.

MORTALITY DECLINE

Nineteenth-century New York City's CDR zigzagged up to an 1849 high of sixty-one deaths per 1,000 population and began to decline from this mid-century high after the third major cholera epidemic had taken its toll in 1854. Even then, it did not fall consistently and below early first-quarter rates until the last decade or two of the century. The CDR pattern among young adult men and women (ages twenty to forty) is similar to that of the general population, although, as we have noted, the 1865 peak among males is more prominent (see Figure 3.2).

The crude maternal death rate pattern is different. It varies over a narrower range (.65 to 1.7 per 1,000 fertile-age women), and though it rises at mid-century, it does not then begin to

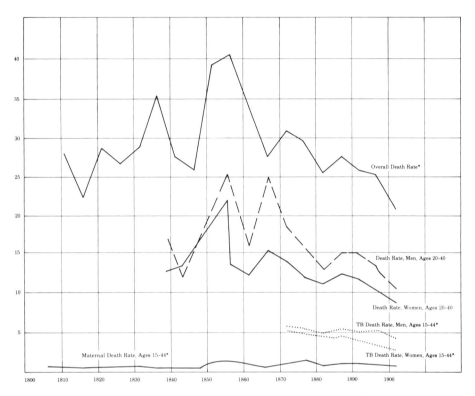

FIGURE 3.3.   Nineteenth-Century New York City Death Rates
per 1,000 Population

*Five-year averages.
Sources: For years 1804-1865: John Duffy, *A History of Public Health in
New York City, 1625-1866* (New York, 1968), App. I, pp. 575-577. For years
1866-1900: Ira Rosenwaike, *Population History of New York City* (Syracuse,
N.Y.: Syracuse University Press, 1972), App. A, p. 177. Tuberculosis death
rates from Columbia University, DeLeMar Institute of Public Health, *Population, Births, Notifiable Diseases, and Deaths Assembled for New York City,
1866-1938* (New York: Columbia University Press, 1941), Vol. 2. Maternal
death rate from annual reports of the New York City Board of Health,
1872-1889; from New York Secretary of State, *1875 Census* (Albany, N.Y.:
Weed, Parsons and Co., 1877): 118-119; and from U.S. Bureau of the Census,
*Eleventh Census. Report on Population of the United States and Report on
Education in the United States,* Vol. 1, Part 2b (Washington D.C.: Government Printing Office, 1893), p. 126.

decline as does the general death rate. Instead, it continues to edge upward, peaking in the years 1870–1874 (see Figure 3.4). Throughout the nineteenth century, New York City's maternal death rate hovered around one per 1,000 women of childbearing age. The overall death rate of women of childbearing age, however, zigzagged in a pattern similar to the general death rate rather than to the maternal death rate (see Figures 3.3 and 3.4).

These patterns demonstrate that the decline in the death rate for fertile-age women was independent of maternal deaths. Maternal deaths, though they averaged somewhat less than 10 percent of all deaths in this age group, did not significantly affect changes in the death rate of fertile-age women. Moreover, the decline in mortality that began at mid-century may not have affected or been affected by maternal deaths, which did not decline until after the period 1870–1875, almost a quarter-century after the CDR had begun to fall.

MATERNAL DEATHS IN NINETEENTH-CENTURY NEW YORK CITY

Why did New York City's maternal death rate begin to decline years after other rates instead of along with the general death rate, as Preston's model suggests it should? Were there special characteristics of the population of fertile-age women in New York City that rendered them particularly vulnerable? Did the great and increasing numbers of immigrant women push up the death rate? Or was something occurring in the conduct of birth that might have stayed any expected decline? As doctors increasingly attended women at birth over the nineteenth century, did they in fact increase rather than decrease the likelihood of death to parturient women?

At first glance, it appears that we could find cause for the unexpected continuation of early-century maternal death rate levels in the immigrant population in New York City, which grew consistently throughout the century. The foreign born were clearly a growing proportion of New York City's population during the century. In 1825 they accounted for only 10 percent of the city residents, but by mid-century, they constituted fully half of the city's burgeoning population. By 1890

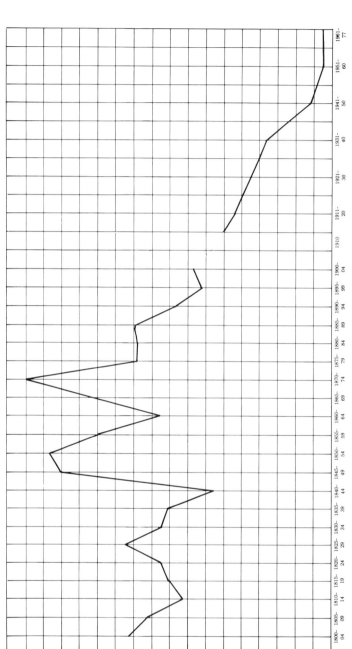

FIGURE 3.4. New York City Crude Maternal Death Rate, 1800–1977: Average Childbirth Deaths per 1,000 Women Ages 15–45.

Sources: Population figures compiled from Federal and New York State Censuses, 1800–1890; Columbia University, DeLeMar Institute of Public Health, *Population, Births, Notifiable Diseases, and Deaths Assembled for New York City, 1866-1938* (New York: Columbia University Press, 1941); and Ira Rosenwaike, *Population History of New York City* (Syracuse, N.Y.: Syracuse University Press, 1972) App. B, Table B-1, p. 188. Puerperal deaths compiled from Thomas K. Downing, New York City Inspector, "Table of Semi-Centennial Mortality of the City of New York, 1804–1853," and from New York City Inspectors' reports, 1836–1865, continued as annual reports of the Board of Health from 1866 to 1893. Figures from 1894 to 1900 from Columbia University, *Population*; figures from 1901 to 1977 from New York City Department of Health, *Summary of Vital Statistics, 1977.*

the foreign born and their children constituted 80 percent of city residents (Rosenwaike, 1972:72; Claghorn, 1901:467). Much has been written about the crowded, dismal, and dirty living conditions typical among nineteenth-century immigrants. Housing, sanitation, and food supplies were generally much worse for immigrant New Yorkers than for the native born. The immigrant lived on the margin. Even as early as 1795, when only 10 percent of the population was immigrant, immigrants accounted for 70 percent of yellow fever deaths (Griscom, 1858:7). Immigrants consistently had high disease and death rates.

In years during which we can calculate maternal deaths by nativity, the foreign born accounted for a far greater percentage of such deaths than the native born. As Table 3.8 shows, foreign-born women accounted for 61 to 69 percent of maternal mortality in New York City between 1872 and 1889. At first glance, these percentages seem high enough to support the argument that it was the great number of immigrant women that kept nineteenth-century maternal mortality rates in New York at levels far beyond what Preston's findings would indicate. However, when we investigate further, we discover that the foreign born in fact represented more than half the fertile-age New York City female population in 1875 and 1890 (56 percent), and two-thirds of those in the most fertile age group (ages twenty to thirty-five) (see Table 3.9).

In addition, studies of nineteenth-century American fertility have consistently shown that the foreign born had higher fertility rates than the native born (Hareven and Vinovskis, 1978:96; Bell, 1963; La Sorte, 1976). Data for New York City

TABLE 3.8. Percent of Childbed Mortality among Native- and Foreign-Born New York City Women, 1872–1889

Years	Foreign Born	Native Born
1872–1875	69	31
1876–1880	61	39
1881–1885	61	39
1886–1889	63	37

Source: Calculated from the annual reports of the New York City Board of Health, 1872–1889.

TABLE 3.9. New York City Female Population, Ages 15-44

	1875		1890	
Age Group	*Native Born*	*Foreign Born*	*Native Born*	*Foreign Born*
15-19	45,501	9,680	56,542	23,626
20-24	32,205	27,723	53,578	43,882
25-29	19,914	35,455	42,355	43,935
30-34	13,532	31,161	31,842	33,239
35-39	10,238	29,142	{ 35,513	{ 61,665
40-44	7,343	26,304		
45-49	5,195	18,809	{ 17,272	{ 47,558
50-54	—	—		

Sources: Calculated from the New York Secretary of State, 1875 Census (Albany: Weed, Parsons and Co., 1877): 118-119; U.S. Bureau of the Census, *Eleventh Census. Report on Population of the United States and Report on Education in the United States,* Vol. 1, Part 2b (Washington, D.C.: Government Printing Office, 1893), p. 126.

demonstrate that women there were no different than their sisters in other parts of the country, where the foreign born regularly had higher fertility rates. Toward the end of the century, years for which we do have accurate New York City data on births by ethnicity, for example, we find that foreign-born women, though only 48 percent of the fertile-age population, accounted for 73 percent of the live births in 1890, 72 percent in 1896, and 66 percent in 1899 (U.S. Bureau of the Census, 1893; New York City Board of Health, 1896, 1899). The percentage of childbed mortality accounted for by the foreign born in those three years, then—an average of 63 percent—was *less* than the percentage of live births attributable to them: 72 percent.

Foreign-born women accounted for the great majority of maternal deaths in New York City hospitals and charity institutions. Of the thirty-one and thirty-five childbed deaths occurring in New York City hospitals in 1858 and 1859, for example, 90 percent and 71 percent, respectively, were foreign-born women. Such proportions suggest that it was because of the foreign born that maternal deaths remained high after mid-century. In fact, these percentages probably reflect the proportional difference in nativity among the women patronizing those institutions. Commonly seen as places to go to die, hospitals in nineteenth-century New York City were only for the desperate. And the foreign born were more often desperate than the native born. In one such institution, The New York Asylum for Lying In Women, the foreign born ranged between 75 and 90 percent of those entering the asylum from the 1830s through the 1850s, about the same percentage range of maternal deaths among the foreign born in hospitals (New York City Inspector's Reports, 1858, 1859; Asylum for Lying In Women, 1832, 1833, 1851, 1856).

It was probably not the continuing influx of poor fertile-age immigrants that kept maternal deaths high decades beyond the time that they could have been expected to decline. What other factors could account for this? Perhaps a look at maternal deaths themselves would reveal some clues about their cause and their eventual decline.

Maternal death can occur during pregnancy, delivery, or in the six-week period following delivery called the puerperium, and it can result from a variety of causes: toxemia, hemorrhage, accidents, sepsis, or from a preexisting condition that the pregnancy or delivery aggravates to the point of death. The early recording of maternal deaths does not reflect this range of causes. Through the first several decades of nineteenth-century New York City tabulations, maternal deaths were listed simply as puerperal fever. By mid-century, five categories of septic and six of accidental death were included in the tabulations, and by 1875 there were twenty-two categories. Beginning around mid-century, then, we can divide New York City maternal deaths into at least two groups: those following septic infection and those following an accident of pregnancy, delivery, or the puerperium. By 1875 we can divide maternal deaths into the standard categories: sepsis, toxemia, hemorrhage, accidents of pregnancy (including miscarriage and abortion), and childbirth accidents (Downing, 1853; New York City Inspector, 1816–1865; New York City Board of Health, 1866–1899).

Septic infection was the major cause of maternal deaths in nineteenth-century New York City.[1] Not until the last five

[1]Present-day Bronx and Manhattan constituted New York City during most of the nineteenth century. In 1898 Brooklyn, Queens, and Richmond County merged with Manhattan and the Bronx to form Greater New York. In this chapter, New York refers to the city before consolidation, unless otherwise noted.

years of the century did the septic portion of maternal deaths drop below 50 percent. By the 1850s, as we can see in Table 3.10, septic causes accounted for two-thirds to three-quarters of New York City's maternal deaths. In the fifteen-year period from 1850 to 1865, that percentage declined slightly. By 1870 the percentage had dropped to around 60, and it hovered there through the next twenty-five years, rising to a high of 64 percent during the period from 1876 to 1880 and falling to 54 percent between 1886 and 1890.

TABLE 3.10. Causes of Puerperal Deaths in New York City, 1819–1940, in Percent

Year	Sepsis	Toxemia	Hemorrhage	Accidents of Pregnancy	Accidents of Birth
1819–1834	14				
1835–1836	—				
1837–1840	65				
1841–1845	93				
1846–1850	86				
1851–1855	73				
1856–1860	67				
1861–1864	71				
1865–1869	—				
1870–1875	59	13	9	8	11
1876–1880	62	12	8	7	11
1881–1885	58	11	9	6	15
1886–1890	54	11	9	12	14
1891–1895	59	12	10	10	8
1896–1900	41				
1901–1905	39				
1906–1910	37				
1911–1915	36				
1916–1920	34				
1921–1925	25				
1926–1930	26				
1931–1935	22				
1936–1940	26				

Sources: Calculated from "Annual Reports of the City Inspector, New York City 1819–1863," and from Columbia University, DeLeMar Institute of Public Health, *Population, Births, Notifiable Diseases, and Deaths Assembled for New York City, 1866–1938* (New York: Columbia University Press, 1941), Vol. 2.

Let us examine infection more closely as a cause of the greatest portion of nineteenth-century New York City childbirth deaths. The labels attached to the various puerperal infections changed over the course of the century. At first grouped under the rubric of puerperal fever, they gradually expanded to encompass a variety of infections: peritonitis, metritis, metro-peritonitis, puerperal cellulitis, and pyemia, to name a few. In the 1890s, labeling changed again and all infections were recorded as puerperal septicemia.

Whatever it might have been called, infection following childbirth has been recognized as a threat through recorded history. However, it was not until women began giving birth in hospitals—maternity wards of general hospitals or maternity hospitals—that puerperal infection appeared in epidemic form. Further, puerperal fever epidemics coincided with the entry of physicians as attendants at normal births.

The first recorded epidemic was in France, the country where male medical attendance at normal birth was initiated. Epidemics grew as such attendance became more and more common. The Hotel Dieu in Paris reported an epidemic in 1664; by the end of the eighteenth century, epidemics occurred in institutions throughout Europe, almost always in hospitals. Hirsch (1885:422–424) reports at least forty-eight epidemics in France, Denmark, Germany, Austria, Sweden, Holland, Ireland, Scotland, and England before 1800. By the beginning of the nineteenth century, epidemics of puerperal infection were occurring not only in institutions caring for parturient women but also in the towns and rural areas of Europe and Great Britain.

Puerperal fever was not unknown in America at the time. Recognized as a threat in the early years of the nineteenth century, it was viewed as an occasional visitor rather than an epidemic disease. Americans cited Europe's ill-kept hospitals and the "filth, and nastiness" in which its poor lived as causes for the devastating fevers like typhus and plague—which periodically swept that continent—and puerperal fever, which settled like a shroud over the poor of city and countryside alike (*Medical Repository*, 1803).

Before long, however, many Americans were faced with repeated occurrences of puerperal fever on their own shores. As early as 1799, upstate New York's Genesee County reported that of thirty-nine adult deaths in the county that year, six, or almost 17 percent, were a result of puerperal fever (Willard, 1854:396).

During the early decades of the nineteenth century, evidence of puerperal fever's increasing presence grew. It was prevalent enough for New Yorker Samuel Bard, author of the first American midwifery text, to admit that some of his patients had indeed died from it, but to deny that it was epidemic in the city (Bard, 1819).

A puerperal fever epidemic struck the lying-in wards of Philadelphia's Pennsylvania Hospital in 1816–1817 (Hodge, 1833:327). During the same years, a rash of cases followed a Philadelphia physician named David Rutter, who, in the four years from 1816 to 1819, saw ninety-five of the women he had attended develop puerperal fever. Not far from Philadelphia, puerperal fever was stalking the patients of Dr. Samuel Jackson wherever he went in Northumberland County. In and around Boston, runs of cases appeared in different doctors' practices beginning in 1817 and increasing through the 1820s (Eights, 1832:154; Holmes, 1843:235–242).

Physicians sometimes were forced to stop attending births or even to close down their practices and move to another city when puerperal fever followed them from one expectant mother to another. By 1820 puerperal fever was an acknowledged threat in America. In hospitals and in private practices, the dread fever threatened to undermine the still shaky faith American women had begun to place in physicians as birth attendants and, as a consequence, to destroy that most important, and often most lucrative, portion of a physician's practice, midwifery attendance.

Puerperal fever deaths had been occurring in New York City from at least the beginning of the nineteenth century. Puerperal fever is one of the original labels on the cause of death statistics kept by the New York City inspector's office, and puerperal fever deaths are scattered during the century's early decades. Although records of early hospitals are scarce, the existing records do refer to puerperal fever, but there is no evidence to indicate its presence in epidemic form. Beginning in the 1840s, however, and continuing to the century's closing decade, epidemic puerperal fever is much in evidence.

Few outbreaks were more harrowing than the one experienced in 1840 by Bellevue, the city's almshouse. Almost half of the fifty-nine women giving birth there in the first six months of the year contracted puerperal fever, and 80 percent of those died. In 1848 Bellevue was again the site of a major outbreak of the infection. Nineteen of twenty-four maternal deaths were attributed to puerperal fever. Similar epidemics during the following decades finally forced the closing of Bellevue's lying-in department in 1873. For the rest of the century, New York's poor gave birth at Charity Hospital on Blackwell's Island (Heaton, 1940:45).

Emigrant's Hospital, a free facility for recent immigrants, opened in the early 1850s, and it too suffered repeated epidemics of puerperal fever. In its first three years in operation, almost 2,000 women were confined, 20 percent of whom contracted puerperal fever. Until the end of the century, puerperal infection regularly invaded the lying-in department of that hospital. Even hospitals with generally low incidence of sickness reported outbreaks of puerperal fever. Opened in 1823, the New York Asylum for Lying In Women saw its first childbed fever death in 1846. The asylum's next outbreaks came in 1857 and 1858, when eight and four women in these years were infected. Two died in 1857 and one in 1858. Off and on through the next few decades, minor outbreaks of puerperal fever would sweep through the asylum, but typically, no more than one or two would die as a result (Asylum for Lying In Women, 1823–1899).

Beginning in the late 1830s, then, and continuing into the last decade of the century, childbed sepsis was the most important problem by far among the various causes of maternal deaths. Sepsis was linked to more than half the childbed deaths in the city during those years. Moreover, between 1841 and 1855, puerperal septicemia was responsible for more than 75 percent of these deaths (see Table 3.10).

It was this high proportion of septic puerperal deaths that kept the maternal death rate higher over the last half of the nineteenth century than we would expect, given both the general mortality decline and the mortality decline among fertile-age women that began by mid-century in New York City. Moreover, a major reason that septicemia continued to be such a problem was because of physicians' escalating practice of intervening in normal births. This practice brought with it the increased danger of infection reflected in the death rate pattern. As a consequence of this increased intervention, septic deaths remained high instead of declining over the course of the century, as we might have expected them to do.

Why would intervention in the birth process carry such a heavy burden of responsibility for the continuing high maternal death rate? Various aerobic and anaerobic bacteria can cause puerperal infection in any of the numerous rents and tears, often tiny, that occur during birth along the birth canal and on the cervix. Most fevers that occur after childbirth are caused by infection of the genital tract, common when labor is accompanied by vaginal or uterine manipulation or when membranes rupture long before birth. But even the womb itself, abnormally thin and vulnerable after birth, and especially the site of placental attachment, is receptive to living bacteria. The offending organisms can be conveyed to the invasion site on the infected hands, instruments, or gloves of the birth attendant. In addition, uninfected hands can carry bacteria already present at the entrance to, or in, the birth canal into the internal cavity. A delivery accompanied by examinations and manipulations within the uterine cavity can easily result in damaged tissue. Such tissue is an excellent medium for bacterial growth. Infective organisms are commonly present in the bowel and lower genital tract and can attack devitalized tissue without help from an attendant's hands or instruments. Once present, infection might travel through adjacent veins (septic thrombophlebitis and pyemia) and invade tissue and organs, frequently including the lungs, outside the reproductive system. In general, then, the more stress and contact to which the womb and birth canal are subjected, the greater the chance of damage and infection (Williams, 1976:758).

As we saw in Chapter 1, increasing intervention in childbirth became the pattern in the nineteenth century. The number and kinds of "treatments" for women giving birth increased, and though certain interventive treatments—such as bloodletting to ease labor pains or hasten labor—gradually fell out of favor, others soon took their place. In general, practices that would expose a childbearing woman to postpartum infection became more common during the nineteenth century.

With anesthesia's entry into midwifery practice in 1846,

"operative interference" to accelerate birth became easier and more frequent (Heaton, 1943:485). With other ways and a willingness to intervene in the birth process came a greater likelihood of infection. Internal examinations, the use of forceps and other instruments, manual removal of the placenta, turning and attempts at turning—all exposed childbearing women to a greater chance of infection as these procedures became more common aspects of birth attendance. Even the position and circumstances in which women gave birth may have increased their susceptibility to infection. In supine or side-lying positions, genitals are more easily, and thus, very likely more often, exposed than when women move around at will and deliver standing, squatting, or reclining in a chair.

In hospitals, the danger of this increased exposure was intensified not only because of the probable concentration of pathogens that a population of sick persons represented, but also because the number of attendants—all likely carriers of such pathogens—was greater: there were more attending physicians, student attendants, and untrained nurses. Moreover, student physicians, as well as attending and visiting physicians, were all likelier to have been involved in surgical or postmortem attendance before attending at birth than physicians not connected with a hospital would have been.

But certainly puerperal infection and epidemics were not confined exclusively to hospitals. In fact, long before the epidemic at Bellevue in 1840, puerperal fever had plagued the practices of physicians in various parts of the country.

Intervention increased for several reasons during the nineteenth century. By and large physicians gained access to the previously exclusive domain of women—childbirth—by claiming that they could intervene in the birth process to provide a safer birth. Asserting that their education, their knowledge of anatomy, and their ability to use life-saving instruments equipped them to provide superior attendance, they took over, as Jane Donegan says, "in the name of safety and implied progress" (1978:132). What previously had been a natural process calling for care by other women trained by experience became, as physicians asserted their claim, a disease calling for cure by physicians trained in medical institutions. The reorientation to birth that such a redefinition re-

quired occurred over the many years of the nineteenth century, and the difficulties that physicians faced in establishing
their hegemony over birth can, in many instances, be traced
to resistance to such a redefinition from parturient women
and their families, as well as from other physicians. The
power to influence was on the side of the innovators, however,
and the notion of birth as disease gradually became dominant.

As early as 1801, the idea that childbearing was a disease
requiring therapies just like any other disease was largely
accepted. When the prestigious Dr. Benjamin Rush wrote
about the painful disease of childbirth, he recommended standard disease therapy to combat it. For the pain of parturition,
Rush recommended that remedies "be the same as for all other
convulsive and spasmodic diseases, taking care to vary them
according to the force of the disease, and the state of the
system" (Rush, 1803:27). "Copious bloodletting" was recommended for pain, seldom less than thirty ounces to start, often
much more. And Rush stated quite plainly the effect hoped for
by both physician and patient, as well as by the patient's
friends: "diminution of pain," and "accelerating the exclusion
of the foetus." Rush suggested other courses of action as well:
a sparse diet during the last weeks of pregnancy, bowel
evacuation, and, most important, opium, an "excellent
medicine" for "destroying useless pains, and shortening the
duration of labour."

Physicians hoped to alter the course of birth—to hasten or
change it—in order to save the parturient from pain and to
save themselves time. Physician attendance was part of a
business, their livelihood, and in general, they practiced an
activist art in this age of heroic medicine. Therapies were
aimed at altering symptomatic difficulties. For example,
cathartics (purgatives), emetics, and bloodletting were all
therapies designed to reduce plethoric systems. For localized
problems, such techniques as blistering, cupping, and leeches
were employed to provide egress for the offending material.
Health was based on the notion of body equilibrium, and
illness was seen as a disequilibrium that could be treated by
affecting the symptoms, harsh though these treatments seem
to us now.

By the beginning of the nineteenth century, physicians had
been attending women in childbirth for about fifty years and

had already established a tradition of intervening in the birth process. To hurry a birth along, a physician might bleed an expectant mother, turn or attempt to turn the fetus in utero, use forceps, order a tobacco enema, or give opium, perhaps in the form of laudanum. Each of these interventions would usually produce visible and dramatic physical results, but at the time, patients expected physiological signs of effect whenever a physician was called upon to intervene. This was the heroic age of medicine, when blistering, bleeding, purging, and puking were but four of the many therapies whose demonstrable effect was both accepted and expected (Bogdan, 1978).

Physicians' predisposition to intervene in birth was not confined to medicines and techniques already a part of medical practice. When a new therapy was introduced, physicians were quick to add it to their interventive arsenal. Their reaction to the introduction of a new drug into the obstetrical pharmacopeia early in the 1800s illustrates this predilection. Ergot, an oxytocic that can increase and intensify the contractions of labor, is a fungus on rye grain that had been used by midwives for centuries. A Saratoga doctor named John Stearns learned from a local Scotch-born midwife about ergot and its effects when given during labor. The midwife apparently gave him the barest instructions for use, because after Stearns went to the fields and gathered some rye fungus for himself, he had to experiment to discover how to prepare it for effective use. After a few years of experimentation, Stearns published his results in a letter to a colleague in a leading New York medical journal. Stearns explained in no uncertain terms how effective ergot was for hurrying labor along and why he found it so helpful: "It expedites lingering parturition, and saves the accoucheur a considerable portion of time. . . . Since I have adopted the use of this powder I have seldom found a case that detained me more than three hours." Stearns also noted in his letter that ergot could be very dangerous because "the violent and almost incessant action which it induces in the uterus precludes the possibility of turning" (Stearns, 1807-1808:309).

Stearns's article met with immediate response. An avalanche of requests for samples and instructions for use poured in from practitioners throughout the East, especially those in remote areas. News of ergot spread quickly from New York to other parts of the country. Jacob Bigelow reported in 1816, just eight years after the publication of Stearns's letter, that a "majority of practitioners in Boston and probably throughout Massachusetts" were using ergot. In Baltimore, A. W. Ives, one of the city's foremost practitioners, could report that all the practitioners who answered a circular he had sent out to physicians in and around Baltimore were using ergot. One replied that he had already used it fifty times (Bigelow, 1816:161; Ives, 1821:408).

Along with the almost immediate indications of ergot's widespread use came evidence of disagreement about its best uses, the wisdom of using it, its side effects, and so on. Despite questions about its safety, however, ergot was used with increasing frequency. New England doctors reported extensive but contradictory results both with the samples Stearns had sent them and with those they had gleaned in nearby fields and grain mills. One anonymous physician/author challenged Stearns's claim that ergot relaxed muscles and could be expected to replace venesection as therapy. Furthermore, he warned ominously, stillbirth often accompanied ergot's use. During the ensuing decade, a few voices of doubt grew into a chorus of protest against ergot and against its use in childbirth even as its use soared. Those asserting that it was harmful would relate their or their colleagues' sad experiences with ergot and stillbirths or ruptured uteri, hourglass contractions, tonic contractions, perineal laceration, injury to the newborn, and so on, and then would counsel banning ergot from the American *materia medica*. Ergot's defenders would counter with contradictory experiences of labors effectively terminated, of babies' and mothers' lives saved, and of physicians' time saved and would recommend the continued, albeit cautious, use of ergot (Bogdan and Kohlstedt, 1982).

Doctors continued to give ergot "to hurry contractions," to speed up a labor, and in place of forceps throughout the century, despite repeated warnings to use it only in abortion or postpartum hemorrhage and despite repetition in article after article of examples of ergot's lethality to the fetus and its damaging effects on the parturient. By mid-century one prominent New York obsetrics professor could say, despite the disagreements and misunderstandings about it, that ergot's use is "so general . . . a disbeliever can rarely, if at all, be found" (Gardner, 1853:209, 214).

Throughout the nineteenth century, the chorus of complaints and denials about ergot's use and abuse continued, if with less frequency and urgency than during the first few decades. Ergot became a standard part of obstetrical *materia medica* used frequently by some physicians and infrequently by others. Distress over the high and rising stillbirth rate continued, but even though physicians generally agreed that ergot could and often did cause stillbirth they successfully shifted blame for the high stillborn rate away from themselves and onto "ignorant and unscrupulous practitioners" (Bogdan, 1978; Bogdan and Kohlstedt, 1982).

Ergot was used despite concern that its effects were potentially very harmful to both mother and child. The ambivalence and contention that accompanied ergot's introduction and use generally characterized other interventive techniques introduced during the nineteenth century. Instruments are a case in point.

Long before the beginning decades of the nineteenth century, physicians had been employing instruments. At first used to destroy and remove an impacted fetus in order to save the mother's life, British and European physicians early in the eighteenth century began using instruments to try to save the fetus's life (Partridge, 1905:766; Thoms, 1933:12).

By the nineteenth century, forceps and other instruments were already a matter of contention among doctors who attended childbearing women. To the conservative physician who stressed art as the basis of superior childbirth attendance, forceps were an instrument to own but to pride oneself on never or very rarely using. To the physicians of more heroic bent who stressed the science of midwifery, the forceps was an important and useful tool for the busy obstetrician. Disagreement continued throughout the century, but as in the cases of other interventionist innovations, the proponents won out.

During the nineteenth century, forceps increasingly became part of the American birth scene. Whereas early in the century physicians usually reported that they used forceps or destructive instruments in fewer than 1 percent of their cases, by the end of the century they were reporting use in anywhere from 1 to 30 percent of their private-practice cases (Bogdan, 1985). Typically, physicians who had begun their practices early in the nineteenth century reported considerably less use than

those beginning after mid-century. William Moore, an early
New York City practitioner, reported that by 1821 he had
attended almost 3,000 births. He had used forceps nineteen
times and other instruments fourteen times, or in just more
than 1 percent of his cases (Bogdan, 1986). Samuel Beach
Bradley practiced in and around Rochester, New York, for
fifty-four years, from 1816 to 1870. Bradley attended more
than 1,000 births during the period, and his records indicate
that he used forceps in fewer than 1 percent of his cases
(Denman, 1821:614; Atwater, 1974:491).

T. C. Wallace, however, reported that in his cases between
1876 and 1881, he used forceps 30 percent of the time, even
more often than did L. B. Tuckerman of Ashtabula, Ohio, who
used the forceps in six of the twenty-eight (21 percent) cases he
recorded between 1877 and 1880 (Wallace, 1881:399; Tuckerman, 1880–1881:113–114). Wallace and Tuckerman represent
the high end of the forceps use spectrum, higher than New
York City hospitals whose records also reflect increased
reliance on instruments at birth.

Indications of instrument use at the New York Asylum for
Lying In Women first appeared in its 1865 Annual Reports.
During the five-year period beginning in 1865, forceps were
used in just over 3 percent of births there. Use increased
during the ensuing years to about 6 percent in the late 1880s
and early 1890s. At Bellevue at mid-century, instruments were
used in 5 percent of births. By century's end at Maternity
(Charity) Hospital—which opened in the 1870s to accommodate
the lying-in patients stranded when Bellevue's maternity
ward was forced to close—records show that 12 percent of
births involved the use of instruments. Other hospital records
reflect use in the range of 8 to 15 percent of childbirth cases
by century's end (Bogdan, 1986).

Forceps use was given a boost in 1847 when anesthesia
came into use. Chloroform and ether made this painful intervention possible in cases in which, before anesthesia, anticipated pain would have counseled caution and instruments
would have been used only under the gravest conditions.
Along with more instruments, as we have said, came a greater
likelihood of postpartum infection, not only because forceps
themselves could be a source of infection but also because
adding one more interventive possibility added one more

means of communicating infection to the many already existing.

Consider the case reported by Dr. J. B. Graves to the New York Medical Society in 1879. Graves was called on to consult on a case by two colleagues, both medical school graduates and both experienced obstetricians, in March 1878. One of the two doctors had begun attending the case three days earlier. Labor had progressed normally, but had slowed toward the end of the first day. First the presiding doctor administered ergot. The response was minimal. He called in the second doctor. Next he gave the patient chloroform and tried the forceps but to no avail. Then the doctors decided to try to turn the fetus in the hope that it would descend. Chloroform was given again and the first doctor

> introduced a hand and brought down one of the feet: and resigned his seat to the counsel, who proceeded to bring down the other foot, and finally extracted the body, but could not the head. He then took a pair of craniotomy forceps and said he would crush the head. He proceeded to introduce the forceps, and wrung and twisted and pulled for some time, until finally the head came away.... (Graves, 1879:189–190).

The doctors continued trying unsuccessfully to extract what they thought was the rest of the fetus and the placenta. Actually they were "portions of the womb." Of course, this was a badly mismanaged case in which the mother died.

The case illustrates the number of interventive possibilities that existed for the mid- and late nineteenth-century physician and how one could follow another, thereby multiplying the means and likelihood of infection transmission. And these were not uneducated doctors. They were medical school graduates and respected men in their Corning, New York, community.

Graves felt that the two other physicians had bungled the birth case badly. Other doctors would not have agreed with Graves. Many nineteenth-century doctors, as we have seen, practiced an activist art and readily accepted innovation. If an attempt at saving the mother or child failed, many would understand this as an heroic attempt to salvage an otherwise

hopeless case. For the most part, physicians accepted intervention and had a variety of explanations for failure.

Physicians' reluctance to assume either individual or collective responsibility for the fate of their childbearing patients
allowed doctors to continue their activism basically unchallenged. Without a widely accepted explanation of cause, the
septicemia that continued to accompany or follow their
childbirth cases could be explained away on a variety of
grounds. Proposed methods of preventing infection could be
dismissed as unrelated to cause. Not until knowledge was
widespread *and* public that puerperal septicemia could be
reduced markedly were physicians forced to acknowledge their
complicity in its production and take steps to prevent it.
Moreover, their efforts at prevention were effective. Both the
maternal mortality rate and the proportion of septic maternal
deaths declined as physicians worked to obviate the dread
postpartum fever.

Nowhere is the connection more apparent between declining
puerperal septic infection and preventive efforts than in the
New York hospitals in which such efforts were chronicled and
even publicly acknowledged. In fact, in these efforts to contain
puerperal fever, strong evidence emerges that it was indeed
physicians' interventive practices, or at least their failure to
take steps to mitigate the septic effects of their interventions,
that kept the septic portion of the maternal death rate high
through the second half of the nineteenth century.

Recognition that success in containing puerperal fever was
possible was apparent in the United States by mid-century,
when Semmelweis's success at the Vienna Lying In Hospital
was reported in the New York and American medical press.
Medical editors reported that Semmelweis's method included
instructions to medical students not to handle "dead matter"
and to wash their hands in chlorine water before and after
every examination they performed on a parturient woman.
American physicians also heard and read about how in the
late 1850s Stephen Tarnier had reduced septic deaths at the
Maternité in Paris from 9 to 1 percent by isolating infected
parturients, requiring clean hands and materials, and insisting
on antiseptic washes of the parturient's genitals.

In Philadelphia, William Goodell was enjoying great success in the Preston Retreat, opened in 1866, a small lying-in

hospital similar to New York City's Asylum for Lying In Women. By a combination of rotating wards, cleaning hands, clothes, and wards with carbolic acid soap and solution, early ambulation after delivery (or what Goodell called puerperal gymnastics), uterine douches, and disallowing autopsies, Goodell was able to maintain a very modest death rate. From the Preston Retreat's opening in 1866 until 1874, only six of 756 women delivered there died, only two from septic causes, making a maternal mortality rate of less than 1 percent (Goodell, 1874–1875).

The same dramatic reductions in the maternal death rate occurred in New York City when antiseptic measures were applied consistently. An illustrative case is Charity Hospital. From its opening, Charity's maternal mortality rate varied from year to year, depending on who was chief of the maternity service. From January to June of 1874, when Bellevue closed, thirty-one women of 166 delivered at Bellevue had died from puerperal fever, a rate of almost 19 percent. Bellevue's maternity patients were transferred to Charity, and only seven of the 389 delivered there during the rest of 1874 died (a rate of 2 percent). The rate increased during ensuing years, however: in 1877 the rate was 7 percent and by 1883 it was up to 9 percent during the first nine months, the highest rate of any maternity service in the city (Bogdan, 1986).

In October 1883, Henry Jacques Garrigues was appointed chief of obstetrics at Charity, and he instituted a plan of "antiseptic midwifery" that revolved around close attention to the cleanliness of attendants, parturients, and any instruments that might be used during birth. Among the next 162 women delivered at Charity, none died. From October 1, 1883, to October 1, 1884, only four septic deaths occurred among the 505 women who delivered at Charity. Three died of other causes, for a mortality rate of 1.4 percent. The following year, mortality was even lower: one septic death out of 541 births, and three other deaths, for a mortality rate of less than 1 percent. In the third year of Garrigues' service, the rate was also less than 1 percent (Garrigues, 1886:21).

News of Garrigues' success at Charity and of his method spread quickly. By 1885 Garrigues could point to the adaptation of his antiseptic method as the main factor in the fall in the death rate, especially the septic death rate, at the New

York Infant Asylum and at the Emergency Hospital. And in Boston, William L. Richardson acknowledged that following Garrigues' suggested regimen had resulted in a dramatic decline in the septic death rate at the Boston Lying In, where a severe epidemic had occurred during the early 1880s (Irving, 1942:170-171).

But success during one chief resident's tenure did not necessarily mean the end of the problem. At a place like Charity, ward policy—especially regarding such matters as cleaning the patient and the attendants—was determined largely by the supervising physicians or by the usually silent agreements arising from the working relationships between the various ward attendants and the supervisory personnel. Garrigues worked zealously to lower and even eradicate puerperal fever on Charity's maternity wards. Those who replaced him took for granted the cleanliness present by the close of Garrigues' service, and the details of enforcement of the antiseptic regimen relaxed. As a consequence, morbidity and mortality rose after Garrigues' departure. By the 1890s, however, the death rate at Charity was again comparatively low, at 1/2 of 1 percent, or 50 per 10,000 births. When a champion of the antiseptic method—like William Goodell at the Preston Retreat or William Lusk at Emergency Hospital—remained a chief force at an institution, backsliding on the details of the method were less likely to occur. Moreover, if cleanliness (or later, antiseptic precautions) were part of an institution's policy, the same was likely to be true, as in the case of New York City's Asylum for Lying In Women.

If, as seems likely from the evidence we have examined, septic deaths continued through the nineteenth century to account for such a great proportion of maternal deaths, and general maternal mortality declined as septic maternal mortality remained artificially high during most of the second half of the nineteenth century, a time when infectious death mortality was declining.

Maternal mortality remained high, not because of the special virulence of any of the infecting organisms, but because *birth attendance grew increasingly interventive at that time,* multiplying the opportunities for infection to enter at a time when there were means neither to prevent its entry nor to treat it effectively once the infection had set in. In fact, the lag between the problems created by intervention and the means with which to deal with these problems spanned the years from the mid-nineteenth century to almost the mid-twentieth century, when infection-killing antibiotics became available.

REFERENCES

New York Asylum for Lying in Women. Annual Reports, 1834-1899.

Atwater, Edward C. "A Rural Practitioner, Dr. Samuel Beach Bradley (1796-1880)." *Bulletin of the Monroe County Medical Society,* Dec. 1974, 483-493.

Bard, Samuel. *A Compendium of the Theory and Practice of Midwifery.* New York: Collins and Co., 1819.

Bell, Wendell. "Differential Fertility in Madison County, New York, 1865." *Milbank Memorial Fund Quarterly* 41(1963):161-182.

Bigelow, Jacob. "The Clavis or Ergot of Rye and Other Plants," *New England Journal of Medicine and Science* 5(1816):156-164.

Blake, John. *Public Health in the Town of Boston.* Cambridge: Harvard University Press, 1959.

Bogdan, Janet Carlisle. "Care or Cure? Childbirth Practices in Nineteenth Century America." *Feminist Studies* 4(1978):92-99.

_____. "The Transformation of American Birth." PhD diss., Syracuse University, 1986.

Bogdan, Janet Carlisle, and Kohlstedt, Sally Gregory. "Not Childbirth, but Obstetrics: The Changing Scope of Medical History." Syracuse: Syracuse Consortium for the Cultural Foundations of Medicine, 1982.

Bolduan, Charles F. *Over a Century of Health Administration in New York City.* New York City Department of Health, 1916.

Claghorn, Kate Holladay. "The Foreign Immigrant in New York City." United States Industrial Commission Reports 15:449-492, 1901.

Coale, Ansley J., and Demeny, Paul. *Regional Model Life Tables and Stable Populations.* Princeton, N.J.: Princeton University Press, 1966.

Columbia University, De LeMar Institute of Public Health. *Population, Births, Notifiable Diseases, and Deaths Assembled for New York City, 1866-1938.* Vol. 2. New York, 1941.

Demos, John. *A Little Commonwealth: Family Life in Plymouth Colony.* New York: Oxford University Press, 1970.

Denman, William. *An Introduction to the Practice of Midwifery,* edited by John W. Francis. New York: Bliss and White, 1821.

Donegan, Jane. *Women and Men Midwives: Medicine, Morality, and Misogyny in Early America.* Westport, Conn.: Greenwood Press, 1978.

Downing, Thomas K. *Table of Semi-centennial Mortality of the City of New York.* Compiled from the Records of the City Inspector's Department, January 1, 1804 to December 31, 1853. New York, 1853.

Eights, Jonathan. "Annual presidential address on puerperal fever, delivered before the New York State Medical Society on February 7, 1832." Medical Society of the State of New York, *Transactions* 1(1832-1833):148-173.

Ernst, Robert. *Immigrant Life in New York City, 1825-1863.* New York. King's Crown, 1949.

Estes, J. Worth. "Therapeutic Practice in Colonial New England." In *Medicine in Colonial Massachusetts, 1620-1820*, edited by Philip Cash, Eric H. Christianson, and J. Worth Estes. Boston: Colonial Society of Massachusetts, 1981.

Gallman, James M. "Mortality Among White Males: Colonial North Carolina." *Social Science History* 4(1980):295-316.

Gardner, Augustus Kingsley. "An Essay on Ergot, with New Views of its Therapeutic Action." *New York Journal of Medicine and Collateral Sciences* 11(1853):206-223.

Garrigues, Henry J. *Practical Guide to Antiseptic Midwifery in Hospitals and Private Practice.* Detroit: George G. Davis, 1886.

Goodell, William. "On the Means Employed at the Preston Retreat for the Prevention and Treatment of Puerperal Diseases." *Obstetric Journal of Great Britain and Ireland*, American Supplement 2(1874-1875):49-53, 65-72.

Graves, J. B. "A Case of Instrumental delivery—with remarks." New York Medical Society *Transactions*, 1879, 188-192.

Greven, Philip. *Four Generations: Population, Land, and Family in Colonial Andover, Massachusetts.* Ithaca, N.Y.: Cornell University Press, 1970.

Griscom, John H. *A History, Chronological and Circumstantial of the Visitations of the Yellow Fever at New York.* New York, 1858.

Hareven, Tamara, and Vinovskis, Maris. "Patterns of Childbearing in Late Nineteenth Century America: The Determinants of Marital Fertility in Five Massachusetts Towns in 1880." In *Family and Population in Nineteenth Century America.* Princeton, N.J.: Princeton University Press, 1978.

Heaton, Claude. "Obstetrics at the New York Almshouse and at Bellevue Hospital." *Bulletin of the New York Academy of Medicine* 16, series 2 (1940):38-47.

_____. "Control of Puerperal Infection in the U.S. during the last Century." *American Journal of Obstetrics and Gynecology* 46 (1943):479-486.

Hirsch, August. *Handbook of Geographical and Historical Pathology*, Vol. 2. London: New Sydenham Society, 1885.

Hodge, Hugh Lennox. "Cases and Observations Regarding Puerperal Fever, as It Prevailed in the Pennsylvania Hospital in February and March, 1833." *American Journal of Medical Science* 12(1883): 325–352.

Hoffman, Frederick L. "American Mortality Progress During the Last Half Century." In *A Half Century of Public Health*, edited by M. P. Ravenal. New York: American Public Health Association, 1921.

Holmes, Oliver Wendell. *On the Contagiousness of Puerperal Fever.* Boston, 1843. Reprinted in *Scientific Papers.* New York: P. F. Collier and Sons, 1938.

Irving, Frederick. *Safe Deliverance.* Boston: Houghton Mifflin, 1942.

Ives, A. W. "Observations on Ergot." *Medical Repository* 21(1821): 403–410.

LaSorte, Michael. "Immigration and Fertility." Paper presented at the Population Association of America Meetings, Montreal, 1976.

Medical Repository. Editorial. 4(1803):440.

New York City. City Inspector's Reports, 1816–1865.

––––––. Annual Reports of the Board of Health, 1866–1899.

New York Secretary of State. *1875 Census.* Albany: Weed, Parsons, 1877.

Norton, Susan L. "Population Growth in Colonial America: A Study of Ipswich, Massachusetts." *Population Studies* 25(1971):433–452.

Partridge, H. C. "History of Obstetrical Forceps." *American Journal of Obstetrics and the Diseases of Women* 51(1905):765–773.

Peller, Sigismund. "Studies on Mortality Since the Renaissance." *Bulletin of the History of Medicine* 23(1943):427–461.

Preston, Samuel. *Mortality Patterns in National Populations.* New York: Seminar Press, 1976.

Rosenwaike, Ira. *Population History of New York City.* Syracuse, N.Y.: Syracuse University Press, 1972.

Rush, Benjamin. "On the Means of Lessening the Pains and Danger of Childbearing, and of Preventing Its Consequent Diseases." *Medical Repository* 6(1803):27–30.

Rutman, Darrett B., and Rutman, Anita H. "Now-Wives and Sons-in-Law: Parental Death in a Seventeenth Century Virginia County." In *The Chesapeake in the Seventeenth Century: Essays on Anglo-American Society*, edited by Thad W. Tate and David L. Ammerman. Chapel Hill, N.C.: University of North Carolina Press, 1979.

Shryock, Richard. *Medicine in America: Historical Essays.* Baltimore, Md.: Johns Hopkins University Press, 1966.

Stearns, John. "Account of the Pulvix Parturiens, a Remedy for Quickening Childbirth." *Medical Repository* 2nd hex. 5(1807–1808): 308–309.

Thoms, Herbert. *Chapters in American Obstetrics.* Springfield, Ill.: Charles C. Thomas, 1933.

Tuckerman, L. B. "An Analysis of the First 33 Cases of Labor Occurring in the Practice of a Country Physician." *Ohio Medical and Surgical Review* 4(1880-1881):113-114.

Uhlenberg, Peter. "A Study of Cohort Life Cycles: Cohorts of Native Born Massachusetts Women, 1830-1920." *Population Studies* 23(1969):407-420.

United States Bureau of the Census. *Eleventh Census. Report on Population of the United States and Report on Education in the United States*, Vol. 1, Part 2b. Washington, D.C.: Government Printing Office, 1893.

_____. *Historical Statistics of the United States, Colonial Times to 1970, Part I*. Washington, D.C.: Government Printing Office, 1975.

United States Department of the Interior. *Statistics of the Tenth Census*. Washington, D.C.: Government Printing Office, 1883.

Vinovskis, Maris. "Mortality Rates and Trends in Massachusetts Before 1860." *Journal of Economic History* 32(1972):184-213.

Wallace, T. C. "On the Use of the Obstetrical Forceps." *Medical and Surgical Reporter* 44(1881):373-376.

Walsh, Lorena, and Menard, Russell B. "Death in the Chesapeake: Two Life Tables on Early Colonial Maryland." *Maryland Historical Magazine* 69(1974):211-227.

Weber, Adna. *The Growth of Cities in the Nineteenth Century*. New York: Macmillan, 1899.

Willard, A. "Mortuary Statistics of the Genesee Country for the Year 1799." *New York Journal of Medicine and Collateral Sciences* 13(1854):395-397.

Williams, J. Whitridge. *Williams Obstetrics*. 15th ed. New York: Appleton-Century-Crofts, 1976.

Wrigley, E. A. *Population and History*. New York: McGraw-Hill, 1969.

Wrong, Dennis. *Population and Society*. New York: Random House, 1977.

PART II
The Conduct of Birth

Childbirth is a biological experience mediated by culture. Anthropologist Brigitte Jordan states that "there is no known society where birth is treated, by the people involved in its doing, as a merely physiological function." Within any given system, birth practices are fairly uniform, systematic, standardized, ritualized, and even morally required (Jordan, 1980:2).

In various cultures, mothers and their new babies are honored with ritual celebrations. This helps mothers adjust to their new status. In American culture, however, childbirth as a rite of passage is downplayed. Despite the extraordinary significance of the act of giving birth to the individual woman, American women generally exercise remarkably little control over the circumstances and experiences surrounding this event. Women give birth in a system that focuses on the most narrow and circumscribed arena of childbirth: the American hospital. In American culture, giving birth becomes fragmented into medical timetables and routines, a framework that may have little to do with a birthing woman's deeper sense of the transformation she is experiencing. Childbirth ritual in the United States is hospital ritual.

Doctors, nurses, and other medical professionals enter the birth environment equipped with an internally consistent symbolic universe that supplies 1) a definition of the event, 2) roles and rules for participants, 3) a specialized setting in which to practice, and 4) a particular set of methods and tools.

When a parturient woman is admitted to the medical system for birth, her decision-making power is automatically transferred to medical and administrative staff. How and why does this transference of authority come about? It begins as an acceptance of expertise in lieu of personal judgment. Surrendering personal judgment and accepting the authority of the doctor and hospital staff can be seen as "a shortcut to where reason is presumed to lead" (Gunn, 1830, as quoted by Starr, 1982:10). In other words, doctors and hospitals presumably have the best interests of the patient at heart. But the transference of authority can also be seen as "a shortcut to where coercion would be presumed to lead" (Starr, 1982:10).

What begins as a question of scientifically determined rationality becomes a question of control embedded in a power structure. As psychiatrist R. D. Laing has noted, women are told where and how they must give birth. Once in the hospital, they may or may not be allowed to move, scream, sing, stand, walk, sit, or squat (Laing, n.d.). In one study, which recorded conversations between doctors and women during birth, a woman with an epidural was acting in a socially unacceptable way, making "too much" noise, and her physician informed her that if she didn't straighten up, he would make her "go natural," in other words, deliver without pain medication. In another study, a woman having a natural birth, also acting in a way considered inappropriate for a patient, was threatened with the use of drugs.

In becoming a patient, a parturient woman must behave in a socially acceptable way *for a sick person.* She is seen as incapacitated, and therefore incapable of making sound decisions. She is therefore exempted from normal responsibilities, surrenders her personal judgment, and transfers her decision-making power to medical personnel.

As we have seen so far, inherent in the symbolic framework of the medicalized world view of pregnancy is a power relationship. Medical professionals, through ownership and exclusive control of highly valued specialized knowledge, acquire the ability to manipulate the situation. The patient may then feel like an outsider, alienated from her own experience.

Part II of this book is about power. It is about the struggle for individual control over institutional demands. Why should we analyze power relations? Because the way we "do" birth in America affects both birth outcomes and women's self-image: the way identity, ability, and self-worth are conceptualized.

We also study power relations because of problems that have arisen within the medical-obstetrical worldview for birth. For example, there is a growing debate, within medicine over the use of the electronic fetal heart monitor and the rising rate of Cesarean section. In addition, women have questioned the system from the outside. There has been a proliferation of "lay" literature criticizing the narrow viewpoint of the medical model. And women increasingly are blaming the medical system, not themselves, for negative birth experiences and outcomes. The best example of this is the rising litigation rate.

In Chapter 4, Barbara Katz Rothman shows how the political struggle for control in childbirth is played out by individuals in the birthplace. She examines how the ability of the medical profession to retain control rests on its power to define and institutionally manage the event. Hospital facilities, for example, require scheduling, and parturition must fit into a specified time frame. Relinquishing control and surrendering personal judgment begin the moment a woman places herself in the care of a doctor and continues through the days after birth. As Rothman says, a baby in a hospital nursery is controlled by the nursery.

In Chapter 5, Sandra K. Danziger scrutinizes the production of asymmetry in the doctor-patient relationship, particularly as it relates to the "illness" of pregnancy. She looks at what doctors and patients say to one another in the doctor-patient encounter, as well as how it is said and in what context. Doctors, states Danziger, first structure the encounter to meet their own needs and then offer advice on appropriate behavior. Finally, they provide the patient with a set of normalizing assurances. All of these behaviors can be seen as postures of dominance on the part of the medical professional that typically go unchallenged by the patient. But the doctor-patient encounter in childbirth involves not only a doctor-patient hierarchical structure but typically a gender-related hierarchical structure as well. The doctor-patient encounter in pregnancy is generally a male-female encounter; thus, it conveys not only patient-appropriate behavior but also gener-appropriate behavior and health stereotypes.

Margaret K. Nelson takes this model one step further in Chapter 6. Not only do we see a doctor-patient/male-female hierarchy in childbirth, but on closer examination we also discover differences in behavior based on social class. The working-class woman's ideal birth is fast, with as little pain as possible, and technologically safe. The middle-class woman's ideal is to apprehend childbirth as an experience, as free from medical intervention as possible, an experience in which she is actively involved but that is also backed by the assurance of medical expertise. Nelson concludes that the middle class can afford to "reject technology" because it has reaped its benefits, while the working class seeks technology because "those who have not yet consistently received these benefits may not be ready to abandon them." Nelson's study shows that women have different desires and goals in childbirth and that we must be careful not to impose class biases when analyzing those desires.

Nevertheless, every woman, regardless of race, creed, or social class, wants to be taken seriously. Historically a major part of women's adult lives has been consumed by pregnancy and the bearing of children. As Pamela S. Summey discusses in Chapter 7, women's version of childbirth and that of the medical model can often conflict. The two main players, doctor and patient, frequently have different perceptions of the scenario they are enacting. The birthing woman, says Summey, is embarking on one of life's most significant and meaningful experiences, trying to face her pain and fear with dignity and courage. But the doctor sees childbirth on the one hand as part of the routine day's work and on the other hand as a potentially dangerous situation that needs to be controlled. According to Summey, Cesarean delivery becomes the epitome of a situation in which "the uncertainty of outcome and the dangers of birth are invoked to control birth and leave women powerless."

As Summey states, a Cesarean section promises a "better baby," but the risk of maternal death from a Cesarean section is twenty-six times greater than with a vaginal delivery. About half of all Cesarean sections result in minor complications, and most women sue doctors for reasons related to technological birth. Nonetheless, it is the fear of being sued that leads doctors to retreat even further into the medical model: to perform ever more tests, diagnostic procedures, and Cesarean sections.

Chapter 8 closes the section with an exploration of medical malpractice by Wenda Brewster O'Reilly, Pamela S. Eakins, Myra Gerson Gilfix, and Gary A. Richwald. As they point out, woman-centered childbirth services are those least often sued. One major underlying variable in whether a lawsuit will follow a problematic outcome is the perception, on the patient's part, of the quality of the relationship between her and the doctor. They call for a new situation of power-sharing in which the public and the legal, medical, and insurance systems are no longer in competition. With shared power comes shared responsibility, and with shared responsibility comes a reduced impetus to sue. People turn to the legal system because they have no voice elsewhere. The power dynamic of competing interests must be replaced by a new dynamic of shared power and trust between provider and patient.

REFERENCES

Jordan, Brigitte. *Birth in Four Cultures.* Montreal: Eden Press Women's Publications, 1980.

Laing, R. D. "The Politics of Birth." In *Active Birth.* Epson, England: n.d.

Starr, P. *The Social Transformation of American Medicine.* New York: Basic Books, 1982.

4

The Social Construction of Birth

BARBARA KATZ ROTHMAN

The history of childbirth is a history of political struggle as different interest groups have worked to gain control over childbirth. That same struggle is re-created in each individual birth as different individuals, representing different societal interests, claim power in the birthplace. The birthing woman, the husband or father, the obstetrician who now calls the fetus his or her patient—each potentially represents different social interests in the birth.

When obstetrics gained political ascendency in American birthing practices, and births were moved into the hospital, the needs and interests of birthing women were subordinated to the needs and interests of the profession of medicine. But the politics of birth have not, for the most part, been made overt. Those who have sought to control childbirth certainly have not done so by the use of armies. Only rarely has the

An earlier version of this paper was published in Stewart and Stewart, eds., *Compulsory Hospitalization—Freedom of Choice in Childbirth?* Vol. 1 (Marble Hill, Mo.: NAPSAC, 1979).

power of the state been openly called into the birthplace.[1] Usually the form that political control has taken has been to shape ideology, the belief systems. In this chapter, I explore the recent ways in which childbirth has been socially defined and organized. I focus on the importance of the institution of the hospital and of the childbirth education movement in the social construction of birth.

Human beings live in a social as well as a physical world. We do not simply see, hear, feel, smell, and taste; we interpret what our senses take in, and our interpretations are based on what we have learned from other people.[2] When we talk to one another, we do not hear just sounds, we actually hear words. As you read this page, you do not see the texture or designs of ink on paper but rather you recognized these as symbols, as words. This social process of interpretation goes on not only for highly abstracted things like language but for physical objects as well. A chair, for instance, may seem to have an obvious purpose. Yet if a Martian viewed a chair, there would be nothing about it to proclaim its use. That it exists is its physical reality; but what it exists as, what its meaning and purpose are, is something that we have created socially in our interaction with one another.

From this perspective, known as symbolic interactionism, birthing can be seen as a social as well as physiological event, a process that is socially constructed and defined. In any social situation, the possibility exists for alternative definitions of the situation, alternative social realities. Which version is accepted and acted on is a reflection of the power of the participants. The consequences of course depend on the definition of the situation. *Those who define, control.*

From the 1950s through the 1970s in the United States, a prepared childbirth movement existed that had as its goal the definition of childbirth as a "natural" and "healthy" phenomenon. Under the heading of the general childbirth preparation movement I include a variety of childbirth educa-

[1]For a discussion of state-ordered Cesarean sections, see Ruth Hubbard, "Some Legal and Policy Implications of Recent Advances in Prenatal Diagnosis and Fetal Therapy," *Women's Rights Law Reporter* 7(Spring 1982): 201-218.
[2]For a classic discussion of this perspective in sociology, see Herbert Blumer, *Symbolic Interaction* (Englewood Cliffs, N.J.: Prentice-Hall, 1969).

tion groups, including Dick-Read, Lamaze, and Bradley. This definition of a universal physiological event occurring preponderantly in healthy women would not seem to be unreasonable. However, even a cursory reading of obstetric texts of the period, and a history of the profession, shows that childbirth in the hands of doctors was perceived as a crisis situation, needing careful medical evaluation and control. In the earlier period of obstetrics, birth was openly referred to as pathological. This is an example of alternative social definitions of a physical event or state: one group calls birth healthy, while the other calls it pathological.

David Sudnow has pointed out that death, clearly a physical state, nonetheless is socially determined and acknowledged, to the extent that two persons in a similar physical condition may be differentially designated as dead or not (Sudnow, 1967). The same physical signs may be death or not-death, depending on what happens next. People who are revived were never dead. Dead people are those who stay dead. Once death is defined as having occurred, attempts at resuscitation stop; thus, the power to define death can indeed be the power over life and death.

Medical power or control over childbirth also rests on the power to define. Consider pregnancy as both a socially determined and a physical state (Miller, 1972). The way pregnancy is dated by the medical profession is an interesting example of a retroactive social definition. A woman who is menstruating considers that menstrual period a sign of her nonpregnant state. Yet if two weeks later she conceives, her pregnancy will be dated from the first day of her last menstrual period. The very date on which she knows she is not pregnant becomes, retroactively, the first day of her pregnancy. It is usually not possible to socially enter a pregnancy before the sixth week, because that is the earliest time to obtain a positive pregnancy test with standard medical testing. Further, the medically defined pregnancy is always approximately two weeks older than the fetus whose existence presumably determines the pregnancy. This is a professional definition, not particularly well suited to the needs or perceptions of women viewing their own pregnancies.

Let us apply this concept of socially determined reality to the physical reality of childbirth and take as an example the situation of a woman who at term is having painful contractions at ten-minute intervals but is not yet dilating. That is, the woman is experiencing "labor pains," but the cervix, the opening of the uterus, has not yet begun to open. Whether she is in labor or not in labor will depend on whether she then begins to dilate, or the contractions stop and then resume days or weeks later. Whether a woman is in labor or "false labor" at that time will depend on what follows.

Inevitably, applying social definitions to physical states will involve a certain amount of bargaining or negotiating between the people involved. If a woman comes to the hospital claiming to be in labor, and yet by professionally established judgments she is not in labor, the client and the professional will have to try to reach an agreement. On the side of the professional is expertise and authority, and on the side of the client is the physical reality of what is happening to her. Perhaps if she cries and pleads the professional will come to think that with so much apparent pain something must indeed be happening, and so she will not be sent home. Similar negotiating processes take place in mental hospitals when patients and doctors negotiate competence (Goffman, 1961) and in tuberculosis hospitals when patients claim that they really are cured enough for a weekend pass (Roth, 1965).

Whatever definition is agreed upon becomes the reality. Let us return to the example of the woman having regular contractions without dilation. If she is admitted when she first requests admission and she does not begin to dilate for twenty-four hours, and she gives birth twelve hours later, that woman will have had a thirty-six hour labor. If she is denied or delays admission, however, and presents herself at the hospital twenty-four hours later for a twelve-hour in-hospital labor, she will have had a twelve-hour labor preceded by a day of discomfort. The physical sensations are precisely the same in this hypothetical example. But the social definitions, calling it labor or not, make the difference between a terribly long labor or a fairly average labor with some unusual contractions beforehand.

What difference would it make in this situation if we did not have to consider the issue of hospital admissions? In a situation in which a midwife is the birth attendant in the home, the midwife comes to see the woman when asked. If nothing much is occurring besides the woman's discomfort, perhaps the midwife will make her a cup of tea and go about her business as the woman goes about hers. The midwife drops in now and again to see how things are going. She stays as needed. The issue of telling a woman that she is not in labor if she thinks she is never arises. It is only necessary to establish a firm definition of her condition if that definition will make a difference in the way she will be handled. Take away the issue of hospital admission, and the question of when labor begins is no question at all.

When obstetrical definitions rule, the pregnant woman must learn those definitions. She needs to be able to accurately define her labor in medical terms for the following reasons: if she gains early admission, she will have helped create the social situation of an overly long labor. In addition to the stress inherent in believing oneself to be in labor for thirty-six hours, hospital treatment of long labor is problematic. Laboring women have been routinely confined to bed, a situation that is as disturbing physically as it is psychologically. Not only is the labor perceived as being longer, but also the horizontal position physically prolongs labor, as may the routine administration of sedatives during an extended hospital stay. In addition to variations in treatment during those first twenty-four hours, treatment is different in the last hours when the woman is hospitalized in either case. Women who have been in a hospital labor room for thirty hours receive different treatment that women who have been there for only six, even if both are equally dilated and have had identical physical progress.

It is also important for the pregnant woman to be medically accurate in identifying her labor because if she presents herself to the hospital and is denied admission, she is beginning her relationship with the hospital and her birth attendants from a bad bargaining position. Her version of reality is denied, leaving her with no alternative but to lose faith in her own or the institution's ability to perceive accurately. Either conclusion has negative consequences for the eventual labor and delivery situation.

The same issue arises when a decision must be made about when to move a woman from the labor to the delivery room. With the hospitalization of childbirth in America, labor and birth, or "delivery," have come to be seen as separate events necessitating separate rooms and frequently separate staff. Women attended by nursing staff throughout their labor may first see their private physician in the delivery room. When a woman is moved from one room to another to mark the transition from one stage of labor to another, the professional staff must make a distinction between laboring and delivering, and then apply that distinction to the individual woman. A cutoff must be named at which a woman is no longer laboring but is delivering. If the point is missed, and the woman delivers in the labor room or the hall, then she is seen as having "precipped," having had a precipitous delivery. If the staff decides that the woman is ready to deliver and the physical reality is that she has another hour to go, then concern is aroused about the length of her delivery because she has spent that extra hour in a delivery rather than a labor room.

Institutional management makes necessary arbitrary decisions in defining labor and its stages, if only because the use of the hospital facilities requires scheduling. For that reason it becomes necessary to periodically examine women, vaginally or rectally, to judge cervical dilation and to predict delivery time. It is usually the function of the nursing staff to make the appropriate predictions so that staff and facilities are ready. Some examinations may be needed to evaluate the physical condition of the laboring woman and fetus, but repeated examinations of cervical dilation are typically more important for scheduling purposes. Such examinations are usually quite painful.

The prepared childbirth movement did not challenge the right of the profession of medicine to define pregnancy, labor, or delivery. For the most part, the movement directed its efforts toward teaching women the medical definitions. Through childbirth education classes, women were taught to apply the medical definitions to their own physical sensations. Time was spent teaching women to recognize "true" (medically defined) labor and distinguish it from "false" (medically not recognized) sensations. Teaching women these definitions can be seen as being in the women's own interests. With some of the other lessons in childbirth education, it is less clear whose interests were being served.

The American Society for Psycho-Prophylaxis in Obstetrics (ASPO) is the original Lamaze organization in the United States. In the 1970s, it was a major source of childbirth education. At that point, the childbirth preparation movement was moving into solidly institutionalized positions. ASPO teachers were being hired by hospitals to teach classes for their patients. The thrust of most childbirth education in America was to prepare women for the experience of a medically managed birth. I will draw upon an early 1970s ASPO publication, "Guideline for ASPO Teachers," though similar material can be found in the original (1961) ASPO training course[3] (Bing, Karmel, and Tanz, 1961) and in other childbirth education material of the period as well. Regarding repeated and painful examinations in the hospital, the ASPO guidelines state:

> It should be pointed out to patients that internal examinations during labor in the hospital can be performed by the patient's own physician, by a resident physician, an intern or a nurse. This depends on the procedures established by hospital policy. Examinations will be given either rectally or vaginally, again depending on hospital rules or individual physicians, but it is not for the parturient to decide who should, or should not, examine her during labor.

Not only is this not in the interests of birthing women, the students of the ASPO teachers (here called "patients"), but it is also in direct opposition to the legal rights of patients. All patients have the right to refuse to be examined by anyone in the hospital setting (Annas, 1975:147).

In her study of maternity care, Nancy Stoller Shaw noted that for a woman giving birth in a hospital, childbirth involves "a continual inability to protect herself and control the access of others to her body" (Shaw, 1974:62). The standard prepping procedures of the 1970s, the period in which Shaw conducted her research, reinforced the idea that the woman loses control over her body and herself, including "a systematic removal of all personal effects as well as parts of the

---

[3] I received the unpublished ASPO teacher guidelines that are cited throughout this chapter from an ASPO teacher I interviewed in 1975-1976. She dates them as having been produced and distributed by ASPO to teachers in 1970.

body (hair, feces) and its extensions (eyeglasses, false teeth)" (Shaw, 1974:69). By the 1970s, the perineal shave had been repeatedly demonstrated to serve no medical purpose at all, having developed (with the invention of the disposable razor) from the clipping of very long pubic hairs to a full shave (Burchall, 1964). While it is a pointless, humiliating, depersonalizing, and irritating experience, the ASPO guidelines stated that "it is not worth while to make an issue out of this." Similar arguments can be made for each of the prepping procedures, with similar ASPO responses.

Health professionals are accustomed to hospitals, adjusted to the sights and sounds and smells. Many childbirth educators are also nurses or other health professionals. Admission to many of the Lamaze teacher training courses of the time frequently required a nursing degree. To the woman in labor, the hospital environment is foreign and quite possibly threatening. When a woman in labor is wheeled and moved around from one unfamiliar room to another, perhaps entering the situation from the emergency room, she is confronted with strange sights, strange noises, and strange smells. She may not even know how to sort out which uniform stands for which kind of worker, may not know whether the person entering her room is there for "good" (e.g., bringing ice chips) or "evil" (e.g., performing a painful physical examination). She is not familiar enough with the situation to sort out legitimate anxiety-provoking cues from those that would not produce anxiety if she understood them. And it is important to remember that the distractions of labor may make such interpretation even more difficult.

For the most part, childbirth preparation classes taught women ways to avoid dealing with external events. For example, with Lamaze training, the woman is taught to distract herself, to take a focal point, a picture or flower she brings from home, or simply a spot on the wall, and focus on that alone, blocking out all other happenings during a contraction. This is preparation or training not for childbirth, but for the hospital experience.

To the woman laboring at home, the background stimuli, far from being anxiety provoking, are actually reassuring. She hears sounds like the refrigerator opening, children playing, someone calling the dog. The sounds are not threatening. She smells the smells of home, cooking and laundry, not medicine and disinfectants. If she takes in outside events, she receives messages of normality.

The cues available to us in a situation include not only physical objects and sensations but also perceived behavior and even how we see ourselves behaving. One of the basic contributions of symbolic interactionist thinking is to point out that human beings can and do take objective account of themselves, and that the cues we get from our own behavior are an important part of how we understand what is happening to us. This has interesting implications for childbirth.

A major element of childbirth education classes, and particularly the Lamaze classes, was learning special breathing techniques. Elaborate patterns of puffs and pants were drilled into the woman during practice sessions in class. The usual explanation for the effectiveness of these breathing techniques in the control of pain in labor is that the concentration on breathing blocks out the sensations of pain. The women were taught, however, to practice their breathing exercises while driving, watching television, or reading, all activities that require some level of concentration. Can the breathing be distracting enough to take one's mind off the pain of late labor, but not distracting enough to take one's mind off the road or a television program?

I suggest that the reason the breathing exercises work in the control of pain in childbirth is that they are presenting the woman with positive cues regarding her situation. If she were not doing the breathing, she might very well be crying, even screaming. Her ability to objectively evaluate her own situation, taking cues from her own behavior as well as that of others, becomes very important. The woman who has just gotten through a contraction without crying out has presented herself with evidence that it is bearable. If it were not bearable, she would be crying. Cognitive dissonance theory offers a framework in psychology with which to understand this process (Festinger, 1957). In a sense, the breathing becomes a more structured version of "whenever I feel afraid, I whistle a happy tune."

The messages that the birthing woman picks up from the cues available to her are not limited to the normality, health, and relative pain of her situation. The definition of the situation goes much deeper than that, to the very heart of what is happening and who controls what is happening. This is best exemplified by the use of the word *deliver*. Both mothers and birth attendants are said to deliver babies. When the mother is seen as delivering, then the attendant is assisting, aiding, attending. But when the doctor (or midwife) is defined as delivering the baby, the mother assumes the passive position of being delivered. The words used are of course the least of the cues that the laboring woman receives regarding the importance of her contribution to the activity taking place, the delivery of her baby. In a classic article, Szasz and Hollender suggested that there are three basic models of patient-practitioner relationships (Szasz and Hollender, 1946). Let us consider each with regard to childbirth.

THE ACTIVE-PASSIVE MODEL

The active-passive relationship is particularly applicable to the unconscious patient in an emergency situation. The doctor makes all decisions, and the patient is "worked on" in much the same way mechanical repairs are made. In the childbirth situation, this relationship is typified by the doctor using forceps or surgery to pull a baby out of an unconscious mother. What is important to remember is that the doctor not only has complete control once the mother is unconscious, but also that the physician has the authority to define deliveries as normal, variations from normal, and obstetric emergencies. The physician in a hospital birth always holds the power to create an active-passive relationship by having the mother anesthetized. The original ASPO teacher training course stated: "If your doctor himself suggests medication, you should accept it willingly—even if you don't feel the need for it—as he undoubtedly has very good reasons for his decision" (Bing, Karmel and Tanz, 1961:33). The 1970s training guidelines stated that "the final decision on the use of drugs has to be with the individual physician." As with the example of cervical examinations, the goal was not the protection of the rights or interests of the birthing woman, but rather the maintenance of medical management. This ASPO policy also contradicted the legal rights of patients to refuse "any medical or surgical procedure from being performed on them regardless of the opinions of their doctors as to the advisability of the treatment" (Annas, 1975:80).

THE GUIDANCE-COOPERATION MODEL

The second model of the practitioner-patient relationship is the guidance-cooperation model. The practitioner guides and directs the patient who, if she is a good patient, takes guidance and direction easily. In childbirth, this is best typified by the in-hospital "prepared" childbirth. The laboring woman is there to be "coached." All of her preparation has taught her to work within the framework of the institutional rules. The ASPO teacher guidelines had this to say about doctor-patient relationships:

> The patient should be encouraged to have a good "rapport" with her physician. If her doctor is not acquainted with the Lamaze technique, she should try and get his confidence, show that she is not fanatic, and perhaps see if he will read the ASPO "Physicians Communique" or the ASPO training manual. It should be pointed out that, quite obviously, physicians do not cherish to be told by their patients how to conduct their labor and delivery. However, it can certainly be tactfully discussed, and from our experience a great deal can be gained from this.

This is hardly revolutionary talk. The childbirth preparation movement accepted professional ascendancy and offered no fundamental challenges to the medical domination of birth. The individual birthing woman, like the movement itself, was to be polite, tactful, and never fanatical.

THE MUTUAL PARTICIPATION MODEL

The third possible relationship is mutual participation, in which practitioner and patient work together toward a common goal. In essence, it is a denial of the "patient" role. In childbirth it is extremely difficult, to achieve this relationship in a hospital setting. The hospital patient is in no position to be an equal participant in her birthing. She is outnumbered and outpowered. She may be allowed to act as though she were an equal participant, even bringing a patient advocate (husband, coach) with her, but should she stop playing by the rules and become disagreeable, difficult, or disruptive, as defined by the hospital staff and physician, her true powerlessness is made clear. Her "advocate" is there only as long as the hospital attendants choose to allow him or her there, only as long as he continues to act in accordance with institutional rules. Lest anyone think that the husband or friend was brought in as social support, to offer loving companionship and protection for the woman at a time when she is relatively defenseless, consider the ASPO teacher guidelines on the subject of husband participation: "ASPO very much encourages 'Family Centered Maternity,' i.e. a husband and wife team during labor and delivery when possible. It is understood, however, that only husbands who have taken a formal course with their wife in the Lamaze technique can be of real help to the wife." The husband is brought in not to serve the interests of the birthing woman but to keep the woman in line with the demands of the institution.

It was perhaps for these reasons that so much emphasis was put on the control of both pain and the expression of pain in childbirth preparation classes. According to the rules of the game, if the laboring woman chooses to deal with her pain by crying or calling out, she has forfeited her right to decision making. Much was made in childbirth preparation classes of being in control during labor, while all that really was meant by that was being in control over expressions of pain. A woman who maintained a fixed, if somewhat glazed, cheerful expression, and continued her breathing patterns regularly, was said to be in control as she was carted from one room to another strapped flat on her back with her legs in the air.

Certainly a woman who was unconscious, semistuperous, amnesiac, or simply numb from the waist down cannot have experienced giving birth as an accomplishment, something over which she had conscious control. But what of the woman who was encouraged in childbirth preparation classes to see herself as a member of a "team" delivering the baby? Though she may help, and watch in a mirror, she is not the primary locus of action. Positioning her and draping her in such a way that she cannot directly see the birth, and not allowing her to touch her genitals and the forthcoming baby tell the mother that the birth is something that is happening to her, or being done to her, and not something that she is doing. The birth is managed by the other members of the team, the ones who tell her what to do, who use their hands on her and the baby. A birth is a thrilling event to watch. But it is an even more thrilling thing to do. Encouraging a woman to watch herself give birth in a mirror moves her from a participant into an observer of the birth. The emphasis on "seeing" the birth came out of the context of prepared, in-hospital, doctor-directed births. The prepared childbirth movement encouraged the woman to be "awake," to see herself as part of the team, and to help the doctor by following suggestions and direction. She was not encouraged to usurp the doctor's dominance, but simply to "be there," to be awake, to observe the birth.

The implications of the active-passive or Guidance-Cooperation model of birth extend beyond the birthing experience and into the mother's relationship with the baby. When the hospital staff is perceived as having delivered the baby, then it is the responsibility and privilege of the staff to present the baby to its mother. The mother thus becomes the recipient rather than the producer of the child.

Before the inroads made by the prepared childbirth movement, it was not uncommon in American hospitals for mothers to be unconscious for the birth and presented with the baby six, twelve, or twenty-four hours later. Feelings of unreality and confusion were common. The jokes about bringing "the wrong baby" home from the hospital attest to the feelings of unease. But even women conscious for the birth, who were not able to perceive it as something that they accomplished through their own efforts, may have some difficulty assimilating what has happened. As one mother, awake but unable to feel the birth because of an epidural block, said, "It's like seeing a rabbit pulled out of a hat." Being the hat is a far cry from being the magician. It is the sleight of hand that makes a magic trick, things done that the audience cannot see. Similarly, continuity is lacking in a birth in which the baby is held up for the mother to see but not touch, and then taken out of her sight for processing, recording, and prophylactic treatment. When the baby is returned, wiped off and swaddled, and in hospital "uniform," it is one step removed from the immediate product of birth. The medical management changed the newborn from being part of its mother's body to being a standard-issue hospital baby.

The issue of control over the baby continues in the days following birth. A baby in a hospital nursery is controlled by the nursery. The mother has access to it only with the approval of the nursery staff. I once saw a mother, her face pressed against the nursery glass, say to her crying infant, "It's ok, baby, I'm here."

In more recent years, childbirth education has moved toward demanding greater access for mothers to their babies, while still accepting the basic underlying ideology of medical management. The desires of mothers to hold their babies is placed as part of a "bonding" process, very much as if the mother was introduced to the baby by the medical staff, and needed time to "greet" and "bond with" the baby.

CONCLUSIONS

This chapter has sought to point out the ways in which the childbirth experience has been socially constructed, from the acknowledgment of labor to the care of the newborn, and to consider the agents that control the definitions used in the childbirth situation. Childbirth education, in order to gain the wide acceptance which it received, had to accept the bulk of professional and medical definitions of childbirth. The preparation, therefore, was for the hospital experience, and not for the birth itself. Unlike the current home-birth movement and the return to lay or empirical midwives, the "natural" or "prepared" childbirth movement's simple desire that the woman be awake, "be there" for the hospital birth, even with her husband, was not a particularly radical request. Medical control over the birthing woman and the baby was not challenged. Consumer pressure for more attractively decorated labor rooms, more comfortable labor-delivery beds or chairs, and rooming-in help make birth in hospitals a more pleasant experience. But these changes do not change the fundamental balance of power between the individual and the institution.

REFERENCES

Annas, George. *The Rights of Hospital Patients.* New York: Discus Books, 1975.
Bing, Elizabeth; Karmel, Marjorie; and Tanz, Alfred. *A Practical Training Course for the Psychoprophylactic Method of Childbirth.* New York: ASPO, 1961.

Burchall, R. Clay. "Predelivery Removal of Pubic Hair." *Obstetrics and Gynecology* 24(1964):272-273.

Festinger, Leon. *A Theory of Cognitive Dissonance.* New York: Row, Peterson, 1957.

Goffman, Erving. *Asylums.* New York: Anchor Books, 1961.

Miller, Rita Seiden. "The Social Construction and Reconstruction of Physiological Events: Acquiring the Pregnancy Identity." In *Studies in Symbolic Interaction,* edited by Norman K. Denzin. Vol 1. Greenwich, Ct.: JAI Press, 1978, pp. 181-204.

Roth, Julius. *Timetables.* Bobbs-Merrill, 1965.

Shaw, Nancy Stoller. *Forced Labor: Maternity Care in the United States.* New York: Pergamon Press, 1974.

Sudnow, David. *Passing On: The Social Organization of Dying.* Englewood Cliffs, N. J.: Prentice-Hall, 1967.

Szasz, Thomas, and Hollender, M. H. "A Contribution to the Philosophy of Medicine: The Basic Models of the Doctor-Patient Relationship." *AMA Archives of Internal Medicine* (1946):97.

5

Male Doctor–Female Patient

SANDRA K. DANZIGER

The emergence of natural childbirth advocacy groups, the feminist health movement, and the trend toward advanced medical technology in obstetrics all imply new and differing conceptions of the doctor-patient relationship. On the one hand, self-help groups aim to develop more symmetrical lay-expert relationships, to reduce the need for professionals and their expertise by advocating alternatives such as home delivery, lay midwifery, nurse midwifery, and birth center services. On the other hand, the increased use of Cesarean sections, electronic fetal monitoring, obstetric anesthesiology, amniocentesis, fetal surgery, and high-risk obstetrics and perinatology subspecialities increases not only technological encroachment in the pregnancy and birth process but also asymmetry between doctor and patient.

The types of relationships exemplified in health care settings reflect the assumptions that both parties hold regarding the sacredness of medical knowledge and authority. My research in this area has focused on the use of "the medical model" of the patient and her "illness" (in this case pregnancy and birth) in the course of the interaction encounter (Danziger, 1978B; 1979B; 1980). The medical model refers to the narrow, restricted aspects of the person that are relevant for the doctor's work concerns, that define the childbearing woman as a medical case. I have investigated what doctors express to patients and how patients respond in the course of the everyday doctor-patient encounter. This entails looking at not only what is said but also how it is said and in what context. In my work, the content and stylistic structure of these clinical encounters are inextricably linked, in that the control doctors have over patients, individually and as a group, appears to be produced by authoritative behavior and routine processing of the patient and her illness.

I have identified three interactional processes occurring in medical encounters throughout childbearing that establish the primacy of the medical model and the status differentials between doctor and patient. Physicians (and nurses who act on their behalf) first *structure the course of the encounter*—that is, they define the relevant topics, set the agenda of the problems to be addressed, dictate the procedures to be done. Second, they *offer advice on appropriate behavior* to follow during pregnancy and birth—establish a course of patient etiquette. This advice may be based in part on current medical theory or popular health practices (e.g., Lamaze training) but may also meet staff needs for routine and convenience. Finally, in their "bedside manner" or style of interaction, doctors *provide a set of normalizing assurances*—that is, suggestions that everything is fine and as expected. These three behaviors occur uniformly across many types of cases and situations, suggesting that they are unwritten rules of patient management. They appear to aid and abet women and their partners in the expression of submissive, conforming roles. All three can be expressed in varying degrees of authoritativeness, from dictatorial to quite subtle and meek. They can be viewed most commonly, however, as postures of social control and dominance on the part of the professional, postures that typically are accepted or unchallenged by the patient (see also Freidson, 1970; Zola, 1972; Fox, 1977; Conrad and Schneider, 1980; Schneider and Conrad, 1980).

In addition, it is well established that sex-appropriate idealized ways of behaving reinforce hierarchical relationships

(Kollock et al., 1985; Goffman, 1979; West and Zimmerman, 1977; Laws and Schwartz, 1977). When a man and a woman interact, as in the typical doctor-patient encounter, traditional sex roles suggest gender dominance of male over female. In many instances, these social conventions of gender-distinguishable behavior approximate the relationship of parent to child, teacher to student, or expert to layperson or novice. In the case of childbearing, the patient's reproductive experiences are to some extent shaped by male medical ideologies. Thus, gender roles come into play in the stylistic way women and/or couples and their doctors interact and in the content of their assumptions about reproduction and women's health. Through both channels, the degree of conformity to gender-stereotypic norms can influence the outcome of health care.

In this chapter, I will utilize the perspective of gender hierarchy to reexamine data on pregnancy and birth encounters. Data from two studies will be used, my own research and that of Ann Oakley, both of which were conducted in the mid-1970s. Each entailed in-depth observation of medical interaction in clinic and hospital settings. In both cases, observations were conducted over about a nine-month period, resulting in extensive systematic notes documenting communication between staff and patients in 906 consultations in Oakley's research and more than 250 encounters in mine. More detailed information on the data collection procedures, participants, and settings of study have been reported elsewhere (Danziger, 1979A, 1979B, 1980:266–267; and Oakley, 1980:105–106).

SETTING THE AGENDA

In dealing with a woman during pregnancy and birth, medical professionals standardize their activities of monitoring and regulating physiological development. This regulation is of primary importance in the medical model; thus, one of their foremost concerns at each prenatal visit is to conduct routine examination and testing to rule out risk factors and indications of abnormality. Although the crisis orientation pervades during birth—that is, the idea that each woman has the potential need for emergency medical or surgical intervention—during pregnancy, there is also a scheduled progression of medical concerns, so that different topics are relevant to the doctor at different points of time. The timing of these priorities does not take into account an individual woman's interests or concerns at any given point and in fact often may have the effect of precluding other topics. In the following instance from Oakley's study of London prenatal encounters, the doctor completely ignored the woman's feelings about the pregnancy by sticking to the medical agenda.

Doctor: This is your first visit in this pregnancy?

Patient: Yes.

Doctor: You were on the pill?

Patient: Yes.

Doctor: Was that period in May the only period you had?

Patient: What?

Doctor: You haven't had a proper period since that one?

Patient: No.

Doctor: Why have you left it so long [patient is about twenty-two weeks pregnant] before coming here?

Patient: Well, I didn't go to the doctor for ages, I was so depressed. I didn't want the baby. I wanted an abortion.

Doctor: Have you ever had diabetes, tuberculosis, rhematic fever, kidney diseases, high blood pressures?

Patient: No.

Doctor: Has anyone in the family ever had any of those?

Patient: No.

(Doctor continues history taking, does vaginal exam.)

Doctor: Okay. All finished. That's fine. Everything's alright. The brownish discharge is from a sore place you've got on the neck of the womb. That's quite common in pregnancy. You're about right for dates, but because you were on the pill, I want you to go to ultrasound.

Patient: Is that date—the third of March—right?

Doctor: When you've been to ultrasound we'll know more accurately (Oakley, 1980:29–30).

A routine feature of the medical agenda for birth that does not reflect patients' interests is the practice of rotating on call for birth attendance. Very few doctors in my study delivered the babies of their patients, even for women who saw them exclusively throughout prenatal care. Yet virtually all of the women, especially those having a first baby, chose the doctor on the basis of wanting that person with them during birth. The doctors were far more cavalier toward who would be present. One said to me, "I'm not going to let prenatals run my life." He went on to describe doctors at delivery as "interchangeable." He considered almost any of his colleagues to be medically competent to deliver any of his patients. Thus, what is relevant to the medical agenda at childbirth is simply the technical mastery of baby catching rather than any dynamic of patient care. For the pregnant women, though, a common expectation of what their in-hospital births would be like is exemplified in one woman's idea: "For me, it's a very personal, private experience, something I share with my husband, my sister because she's a nurse and will be with me, and with my doctor" (Danziger, 1978A:126).

The assertion of the medical agenda leads not only to occasionally brushing aside patients' concerns but also to presuming that the women's concerns ought to coincide with the medical model of pregnancy. In the following example, a doctor explains to the researcher what patients should and should not be thinking about at various times in the pregnancy.

Doctor: Are you looking to give her the early pregnancy stuff or the you're-almost-there literature on babies? It must be one of those times. (To observer.) There are two stages when we bombard prenatals with things to read. So, Marge, is this a beginning or an end?

RN Marge: Beginning.

Doctor: (To observer.) Yes, see we don't like to give them the reading on actual babies until their pregnancies are pretty well established. Before the seventh month, there's a good chance of miscarriage, and what a disappointment. After that they can begin learning about how to care for the child, how to childproof your house, child safety in the car, and whatnot. What people don't realize is that before that, 15 percent of all pregnancies are lost. Now that includes losing it before you even have any idea that you're pregnant (Danziger, 1980:282).

Finally, much of this activity appears to have very little physiological basis yet clearly serves to enhance the doctor's control. Two examples are the methods used in late pregnancy to detect onset of labor and the routine times of day in which birth interventions are begun in the hospital.

A major part of the prenatal visit in the last month of pregnancy involves the scrutinizing for signs of the onset of labor. Patients may ask for predictions, and doctors regularly conduct either internal examination or external palpation and then discuss the findings in combination with the due-date estimate. However, the findings regarding "dropping," "changes in the cervix," "false labor," or Braxton-Hicks contractions, and their relation to labor onset are presented to patients in often contradictory or confusing ways. The following case typifies this lack of clarity. The patient claimed that her pains were not the false Braxton-Hicks, but rather the real thing. The doctor said that he would verify her feelings by seeing whether any internal changes relevant to labor had taken place. Upon examination, however, he was not optimistic but then disclaimed the predictive value of the exam. Even though her pains were labeled as inefficient and therefore not the "real thing," she still could go into labor any time. So, why, one may ask, did he scrutinize for signs of labor?

(The patient is describing the contractions she had the previous night.)

Patient: They weren't Braxton-Hicks, either, they were the real thing. I'm sure they were labor contractions. They were coming often enough over a couple of hours that I thought perhaps I should start timing them. Mike woke up and I said, "This is it, now, we better get some sleep while we can." Then I woke up this morning and they were gone. Nothing.

Doctor: Well, we'll check you today and see if anything is happening. . . . (Puts on glove and lubricant.) Okay, cold wet jelly. I have to push a little here. Here's the cervix. Is it open? Aha, hole in cervix. Okay, you're just about a fingertip dilated. And baby's head... is not quite engaged. I'd say at a minus 1 or even minus 2.

Patient: What does that mean?

Doctor: Well, ladies with second babies or more don't have much dilation before they go into labor, so it doesn't mean you still couldn't have the baby before 6 A.M. tomorrow.

Patient: It doesn't? But I thought you always... they said in class....

Doctor: Well, that's true for first babies, but not at all for second.

Patient: Oh, well that's a relief to hear. I thought I still had 2 weeks more for a minute. Well, I guess it still could be right? It still could be anytime from now on. But what about those contractions? I'm sure they weren't the Braxton-Hicks.

Doctor: Well, the difference is really in what they do, their efficiency in getting the work of the uterus done, not in how they feel so much.

Patient: I see. Oh, well... (Danziger, 1978A:84).

In the course of my research, one doctor questioned the practice of conducting routine internal physical exams to check for changes in the cervix.

Doctor: Do you know there are some doctors who do a vaginal every single time? Do you believe it?

Observer: They really do? Why is that, do you think?

Doctor: I don't know. I suppose they think it's good obstetrics. To examine cervical changes, I guess.

Observer: Is that important?

Doctor: Not really. Dr. X does it every time. I know he does, I've worked with him. The other doctors here do it more often than I do, I'm sure (Danziger, 1978A: 87).

What doctors accomplish by routine checking in late pregnancy is not a prediction of when onset will occur but a determination of whether labor has already begun. The earlier the doctor can catch the labor as it begins and can pronounce this status change, the better for the medical staff's scheduling purposes. Whether it is necessary or desirable from the patient's perspective, whether she needs it to tell her whether she is in labor, is a different consideration.

The final example of procedural agenda setting for other than strictly clinical reasons is the scheduled manner in which birth interventions sometimes occur. At one hospital in my study, nurses on the labor and delivery unit knew that pitocin augmentation of a course of labor would be detained until the primary doctor's office hours were finished for the day. At another unit, the nurses knew that the decision to perform a Cesarean section was likely to come after office hours. It is not that after 5 or 6 P.M. the rhythms of labor in patients can be more clearly established but rather that this was a more convenient time for the doctor to begin a course of action that demanded closer and more concerted medical attention. The laboring women were not typically made aware of the extent to which things other than their own physiological progress were taken into account in the scheduling of these interventionary measures.

Thus, one major control-producing aspect of obstetrical care involves applying routinized conceptual versions of the woman and the course of pregnancy and birth. These may entail attention to certain topics over others and can result in the doctor's disregarding patient interests in favor of medical priorities. In addition, the medical model implies a schedule of appropriate pregnancy and birth events that is applied somewhat arbitrarily to individual cases. In terms of how gender roles may influence this process, one obvious way is through mediation of patients' reaction to the routine control maneuvers and through the level of flexibility in the doctors' behavior.

For example, the fact that most of this patient processing goes unchallenged in the doctor-patient encounter appears to fit with traditional expectations of female submission to male initiative-taking and assertive behavior (Goffman, 1979; West and Zimmerman, 1977; West, 1982; West, 1984; Fishman, 1978; Kemper, 1984). The style of agenda setting (with routines being unilaterally imposed with little or no discussion or opposition) parallels male-female interaction in general.[1] Thus, it is not atypical or remarkable for women to find themselves being ignored, labeled, or mildly coerced into modes of behavior men define as appropriate. Nor is it extraordinary for men to find themselves initiating and structuring encounters with such leverage and deference from women.

The content of agenda setting in the doctor-patient encounter in pregnancy and birth, however, probably has more to do with the professional-layperson dynamic than with the fact that doctors are typically men and the patients in this instance, women. Most of this type of dialogue focuses on issues of processing cases, identifying relevant signs of trouble, scheduling work routines, juggling caseloads, setting work priorities, and selectively attending to problems for which medicine can be effective. The resulting patient alienation is not without a potentially negative impact on health outcomes, but the underlying concerns of the doctor in these instances seems to be to structure the work routines and achieve some sense of order in the everyday clinical practice (see also Danziger, 1980; Scully, 1980; Zola, 1973; Haug and Sussman, 1969).[2]

GIVING BEHAVIORAL ADVICE

Another major activity in doctor-patient relationships that reinforces the medical model is counseling on how to take care of oneself (i.e., behave) as a mother-to-be. The extent to which doctors or their designated patient educators provide this information varies a great deal throughout pregnancy. Both

[1]While not all the doctors in my study were male, the few women doctors did not differ from the men in their behavior (see also Carver, 1981). However, West's recent study found that, according to the number of times the doctor interrupted the patient as opposed to the number of times the patient interrupted the doctor during the encounter, women doctors were accorded lower or less dominant interactional status than the typical male doctor (West, 1984:93).

[2]The analyses of these data do not include a quantitative assessment of the relative proportion of time spent on agenda setting rather than some other activity, such as applying a treatment, explaining a diagnosis or prognosis, counseling, etc. I mean to suggest only that agenda setting, giving advice, and providing assurances are three very frequent and dominant themes in these encounters.

physical and dietary activity are considered from the point of view of keeping one's health level up, preventing the onset of illness, and taking extra precautions for the state of pregnancy. It is interesting that what is considered especially healthy for pregnancy is highly variable in obstetrical custom. Only within the past decade have most doctors felt it healthful for women to gain twenty or more pounds and in some instances more than thirty pounds for the entire course of the pregnancy. Before this time, doctors advocated strict limitations for what was considered a healthy weight gain.

The same turnaround seems to be true for physical activity, although this may break down at different stages of the pregnancy. Most doctors now encourage women to continue being as active as they wish, although they advocate that women refrain from doing irregular, extraordinarily rigorous exercise. I observed very little emphasis on the "delicacy" of the state of being pregnant, whereas in other eras, typical prenatal advice may have included confinement and bed rest. An example of this latest trend in "natural health" obstetrics is illustrated in the following excerpt:

Doctor: Are there any other problems?

Patient: Just this low back pain. It's not from swimming, I know, but maybe from biking or standing for long stretches at work. What can I do?

Doctor: Massage it, it's the greatest thing. Get your husband to massage you. You can get this book that's the best authority . . .

Patient: Are there any calisthenics I can do in particular that are good?

Doctor: Anything is good. Really, the better tone your cardiovascular system, the stronger you'll be and the easier labor will be for you. Like women in the fields, right? (Danziger, 1978A: 57).

Note that here the doctor conveys a somewhat limited authoritativeness of the medical perspective. The doctor is, for these matters and of his or her own admission, not the only source of advice. In the case of potential difficulty, however, the doctor may become more patronizing, provide advice on a broader range of behavior, and invoke images of women's motherly mandate to ensure obedience. One example of advice on a multiple pregnancy in Oakley's study and one on managing elevated blood pressure in my study illustrate the doctor's view of the obligation to comply.

Doctor: This is twins. They're growing well, but you need more rest. I'd advise some good books and a quiet life for three months. You're not working?

Patient: No.

Doctor: Just normal exercise—I want you to have a walk every day, but no gardening, no heavy work, postpone moving or decorating the house. If you do rest, you'll grow yourself slightly bigger babies. After all, it's this (pats her abdomen) that's your most important job, isn't it? (Oakley, 1980:39–40).

Doctor: You obviously didn't do any of the things I told you. Your pressure's up.

Patient: (Sheepish.) I guess I didn't.

Doctor: I'll tell you, you keep this up and I'll put you in the hospital. And if you think that's a threat, it's because it is. I'm threatening you to make you realize that you just cannot continue like this. Now what kinds of excuses are you going to give me for not doing what you're supposed to? (Pause.) No excuses?

Patient: I've been busy? (Sheepish giggle again.)

Doctor: Busy? You should be busy reading and that's all you should be doing! Did you have high blood pressure with your last pregnancy?

Patient: No, I don't think so. They didn't make a big deal out of it, so I would think not.

Doctor: Well, it is a big deal. It's the way mothers and babies die. Does your husband know you're supposed to be taking it easy?

Patient: Well, yes, but. . . .

Doctor: This has got to stop. You are to do absolutely nothing except rest two hours in the morning, two hours in the afternoon, and be in bed every night by 9 o'clock.

Patient: My little girl isn't even in bed by then.

Doctor: Well, her father will have to stay up with her but not you. And if you can't do this, I'll put you in the hospital and put nurses on you who won't let you out of bed (Danziger, 1980:368).

During birth, behavioral admonitions—when they do occur—come in the form of staff attempts to control the birth process. An example of how such control is exerted is given in the nurse-patient interaction regarding the woman's responses to her labor pains.

Patients who, instead of being quiet and withdrawn during labor, displayed screaming, writhing, or thrashing about the bed were highly criticized. Such labor behavior was not tolerated, but was instead taken as grounds for procedural action, usually in the form of verbally chastising the behavior or administering tranquilizing or pain-relieving medication. Among themselves, staff members looked on such patients with hostility or pity for "not being able to take it." Usually, an expressed low pain threshold was attributed to a person's weakness, not to the possibility of her labor being extraordinarily difficult. Whether or not analgesic medication was appropriate at the time, a staff member often intervened with harsh reprimands to quiet the patient, as in the following remarks.

Don't get so excited. C'mon. Don't let them overtake you.

Look, breathe with me. Blow the air out like you're blowing out a candle. Concentrate on it. That's it.

Slow down on your breathing, Irene.

Are you breathing that hard because it makes the contraction easier for you? You're breathing awfully hard, almost like you're not getting enough air.

Grow up, Diane.

You've got to help yourself, honey (Danziger, 1979B:898).

The talk that occurred with the women during contractions was primarily encouragement of one particular form of behavior as opposed to another. It was routinely suggested that the appropriate response to contractions was to be calm and quiet. Whether or not it is indicative of one's tolerance, it clearly means less work for the staff members. Acting excited, however, signified that the women were not tolerating the pain well. Thus, they needed instruction, medication, or something to help them.

Nurses argued (as does Lamaze training) that fighting labor instead of being passive toward it makes it harder and brings on fatigue and tension, which not only makes contractions hurt more but also can perhaps slow the physiological progress of labor. They do not, however, publicly state that Lamaze-trained women have faster and less complicated courses of childbirth. Thus, the actual therapeutic benefits to remaining quiet are not clear, although patients are given to believe that they "do better" by acting in such a fashion. In one instance, a nurse and doctor were talking to a woman about how well she was doing her Lamaze breathing. They emphasized that the "correct way to do it is the quiet way. We don't need to hear 'em down the hall."

Advice giving to encourage compliant and medically convenient behavior appeared to be fairly lax, more or less suggestive, throughout most of the routine courses of pregnancy. Nevertheless, doctors typically invoked women's moral obligations to obey them 1) when the potential of prenatal risk factors was present and 2) during childbirth, when the medical model of "correct" labor behavior was applied. The appeals to comply usually focused on the women's "desire" to exhibit traditional femininity and/or ideal maternal "instincts." Many women no doubt participate in reinforcing these attitudes in their doctors. For example, in Bromberg's study of women who had babies between the 1950s and 1970s, women recall asking their obstetricians to be paternalistic with them.

> And I said, "I am just really panicked. I hate it. I want to have another child but the whole idea of going through this (so I think in a way he thinks that he's the daddy of them *all*) again just absolutely terrifies me." And he said, "Wipe it out of your mind." (This is the God complex.) He said, "You might not believe this but having a baby with me is like having *no other* obstetrician. *Anywhere!* And it's going to be a wonderful experience." And you know, I said, "Oh yeah?" And he was right, he was right. It *really* was.

> And I remember going to this obstetrician and saying, "Well

now. My friends tell me that I should ask for natural childbirth. What do you say?" And he said, "I will be glad to go along with whatever you like *up* until the moment when *I* think that you might be in difficulty. And at that moment *I* become the person in charge and I make the decisions. How do you feel about that?" I said, "I feel wonderful" (Bromberg, 1981:42-43).

It would be interesting to compare doctors' appeals for compliance to male versus female patients, and to the patient responses in both cases. It seems highly improbable that a grown man would be told (and would take passively being told) to "be a good boy and get some rest." Nor would he be made to feel that it is his altruistic duty, indeed, his biologically imposed destiny, to follow the doctor's orders. Finally, assumptions regarding what becoming a mother "naturally" means for women are often presumed. A personal anecdote from my own childbearing experience reveals such assumptions.

My doctor came to visit me the day after a difficult delivery. I was lying on my side in bed, gingerly avoiding pressure on my episiotomy. I was breathless from having nervously changed my baby's diaper for the first time and having just settled him down in his crib. I was feeling exhausted from the birth, worried about how I would ever get my strength back, overwhelmed by the total dependency and vulnerability of a new infant, and in he strolled. He took one quick visual sweep and proclaimed, "Ah, the picture of maternal peace!"

In advice giving, gender roles may figure prominently in both style and substance. Increased awareness because of the feminist health movement has perhaps reduced the frequency of the most obvious forms of sexism in doctors' behavioral admonitions and the frequency of women's acceptance or reinforcement of these attitudes. However, a more subtle and therefore more intransigent form is the appeal to motherhood as idealized destiny. Oakley refers to this as the feminine paradigm in medical attitudes to reproduction (1979; 1980:7-49). In this model, normal adjustment to childbearing implies complete acceptance of and enthusiasm over prospective motherhood and, by extension, adjustment is best demonstrated by complete dedication to doing whatever the doctor says.

NORMALIZING ASSURANCES

A major by-product of the business of monitoring physiologi-cal changes and screening for abnormalities in both preg-nancy and birth is the need to communicate the findings to the patient. In these encounters, the most common manner in which this information is conveyed takes the form of reas-surance. Doctors in my study seemed to presume that many women needed the comfort of reassurance more than the specific details or a clear understanding of their situation. In prenatal care, this tended to take the form of trivializing a woman's concerns and reminding her in subtle ways that "doctor knows best." In birth, normalizing statements often served as a smokescreen while alternative crisis management strategies were planned. Oakley found in her research that of 677 statements made by pregnant women to their doctors, 12 percent involved symptoms of pain or discomfort, to which the doctor responded by normalizing, such as in these examples.

Doctor: Feeling well?

Patient: Yes, but very tired—I can't sleep at all at night.

Doctor: Why is that?

Patient: Well, I'm very uncomfortable—I turn from one side to the other, and the baby keeps kicking. I get cramp on one side, high up in my leg. If I sleep on my back I choke myself, so I'm tossing and turning about all night long, which isn't very good.

Doctor: We need to put you in a hammock, don't we? (Reads case notes.) Tell me, the urine specimen which you brought in today—when did you do it?

Patient: I've got a pain in my shoulder.

Doctor: Well, that's your shopping bag hand, isn't it?

Patient: I get pains in my groin, down here, why is that?

Doctor: Well, it's some time since your last pregnancy, and also your center of gravity is changing.

Patient: I see.

Doctor: That's okay. (Pats on back.) (Oakley, 1980:15-16).

Most striking about the normalizing conversation that occurs during birth is the comparison between what is said
directly to or in the presence of patients and fathers and what
is said among staff or to the observer when out of the hearing
range of the patient. One case demonstrates the discrepancy
between the two versions of the situation and the overall
thematic emphasis of each. In the talk with parents, what is
delivered is the general assurance that either the labor is
going well or that the staff is perfectly capable of handling
the minor problems in the labor. What is otherwise indicated
is a more complex version of the situation with strategies
being formulated and predictions being revised. In the latter
assessment, the range of matters taken into consideration
that affect how the case is managed is far more evident.

THE CASE OF URSULA'S BIRTH

Ursula entered the labor and delivery unit early in the morning with ruptured amniotic membranes. Her doctor said that
they would wait to see what she would do until about 2 P.M.
that afternoon. Then, if her labor had not begun, they would
have an X-ray series of her pelvimetry and possibly induce
her labor. The nurse told me as observer, "Her spines are
narrow. If Dr. ____ thinks there's a good chance of no problem,
he'll 'pit' her for a 4 to 5 hour trial, see how she does."

Her labor did not begin before this time, and after she had
the X-rays, several nurses brought in the IV equipment to her
labor room and began to set up the apparatus for the induction. The doctor came in to tell Ursula, "Okay, it's time you
had some contractions." The implication was that the report
of her pelvic and baby proportions was favorable, but this was
not mentioned directly. During the process of setting up the
machine, Ursula asked the staff people, "How long will I have
to be on the machine?" One of the nurses explained, "Until
your labor gets good and well established. They'll keep upping
the medication 'til they can see your contractions at two to
three minutes apart. You can't even feel these, so they aren't
doing the work yet."

After the 3 P.M. shift change, the new nurse came in to
monitor the fetal-labor monitor and pitocin drip apparatus.
She escalated the frequency of the drip, thus increasing the

medication and asked if Ursula could feel her contractions. She chatted with her and the expectant father about her own three children. As this was their first baby, she assured them, "Let me tell you, you're going to enjoy having a baby...." They continued to talk and watch a football game on the television. Although things had begun in terms of initiating the labor, they were in effect waiting for her uterus to start contracting in response to the medication.

A couple of hours later, after she had begun to feel contractions, the nurse told her, "I'm going to keep real close tabs on you now." What she did not say is that the stricter attention was in part because the doctor was temporarily out of the hospital and out of reach, so he had ordered that she stay in careful contact. Ursula attempted to describe her pains, "I feel them way down here now," and gestured to her groin area. The nurse responded with information, "Those contractions are effacing your cervix." A couple of hours went by and the nurse announced to them that she would like to "check" her "to see if she's progressed far enough to get medication." She needed to be dilated five centimeters.

The nurse did a vaginal examination and provided the assessment, "Well, the baby has come down some. It's a good minus one." She told them nothing further, and neither of them asked for elaboration or interpretation. An understanding of the process would have indicated to them that the assessment provided no information on dilation or on whether or not she could yet receive medication. The nurse told me when out of earshot of the parents, "she's not dilated yet." In other words, the relevant marker for medical work had not been attained, although another sort of progress could be conveyed to the parents. She further expressed some worry to me that the woman's contractions were possibly too rough judging from the graphic representation of them on the monitor printout. She thought that such contractions should be effective in producing cervical dilation if everything was going well, but she refrained from assessing the severity of the situation until the doctor's return.

Later, he and the nurse discussed the matter and he assured everyone—nurse and patient—that the contractions were "fine. It's just taking awhile for the cervix to get effaced." He watched the monitor himself and then explained to the nurse that what is provided in the printout is not an accurate picture. He told her what things to look for that are indications for worry. The concern here was how to interpret and act on the readings obtained through the instrumentation. The controversy and potential misreading of signals was not something about which the expectant parents were informed.

Almost two hours later, Ursula began to feel rectal pressure and complained of it to the nurse. This is usually an indication of progressive active labor, if not well-advanced labor, and thus it calls for a vaginal exam. The doctor came to check her and announced to everyone in the room, "She's zero to minus one and four centimeters. You can have medication in about a half-hour or so, if that sounds good. We're definitely getting someplace now, but you won't have the baby before Nurse ⸻ here leaves, I don't think. Okay, then?"

For the patient, this temporal marker of "not before shift change" put off the time of delivery to a vague future point, clarifying only that it was not likely to occur soon. It indicated to the nurse an entire set of meanings by assigning the current point in this case in relation to other activities and other cases that she and the doctor were managing. Before she went off duty for the night, I asked the nurse whether the amount of pitocin being administered was excessively large in this case or usual. She claimed that her dosage is "an average amount of pit, not an excessively large amount. It can get up to 100 [cc's per minute]. And considering that she started from scratch, literally, with no effacement and no contractions, it's coming along well, although so, so slow." She predicted to me that Ursula would deliver around 3 A.M.

Ursula expressed some discouragement to the nurse when she asked her how long the nurse would stay. "About 15 minutes more," she replied. "Aw, hon," Ursula pleaded, frowning, The nurse responded with an attempt to provide comfort. "Well, listen, you have a couple of more hours to go, or else I'd stay with you." Then, she brought her the medication, telling me, the observer (who was aware that she may not have been dilated enough yet), "It can't hurt at this point." Giving the medication supplied a sense of progress in terms of the physiological "time" being made. It provided the assurance that advances were occurring at a normal or good pace.

Before and during the next shift change, Ursula's labor picked up speed and she was almost completely dilated, nine centimeters, before the next night nurse arrived. She came in at 11 and announced, "Well hello, you're almost done here. I'm ____, I'll be with you in delivery." Within another half-hour, Ursula began pushing and the baby was born very quickly then, within another half-hour. The tempo of the course of labor thus differed from most estimates given beforehand. Signs of potential trouble were withheld from the parents, who were offered only bare tidbits of information throughout the day.

Thus, in the process of providing assurance, the doctor or nurse in these studies typically displayed a presumption of the patient's relative incompetence. They exhibited very little appreciation of or patience with the women's views of symptoms and possible desire for information. Instead, the staff appeared to prejudge that most patients were better off not knowing all the potential implications and possible interventions at the doctor's disposal. As in agenda-setting encounters, gender roles may affect the style of these interactions, in that professionals give normalizing interpretations in patronizing not-to-worry tones, and the women defer by rarely asking for clarification or expansion and by rarely expressing dissatisfaction with their treatment. As in the advice-giving sessions, gender affects the presumptions the doctor or nurse makes about women's needs (leading to restricting their information giving), with the result that they seek to convey the impression that no matter what, the staff is in charge, can control the situation and respond effectively. Another way in which gender roles may influence this normalizing interaction is the extent to which both parties presume a woman's psychological vulnerability to illness, her need to be protected from stress, and anxiety.

A portion of the literature on sex differences in health converges with studies on sexism in health care in its emphasis on why women go to doctors more frequently than men and what may occur in those visits to reinforce women's excessive "demand" for medical care (Clarke, 1983; Nathanson, 1975; Ehrenreich and Ehrenreich, 1974; Scully and Bart, 1981; Waldron, 1976; Verbrugge, 1979, 1984; Maracek, 1978; Marcus et al., 1983; Marieskind, 1980: esp. 4-35, 287-295). Many people in our culture express the hypothesis that women are particularly prone to 1) thinking they might be ill or that their symptoms are serious and 2) becoming ill because of such emotional reactions. It follows, then, that much of what women need in medical encounters is assurance; in fact, assurance may be a preventive medical treatment.

The corollary would be that too much information may result in illness-inducing anxiety or stress in a woman. That women's emotional fragility may be heightened during pregnancy is also a popularly accepted assumption in lay and health care circles. It would be intriguing to research the differential presentation and management of complaints from male and female patients to ascertain the relative frequency of assurances versus informational responses from doctors.

CONCLUSIONS

In sum, I argue that three types of interactional processes exemplify the routine uses of the medical model for maintaining power and authority over pregnant and birthing women. They have been observed in two studies of prenatal and birth care as typical, recurrent behavior on the part of doctors and nurses—behavior that is routinely accepted or at least unchallenged by the women and their accompanying spouses or coaches. At the time of the encounters, there was little variation in the women's responses. Both studies provided data on primarily middle-class patients, but the varying assumptions that different women bring to their care situation seemed to be of little relevance in the face of the imposition of the medical model. These studies have critically examined how this medical model is produced in the doctor-patient relationship and what it conveys regarding gender-appropriate behavior and health stereotypes. Both professional social control maneuvers and gender dynamics reinforce the conception that the childbearing woman is in need of the doctor's protective guidance and comfort in order to become a happily-ever-after new mother. This stereotype may be quite incongruent with the needs of many women, and recent studies are beginning to document that nontraditional attitudes may be helpful in adjusting to motherhood (Jiminez and Newton, 1982; Pistrang, 1984; Bassoff, 1984; Hock et al., 1984).

Numerous other aspects that occur in obstetrical care are not the object of my attention or criticism in this paper. I do not mean to suggest that many very serious health crises are not averted in obstetrics. Indeed, a good deal of modern medicine is beneficial to women and families, and there may in fact be cases in which the imposition of the medical model is justified. It may also be true that a growing number of doctors and clinic and hospital settings are relatively humane and flexible, less inclined to overstructure encounters with patients and to exhort these women to behave with traditional feminine deference. The following factors, however, are still problematic: 1) the lack of alternative types of care for childbearing women; and 2) the medical profession's monopolistic control over the right to administer care for all patients and to define how that care will be provided. The "natural" childbirth movement demonstrates that the archetypal traditional ways in which doctors and patients relate to one another have become increasingly untenable to many women in our society.

REFERENCES

Bassoff, Evelyn S. "Relationships of Sex Role Characteristics and Psychological Adjustment in New Mothers." *Journal of Marriage and the Family* 46(1984):449–454.

Bromberg, Joann. "Having a Baby: A Story Essay." In *Childbirth: Alternatives to Medical Control,* edited by Shelly Romalis. Austin: University of Texas Press, 1981.

Carver, Cynthia. "The Deliverers: A Woman Doctor's Reflections on Medical Socialization." In *Childbirth: Alternatives to Medical Control,* edited by Shelly Romalis. Austin: University of Texas Press, 1981.

Clarke, Joanne N. "Sexism, Feminism, and Medicalism: A Decade Review of Literature on Gender and Illness." *Sociology of Health and Illness* 5(1983):62–82.

Conrad, Peter, and Schneider, J. W. *Deviance and Medicalization: From Badness to Sickness.* St. Louis: C. V. Mosby, 1980.

Danziger, Sandra K. "The Medical Context of Childbearing." Boston: Boston University dissertation, 1978.

_____. "The Uses of Expertise in Doctor-Patient Encounters During Pregnancy." *Social Science and Medicine* 12(1978):359–367.

_____. "On Doctor Watching: Fieldwork in Medical Settings." *Urban Life* 7(1979):513–522.

_____. "Treatment of Women in Childbirth: Implications for Family Beginnings." *American Journal of Public Health* 69(1979):895-901.

_____. "The Medical Model in Doctor-Patient Interaction: The Case of Pregnancy Care." In *Research in the Sociology of Health Care*, Vol. 1, edited by Julius Roth. Greenwich, Conn.: JAI Press, 1980.

Ehrenreich, Barbara, and Ehrenreich, John. "Health Care and Social Control." *Social Policy* 5(1974):26-40.

Fishman, Pamela M. "Interaction: The Work Women Do." *Social Problems* 25(1978):397-406.

Fox, Renee C. "The Medicalization and Demedicalization of American Society." *Daedalus* 106(1977):9-22.

Freidson, Eliot. *Profession of Medicine: A Study of the Sociology of Applied Knowledge*. New York: Dodd, Mead, 1972.

Goffman, Erving. *Gender Advertisements*. New York: Harper and Row, 1979.

Haug, Marie R., and Sussman, Marvin B. "Professional Autonomy and the Revolt of the Client." *Social Problems* 17(1969):153-161.

Hock, Ellen; Gnezda, M. T.; and McBride, S. L. "Mothers of Infants: Attitudes Toward Employment and Motherhood Following Birth of First Child." *Journal of Marriage and the Family* 46(1984):425-431.

Jiminez, Marcia J., and Newton, N. "Job Orientation and Adjustment to Pregnancy and Early Motherhood." *Birth* 9(1982):157-163.

Kemper, Susan. "When to Speak like a Lady." *Sex Roles* 10(1984): 435-443.

Kollock, Peter; Blumstein, P.; and Schwartz, P. "Sex and Power in Interaction: Conversational Privileges and Duties." *American Sociological Review* 50(1985):34-46.

Laws, Judith L., and Schwartz, P. *Sexual Scripts: The Social Construction of Female Sexuality*. Washington, D.C.: University Press, 1977.

Maracek, Jeanne. "Psychological Disorders in Women: Indices of Role Strain." In *Women and Sex Roles: A Social Psychological Perspective*, edited by Irene H. Freize et al. New York: W. W. Norton, 1978.

Marcus, Alfred C.; Seeman, T. E.; and Telesky, C. W. "Sex Differences in Reports of Illness and Disability: A Further Test of the Fixed Role Hypothesis." *Social Science and Medicine* 17(1983): 993-1,002.

Marieskind, Helen I. *Women in the Health System: Patients, Providers and Programs*. St. Louis: C. V. Mosby, 1980.

Nathanson, Constance A. "Illness and the Feminine Role: A Theoretical Review." *Social Science and Medicine* 9(1975):57-62.

Oakley, Ann. "A Case of Maternity: Paradigms of Women as Maternity Cases." *Signs: A Journal of Women in Culture and Society* 4(1979):607-631.

_____. *Women Confined: Towards a Sociology of Childbirth.* New York: Schocken, 1980.

Pistrang, Nancy. "Women's Work Involvement and Experience of New Motherhood." *Journal of Marriage and the Family* 46(1984): 433–447.

Schneider, Joseph W., and Conrad, P. "The Medical Control of Deviance: Contests and Consequences." In *Research in the Sociology of Health Care*, Volume 1, edited by J. Roth. Greenwich, Conn.: JAI Press, 1980.

Scully, Diana. *Men Who Control Women's Health: The Miseducation of Obstetrician-Gynecologists.* Boston: Houghton Mifflin, 1980.

Scully, Diana, and Bart, P. "A Funny Thing Happened on the Way to the Orifice: Women in Gynecology Textbooks." In *The Sociology of Health and Illness*, edited by P. Conrad and R. Kern. New York: St. Martin's Press, 1981.

Verbrugge, Lois M. "Female Illness Rates and Illness Behavior: Testing Hypotheses about Sex Differences in Health." *Women and Health* 4(1979):61–79.

_____. "How Physicians Treat Mentally Distressed Men and Women." *Social Science and Medicine* 18(1984):1–9.

Waldron, Ingrid. "Why Do Women Live Longer than Men?" *Social Science and Medicine* 10(1976):349–362.

West, Candace. "Why Can't a Woman Be More Like a Man? An Interactional Note on Organizational Game-playing for Managerial Women." *Work and Occupations* 9(1982):5–29.

_____. "When the Doctor Is a 'Lady': Power, Status, and Gender in Physician-Patient Encounters." *Symbolic Interaction* 7(1984): 87–106.

West, Candace, and Zimmerman, D. H. "Women's Place in Everyday Talk: Reflections on Parent-Child Interaction." *Social Problems* 24(1977):521–529.

Zola, Irving K. "Medicine as an Institution of Social Control." *The Sociological Review* 20(1972):487–504.

_____. "Pathways to the Doctor—From Person to Patient." *Social Science and Medicine* 7(1973):677–689.

6

Birth and Social Class

MARGARET K. NELSON

It has often been reported that middle-class women receive better medical services than working-class women. It follows from this literature that the chances of being provided with the optimal birth experience are greatly enhanced if one enters the hospital as a middle-class client. Based on this assumption, my research, which examines class differences in childbirth procedures, began as a critique of 1) birth practices in a modern New England teaching hospital, and 2) class biases implicit among medical personnel. What emerged was the discovery of a complex interaction between social class, perception of ideal birth situation, and birth experience.

Responses to my questionnaires and interviews suggested that women can be divided along certain significant social dimensions that correspond to kinds of birth experiences. One group of women experienced birth in a relatively active and involved way. Another group had more passive births involv-

© 1983 by The Society for the Study of Social Problems. Reprinted with revisions from *Social Problems* 30 (Feb. 1983):284–297, by permission.

ing more monitoring, medication, transfers to the delivery room, and use of forceps.

I then went one step further: were the women within each of these groups having the kind of birth experience for which they had indicated preferences during the prenatal period? I hypothesized that middle-class women would be more likely to have their choices respected in the hospital than working-class women. I suspected that doctors would use low social status as a justification for disregarding client preferences and select the procedures *they* deemed necessary for working-class women.

I was wrong on two counts. First, in neither of the two groups that I studied did women receive the precise treatment they wanted. Second, there were few differences between the two groups in the extent to which the women got what they wanted. What I found instead was that the middle-class women generally wanted active, involved births free from medical interventions; some of their requests were respected in the hospital. The working-class women wanted more passive birth experiences with more medical intervention; some of their requests also were met within the hospital.

The data thus suggested that within the hospital at least three different models of an appropriate childbirth were operating: two different client models and a medical model. My initial approach to this topic had overlooked the existence of more than one client model distinct from that of the doctors' model.

The literature on women's control over childbirth had highlighted the importance of this life event for women. It has also used a set of implicit assumptions: 1) women share a set of common desires and make choices about childbirth independent of their social backgrounds; and 2) women's desires are different from those of doctors. In short, the literature assumes that women all want (or will come to want) conscious control over a basically "natural" childbirth experience and that doctors have resisted those demands. However, my data suggest that these assumptions are not entirely accurate. There is clearly more than just one client model of childbirth: not all women want the same kind of birth experience. And doctors, in fact, appear to resist and reject aspects of each client model in favor of their own approach.

SOCIAL CLASS IN CHILDBIRTH RESEARCH

Three traditions of research and theory on childbirth have, each for its own reason, ignored social class differences. These are 1) the feminist literature; 2) the general medical sociology treatment; and 3) studies that focus on the effects of preparation for childbirth.

Middle-class feminists, eager to take childbirth out of the hands of male obstetricians, seem more intent on describing how childbirth has become distorted over the years than in examining whether the "warping" (Haire, 1978) has affected all groups in the same way. Numerous historical studies document how male physicians wrested control of childbirth from female midwives, and enumerate class biases in the way in which new technologies were distributed (Ehrenreich and English, 1973; Kobrin, 1966; Wertz and Wertz, 1977). They do not tell us whether women of different social classes felt the same way about the changes—or whether there are class differences in attitudes toward childbirth today. (For an exception, see Hubert [1974], who explicitly notes the lack of homogeneity in attitudes about childbirth.)

Shaw (1974) found class differences in treatment during the prenatal and hospital periods: the medical staff was aware of the class origins of its clients and treated them according to preconceived notions of what was most appropriate for each group of women. However, the solutions that Shaw offers at the end of her book suffer from the opposite type of discrimination and ignore social class differences. She assumed her solutions would be equally acceptable to all clients, but never asked how they—as individuals or as representatives of social categories—would like childbirth to proceed.

The heavy emphasis on personal experience in much of the childbirth literature has resulted in the emergence of a single critique that presumes to speak for all women (e.g., Brinley, 1981; Comaroff, 1977; Hart, 1977; Rothman, 1982). (Oakley [1979:627] makes a similar point.) Most of those who write about childbirth are middle-class women. They are motivated by a feminist consciousness and possess the verbal ability that is part of class privilege. Thus, those who are most interested in women defining for themselves the nature and meaning of childbirth are, perhaps, guilty of prescribing a perfect birth for all women, regardless of individual needs or motivations. The less explicitly feminist literature has also ignored social class, albeit for different reasons. First, the ahistorical bias in much social science has inhibited attention to the social history of childbirth movements, a history that is important for understanding different class attitudes toward childbirth. Second, the use of some of the major sociological concepts might also inhibit a consideration of social class. For instance, although Stewart and Erickson attack mainstream sociology for failing to seriously consider childbirth, their own emphasis on roles as the best possible approach to understanding pregnancy and childbirth leads them to ignore social class. They note, for example, that "the manner in which women describe their labor and delivery varies by many factors including the setting, the difficulty of the labor, their definitions of themselves as sick or healthy, their expectations and how well these were met" (1977:41).

The view of childbirth expounded by middle-class feminists has been the best articulated and, therefore, has frequently been adopted by academic writers as the only view. Thus, as feminist critiques of contemporary obstetric care became more frequent and solidified, they were adopted by academic writers as representative of a single model or paradigm of childbirth that conflicted with that offered by the medical establishment. Nash and Nash (1979:493), for example, argue that "in American society at the present time there exist two primary interpretations of the meaning and practice of childbirth: the medical and the 'natural' view." Romalis (1981:5) similarly groups all women together when she asserts that "the nub of the problem is that doctors and patients can be said to hold very different models of reality."

Oakley (1979) offers by far the most sophisticated exploration of competing childbirth paradigms. She notes the paucity of client-oriented studies and emphasizes the different models at work in medical science, clinical psychiatry and psychology, and academic psychology and sociology. Until recently the sociologist's contribution had not been "to investigate the women's experience but to extend the limits of the medical model and propose a more elastic conception of the variables which can be seen to influence the biological outcome of maternity" (1979:624). However, Oakley emphasizes the "natural" model of childbirth as the principal one in conflict with the various medical models. Danziger (1978), in a paper on prenatal encounters between physicians and clients, also assumes that there is only one *client* paradigm.[1]

Some research on childbirth has ignored social class by matching or controlling independent variables too rigorously. Studies on preparation for birth clearly fall within this category. Most research shows that preparation for childbirth has both physiological and psychological effects on the birth process (Doering et al., 1980; Norr et al., 1977), though some studies indicate little or no effect (Zax et al., 1975). Motivation to learn about birth does not appear to be the key factor at work here: studies that compared women who wanted to take classes in childbirth preparation but could not, on the one hand, with women who did take classes (or were randomly assigned to classes) on the other found that preparation was the critical variable (Enkin et al., 1972; Huttel et al., 1972). To test whether preparation is a significant factor in the birth process, researchers have been careful to control for socio-economic status and education in experimental and con-trol groups. For example, Doering and Entwisle's (1975) work on the effects of preparation on the ability to cope with labor and delivery dismisses social class after noting that there were no significant social differences between trained and untrained subjects, even though only 18 percent of the total number of subjects were working-class women. Both Gaziano's (1979) study and the Greenfield-Tepper (1981) study examined working-class women who used a clinic and therefore could not compare clients at different levels of income or education. Other researchers who compare the effects of different kinds of preparation for childbirth also controlled for the class

[1] Comaroff (1977) offers an alternative approach. She notes that within the medical world, midwives and physiotherapists have different paradigms of pregnancy, and that clients adopt one or the other of them (though sometimes sequentially). The clients are assumed not to bring with them their own paradigms of pregnancy but rather to be tabula rasa upon which competing health personnel write a script. Comaroff does not see social background as determining which script is adopted, although she does acknowledge the influence of psychological factors.

origins of the client groups (e.g., Zimmerman-Tansella et al., 1979). Researchers have given only cursory attention to the issue of who chooses to attend childbirth classes and why.

Much of this research assumes that the outcomes of preparation—knowledge, control, cooperation, and an avoidance of medication—are definite, clear-cut, and desirable goals. That is, the studies assume that everyone wants an identical birth. Yet not all women perceive the outcome of preparation as a benefit. In fact, the data I collected for this paper suggest otherwise: we can no longer assume that all women want the same kind of birth.

METHOD

Background

In response to the declining U.S. birth rate, the movement for home birth, and the criticisms of women committed to hospital birth without extensive intervention, the Department of Gynecology and Obstetrics of the Medical Center Hospital of Vermont (MCHV) in Burlington, Vermont, decided in 1979 to revamp its maternity services. It hired certified nurse midwives to work with clients (both alone, for low-risk clients, and in conjunction with obstetricians for all other clients), opened a labor lounge, altered labor rooms to do double duty as delivery rooms, and stated that clients could choose their own birth style. It immediately hired two social scientists to evaluate whether these changes were satisfying the demands of knowledgeable, consumer-conscious, low-risk clients. I was one of those hired.[2] We thus collected the data on which this paper is based within the context of a specific mandate. The sponsors of the project were not interested in the particular issues underlying my present concern.

---

[2]The other was Helen McGough, who became director of the Mary Johnson Day Care Center in Middlebury, Vermont. Our evaluation of the maternity services (McGough and Nelson, 1981) showed that although most clients were pleased with the treatment they received, those clients who did not have the treatment they anticipated were less satisfied than those who got what they wanted. We also found that the medical staff was not giving full support to the innovations and that there remained a high level of medical intervention in childbirth.

The Data

We collected data in three stages from all clients who were served by a private group of obstetricians in MCHV; this group accounted for 80 percent of all births in the hospital during a six-month period in the winter of 1979–1980. During the ninth month of their pregnancy, we gave the women questionnaires about their previous birth experiences, their feelings about pregnancy and childbirth, and their choices for childbirth procedures. Three or four days after the women gave birth we interviewed them in the hospital, asking them about the birth itself. When the women returned to the doctor for a postpartum checkup (generally six weeks after birth), we gave them a second questionnaire, which asked about their feelings about the birth. A total of 322 women completed the first questionnaire (94 percent of those asked to participate in the evaluation study); 273 were interviewed in the hospital; and 226 completed the second questionnaire. The attrition rate of 30 percent was the result of various factors, including early hospital discharges and client failure to keep scheduled appointments. Equal proportions of working-class and middle-class women were lost in this process.

Independent Variables

There are three independent variables in this study: social class, preparation, and parity. The first of these is the most important.

Social Class

Because I suspected that social class affected choices about childbirth, I sought a way to distinguish class position among the clients. I chose education as the best indicator: women with no more than a high school diploma were categorized as working class; those with at least four years of college were categorized as middle class. Women with some college education or vocational training beyond high school were assigned to a category on the basis of the type of job they held at the time of participation in the evaluation study, or their prior work experience.[3] These procedures resulted in a total of 127

[3] I excluded all nurses and allied health workers from the study on the grounds that their perspective on birth would reflect their training and level of knowledge, rather than their class position. In fact, most of the women in the sample had some college education (but not four-year degrees) or were nurses.

working-class women and 124 middle-class women in the analysis.

Information on client income was not available. In any case, the fact that my sample includes a small proportion of "voluntary poor"—highly educated women who chose subsistence farming or craft work as a way of life—made income a poor indicator. Nor could occupation alone be used. I found that differences in education made a significant difference in the kind of occupations the women held, either at the time of the study or before it, and the pattern of their work involvement. However, not all the women were working or reported ever holding jobs. Occupations of the husbands were also unhelpful, because I wanted a variable that would reflect the background experiences of the women themselves. Furthermore, whether a woman had a college education made a difference along a range of other experiences, such as whether or not she was a native of Vermont, her religion, and her age at the birth of her first child. I wanted to investigate whether education also made a difference in women's attitudes toward, and experiences during, childbirth. If it did, I could at least argue that childbirth, for these women, was experienced through a set of social mechanisms. I use the notions of middle class and working class to denote the two groups in my sample, although I am aware of the weakness of my indicator for examining social class.

Preparation

A strong relationship exists between social class and formal preparation for childbirth. Seventy-nine percent of the middle-class women in my sample took childbirth classes, compared with 50 percent of the working-class women. The middle-class women also read an average of three books about pregnancy and childbirth, compared with an average of one for working-class women. These two kinds of preparation were themselves related: women who took childbirth classes were likelier to read about pregnancy and childbirth than women who did not. This naturally raises the question of whether I am, in fact, examining differences in knowledge rather than class differences. My data do not support this conclusion. Among middle-class women, preparation for childbirth made little difference in the kinds of attitudes I am examining in this chapter. Among working-class women, however, preparation for childbirth was extremely important: the attitudes of working-class women who were prepared for childbirth—whether through classes, reading, or a combination of both—were closer to those I defined as middle class than the attitudes of their unprepared peers. Had I examined the unprepared women in each social class I would have found even greater differences between the two groups than I did when I combined the prepared and unprepared women. Therefore, preparation is not relevant to the issue of attitude, except insofar as the findings about class differences in preparation reinforce my fundamental conclusions. When preparation is relevant to my analysis, I mention it below.[4]

Parity

One would expect women who have given birth before (multi-paras) to have different attitudes about childbirth compared with women who have never given birth (primiparas). Surprisingly, this was not the case. There were relatively few instances in which multiparas and primiparas had different attitudes during the prenatal period about what they wanted, although parity was an important determinant of what actually happened once a woman entered the hospital: multiparous women were less likely to have births marked by extensive medical intervention. In those cases in which parity was important, it had the same effects among middle-class women as it did among working-class women. Therefore, since parity—like preparation—is not crucial to most of the issues under consideration, I will discuss it only when it can help clarify my findings.

MODELS OF CHILDBIRTH

The middle-class and working-class women I studied became pregnant within different contexts and had different attitudes toward childbirth during pregnancy, different experiences during childbirth, and different postpartum evaluations of their experiences.

---

[4] When I did include childbirth preparation as a variable, I measured it by attendance at a series of childbirth classes for the latest, or an earlier, pregnancy. (For a more complete discussion of these issues, see Nelson, 1982.)

The Context of Pregnancy

The working-class women in my study grew up in larger families than did the middle-class women, and they were more likely to be Catholic. For both of these reasons, I expect that they began their adult lives with different attitudes toward optimum family size and structure. And, in fact, although the two groups did not differ significantly in response to a question about how many children they wanted to have, actions speak louder than words. The working-class women started their families at a younger age and at every subsequent age level had more children living in the home than did the middle-class women.

Given the greater likelihood of a large family size among working-class women than among middle-class women, it is not surprising to find that the two groups of women entered a single pregnancy differently. When asked why they became pregnant this time, more than a third (39 percent) of the working-class women responded that they did not have any choice in the matter, that the pregnancy was accidental. This response occurred for less than a quarter (22 percent) of the middle-class women.

But even when I exclude from my analysis of the reasons for entering a pregnancy those women who stated that the current pregnancy was accidental, differences remained in both content and number of reasons.

Working-class women emphasized only those factors related to family formation: they said that they have children because they feel it is an appropriate amount of time since the last child, because they can afford to start or enlarge a family now, and because their partner wants them to. Among middle-class women these same concerns compete with two others. They time childbirth so that it will not interfere with their work, and they are concerned about age. (These latter concerns are more relevant for the middle-class women who are more likely to be working at the time they become pregnant and more likely to be engaged in jobs that constitute a "career." They are also having their first babies at an older age.)

In addition, the proportions of women who indicated that any given factor was taken into consideration differed for the two groups. Middle-class women gave more responses than did

working-class women and a larger proportion of them responded to a single factor. Pregnancy for these working-
class women was either accidental or motivated by a single
concern: to create a family. Pregnancy for middle-class women
was motivated by a larger number of concerns. Their delibera-
tions included factors relating to personal needs as well as
family structure.

Working-class and middle-class women also gave different
reasons for reaching a decision about the number of children
that they felt constituted an ideal family size. As with the
factors relating to the current pregnancy, differences can be
found with respect to the emphasis with which issues were
cited as being relevant. Again, the working-class women
stressed family-related issues: money, the amount of time
available for each child, and the provision of siblings for
children. Middle-class women stressed the same family-centered issues, but those issues competed with others: concerns
about a career, overpopulation, and the availability of child
care facilities. Working-class women were also more single-
minded in their considerations than were middle-class women:
half of the former group gave fewer than three reasons compared with a quarter of the latter group (see Table 6.1).

Attitudes Toward Pregnancy

Working-class women were more likely than middle-class
women to have negative feelings about pregnancy. They
were less likely to say they felt good about the way they
looked or felt, and they did not feel they received sufficient
consideration from others. Pregnancy was not an unambiva-
lently positive state for working-class women. There were
obvious material causes for this attitude: not only were the
working-class women more likely to become pregnant by accident than the middle-class women, but they were less likely
to have the resources with which to find space to rest and
relax. Ideological issues may also have been at the root of
these differences. Middle-class women felt that pregnancy,
labor, delivery, and the postpartum presence of a baby were
interrelated pleasures, and this was true regardless of either
their preparation for childbirth or parity. Working-class
women made a greater distinction between the stages that led

TABLE 6.1. The Context for Pregnancy

Context	Working-Class Women (%)	Middle-Class Women (%)
*Reasons for Current Pregnancy**		
Reasons		
Appropriate time since last child	37	39
Financially feasible	24	38
Partner's desire	19	25
Appropriate time in work or career	8	40
Age	6	26
Other	0	2
	(N = 98)	(N = 103)
No. of Reasons		
One	75	45
Two	17	35
Three	8	13
Four or more	0	7
	(N = 98)	(N = 103)
Reasons for Desired Family Size		
Reasons		
Financial constraints	85	78
Enough time for each child	62	85
Provide siblings	37	49
Career	28	62
Overpopulation	13	39
Available child care	12	22
Care in old age	8	3
Family pressure	5	2
Church	4	8
	(N = 125)	(N = 117)
No. of Reasons		
One	22	3
Two	28	23
Three	27	24
Four or more	23	50
	(N = 125)	(N = 117)

*Among those whose pregnancy was planned, not accidental.

to birth and the presence of the baby itself: the former was not necessarily desirable, though the latter was. As with middle-class women, these attitudes were unaffected by parity and preparation.

Furthermore, during pregnancy working-class women were more apprehensive than middle-class women about labor and delivery. They worried about their own knowledge and competence; they worried that they wouldn't know when they were actually in labor; and they worried that they did not know what would happen in the hospital. Clearly, the context in which birth occurred was seen as somewhat threatening. In addition, working-class women were more worried than middle-class women about the discomfort of labor and delivery, and whether or not their personal physician would be present for the birth.[5] However, working-class and middle-class women had almost identical attitudes toward one birth issue and one issue pertaining to the baby itself: they all expressed strong concern about whether the birth would proceed according to personal desire, and they all felt certain that they would love the baby once it was born.

Among both groups, parity was irrelevant for all issues except concern about whether or not the baby would be healthy, and whether or not the mother would love it; those who had given birth before were less anxious. Yet among the primiparas the differences between the two social groups remained. Moreover, preparation for childbirth was related to concern about two issues: bearing the discomfort and having the birth as planned. However, in both groups those with more preparation were more concerned about these issues than were those with less preparation. Different levels of preparation did not account for the differences between the two groups.

Two additional questions in the questionnaire that I gave to women in their ninth month of pregnancy were designed to elicit their general attitudes toward childbirth (see Table 6.2). The first of these asked clients whether they agreed with the statement: "I feel that the birth experience can affect the

---

[5]This is not related to the fact that more working-class women than middle-class women see doctors in a clinic rather than in a private office, since clinic patients, like private patients, are assigned a regular doctor whom they see at each prenatal visit. In fact, no client in the group practice was promised that her doctor would be present at the birth.

TABLE 6.2. Client Attitudes Toward Pregnancy, Labor, and
Delivery during the Ninth Month of Pregnancy

	% Women in Agreement	
Statements	Working-Class	Middle-Class
Attitudes toward pregnancy:*		
When I'm pregnant people don't take my feelings seriously.	25	14
I like the way I look when I'm pregnant.	27	40
When I'm pregnant I feel well most of the time.	67	77
When I'm pregnant I feel depressed a lot of the time.	35	17
Concerns about labor and delivery:†		
I worry that I won't know when I'm in real labor.	50	30
I worry that I won't be able to bear the discomfort.	43	33
I worry that I don't know what is going to happen to me in the hospital.	36	25
I worry that I don't know enough about the process of childbirth.	32	17
I worry that my doctor won't be there for the birth of my baby.	49	31
I worry that the birth of my baby won't be the way I want it to be.	52	58
I worry that there will be something wrong with my baby.	49	31
I worry that I won't love the baby.	7	6
General attitudes toward childbirth:*		
I feel that the birth experience can affect the quality of the parent's relationship with the baby.	48	78
I feel that a natural childbirth will be best for my baby.	54	69
	(N = 127)	(N = 124)

*Five response options were offered for these statements: "Strongly Agree," "Agree," "Neither Agree Nor Disagree," "Disagree," and "Strongly Disagree." Percentages include those who gave either the "Agree" or "Strongly Agree" responses.

†For these statements, four response options were offered: "Very Important," "Pretty Important," "Not Too Important," and "Not Important At All." Percentages include those who gave either the "Very Important" or the "Pretty Important" responses.

155

quality of the parent's relationship with the baby." Seventy-eight percent of middle-class women agreed with this statement, compared with 48 percent of working-class women. This indicates that middle-class women place more emphasis on the birth experience itself as a critical stage in becoming a parent. In response to a second question, 69 percent of middle-class women and 54 percent of working-class women agreed with the statement: "I feel that a natural childbirth will be best for my baby." This suggests not only that middle-class women believe the birth experience to be significant in and of itself, but also that they have a specific idea about what kind of experience will be most appropriate.

Parity was not relevant to either of these attitudes. Among working-class women, preparation altered both attitudes; among middle-class women, only the feeling about a natural childbirth was affected by preparation. The class differences remained when I compared prepared women in each group (Nelson, 1982).

Similar differences between the middle-class and working-class women emerged when the multiparas within each group commented during pregnancy about how they would like the impending birth to differ from past ones. Middle-class women and working-class women shared a desire to have a spouse or partner present during the birth if he had not been present before. Women in both groups complained about the treatment they had received, but the content of their complaints was not the same. Middle-class women complained in detail about personality conflicts with their doctors, mismanagement (by the staff) of various aspects of labor, and the fact that medication was offered too frequently. Working-class women complained mostly about the lack of information offered to them during labor and delivery.

There were other differences as well. Working-class women often mentioned medical complications and the discomfort of labor and delivery. They expressed a wish that the next birth be faster and easier—if necessary, through the use of more intensive medication. Two comments were typical: "I would have liked to have been put to sleep—it was a long and painful labor"; and "Next time I want a quicker labor—my first was only eight hours but the pains were hard and came every two minutes." Middle-class women rarely mentioned either the intensity of pain or the length of labor. They stressed instead obstacles to a pleasurable experience: "I did not see my baby being born"; and "I would have wanted a more creative delivery."

Both working-class and middle-class women felt that they had a right to evaluate the past performance of medical personnel: if any of the women felt intimidated by the professionalism of the staff, they were not so intimidated as to totally inhibit subsequent evaluation. Women in both groups felt that the medical structure could be modified. However, there were significant differences between the groups. Working-class women felt that the responsibility for providing information rested with the doctor. In addition, they wanted to reduce the length of labor and avoid medical complications. They wanted a birth marked by less pain. In contrast, middle-class women were looking for a pleasurable, and often "natural," experience, and a more cooperative—rather than instructional—relationship with the physician.

Two issues must be considered in evaluating the women's responses to concrete questions about what they had wanted to happen when they entered the hospital to give birth: 1) whether the women even thought about the birth experience in detail during their ninth month of pregnancy; and 2) if so, what they wanted to happen to them.

With respect to the first issue, we can clearly divide the women into two groups: those who knew about and had already considered the different aspects of the birth process and those who had not. In fact, more middle-class women than working-class women considered each of the procedures surrounding birth. However, differences between the groups were not found for those procedures directly related to family formation: having the husband present, watching the birth, and holding the baby after it was born. More than 90 percent of the women in both groups considered each of these procedures. Middle-class women as a group thus considered each step of the birth process; a substantial number of working-class women focused only on the final stage—the creation of a new family.

Parity was not relevant here, with the exception that those who had given birth before (in both groups) were less likely to say that they wanted medication during labor than those who had never given birth. Preparation for childbirth was important here but, as indicated earlier, preparation changed the attitudes of working-class women but not the attitudes of middle-class women. Most of the unprepared working-class women, those who had wanted medical intervention, had not thought about the issues (Nelson, 1982). (See Table 6.3.)

Among the women who thought about what they wanted to happen, there were differences in the content of their choices—differences that again corresponded to class. Working-class women selected medication during labor and delivery, artificial rupture of membranes, delivery room births, and fetal monitoring more often than middle-class women did. The differences between the two groups on these issues ranged from 35 percent for delivery room births and fetal monitoring to 55 percent for the artificial rupture of membranes. Differences between the two groups with respect to the "social" aspects of birth were never more than 7 percent. More than 90 percent of both the middle-class and the working-class women chose to have the birth become an event in which they could participate by having a partner present during labor and delivery, watching the birth, and holding the baby as soon as it was born.

The working-class women seemed to be striving for speed (enema, episiotomy, artificial rupture of membranes), less pain (medication) and technological safety (delivery room birth, monitoring). They favored intervention because they thought it could help achieve the birth easily, quickly, and safely. The middle-class women favored a process that entailed safety (as they defined it) and personal participation but excluded medical intervention in a "natural" process.

In sum, the content of middle-class choices was noninterventionist. When middle-class women did not make choices, it was often because they were willing to leave some control in the hands of the physicians—not because they had not thought about the issues. "I'll let the doctor decide" was often how they responded to questions about their attitudes to specific procedures. In contrast, when working-class women made choices, they favored intervention; when they didn't make choices it was more often because they had not thought about the issues.

Among working-class women, there was a tension between

TABLE 6.3. Planning for Childbirth: Choices about Procedures

Procedures	% of Clients Who Considered Procedure		Clients Who Wanted Procedure*				Physicians Who Wanted Procedure†	
	Working-Class	Middle-Class	Working-Class		Middle-Class			
			%	No.	%	No.	%	No.
Shave	85	97	20	47	20	67	33	15
Enema	85	98	42	55	46	68	50	12
Labor medication	81	98	57	51	11	55	22	9
Delivery medication	84	96	58	55	17	64	33	9
Artificial rupture of membranes	44	68	59	17	4	25	—	9
Episiotomy	64	95	64	14	62	37	55	8
Fetal monitoring	53	86	90	31	55	44	63	8
Lithotomy position	64	77	—	—	—	—	—	11
Delivery room birth	90	95	80	89	45	76	54	18
Support person present during labor	96	100	88	116	98	107	100	18
Support person present during delivery	93	100	83	112	96	108	100	18
Watching the birth	91	92	89	112	93	99	—	—
Holding baby at birth	94	99	92	106	97	111	100	15
	(N = 179)	(N = 119)						

* Based on the number of clients who made a choice—either positive or negative—with respect to the procedure.
† Based on what the practitioner said would be desirable for self or spouse if hospital birth was planned.

not thinking about the impending event and preparing for it by making decisions; between avoidance and self-determination. For the middle-class women, the tension was between self-determination and reliance on professional expertise. Moreover, the goals of self-determination were also different for the two groups. Among middle-class women, the goal was a definition of childbirth free from the prevailing medical and technological model embodied in the authority of the male physician. Working-class women sought freedom from the birth process itself through the use of strategies that would reduce pain and effort. Working-class women were not trying to give the experience a unique definition. They were trying to survive it with a minimum of embarrassment, discomfort, and isolation. Of course, there were exceptions to all of these generalizations. We can speak about models only in the most general terms.

Although my concern here is those clients who made choices about what they wanted to happen to them when they entered the hospital, it is possible that these clients had been effectively socialized by the staff members with whom they had contact during the prenatal period. If they were expressing preferences that corresponded to practitioner preferences or established protocol, they were, perhaps, acting no more independently than if they had made no choices at all. In fact, however, neither working-class choices nor middle-class choices were entirely congruent with either what physicians said they would want for themselves or what actually happened in the hospital. The content of the discrepancies was different for the two groups of women.

When physicians were asked what they would want for themselves (or their spouses) if they were to give birth at MCHV, they chose a model of birth that can be characterized as a safe delivery with active management by an attending physician. (Most physicians who did not make a choice said that they would let a doctor decide.) Physicians were more likely than middle-class clients to opt for monitoring and medication. They were less likely than working-class clients to opt for these procedures. These findings suggest that at least three different models of what constitutes an ideal birth exist. Neither working-class women nor middle-class women have concepts that are purely the result of intensive socialization before delivery or purely the result of an awareness that they had better avoid a confrontation with hospital personnel. The style of birth selected is different for the two groups of women, and both styles differ from the one physicians say that they would want for themselves or their spouses. I do not mean to imply that socialization is irrelevant, but that it alone cannot explain the content of the women's choices.

Childbirth Events

Not only did working-class and middle-class women have different ideas about what they wanted to happen during childbirth, but they also had different experiences during the actual birth. Working-class clients had births marked by more medical intervention and less client participation than did middle-class women. To a certain extent these features are interrelated: the use of medication during labor and delivery makes it more likely that the delivery will take place in the delivery room and that forceps (or vacuum suction) will be required; the use of forceps ensures that an episiotomy will be necessary and that the client will have to be in a prone rather than sitting or semisitting position. And the more intervention, the less likely the woman is to be able to respond to the baby immediately.

Many middle-class women also had a great deal of intervention during labor and delivery: more than 70 percent of them experienced an artificial rupture of membranes, an episiotomy, fetal monitoring, a delivery room birth, or forceps or vacuum suction. The proportion of middle-class women who had such intervention was smaller than that for working-class women by more than 10 percent for the issues of labor and delivery medication, lithotomy position, delivery room birth, IV attached during labor, and forceps or vacuum suction. The middle-class women were better able to be active participants in the birth: they controlled the contractions with breathing techniques, pushed the baby out themselves, and held the baby as soon as it was born. Ninety-eight percent of them had a partner present during labor and 94 percent had a partner present at the birth (see Table 6.4).

Parity was relevant to the birth experience in the same way within each group: primiparas had births that involved more

TABLE 6.4. Hospital Events: Percentage of Clients Having Each Procedure

Procedures	All Clients	Working-Class	Middle-Class
Shave	65	61	67
Enema	49	54	47
Labor medication	44	50	35
Delivery medication	41	52	30
Artificial rupture of membranes	70	69	75
Episiotomy	85	83	88
Fetal monitoring	85	87	80
Lithotomy position	75	84	67
Delivery room birth	87	96	82
IV attached during labor	85	91	74
Forceps or vacuum suction	20	24	13
Support person present during labor	94	96	98
Support person present during delivery	87	83	94
Watching the birth	45	44	46
Holding baby at birth	85	81	88
	(N = 203)	(N = 105)	(N = 98)

extensive medical intervention. Preparation for childbirth influenced only the use of medication and the presence of a support person—and these only among working-class women. Therefore, preparation cannot explain the class differences (Nelson, 1982).

The difference between the births of middle-class and working-class women corresponded roughly to what the women selected during pregnancy—although not, perhaps, to the motives behind the choices, in the case of working-class women. Working-class women wanted a speedy delivery and immediate access to the baby. They didn't necessarily get speed, nor did they get the baby immediately. In fact, the more typically middle-class concern with the entire process might have ensured a speedier labor and delivery and more immediate access to the baby (Doering et al., 1980; Huttel et al., 1972; Zax et al., 1975).

Neither working-class nor middle-class women had all their choices met during labor and delivery. The extent to which client choices about shaves, labor medication, episiotomies, watching the birth, and holding the baby were respected was about the same for both groups. But the two groups differed in the extent to which other choices were respected. More middle-class women than working-class women had their wishes met with respect to enemas, delivery medications, and the presence of a support person during labor and delivery. More working-class women had their way with respect to fetal monitoring, artificial rupture of membranes, and the delivery site.

When we focus on the causes of these discrepancies, the issues become even more complex. With respect to enemas, the greater discrepancy among the working-class clients derived from their having had an experience imposed on them that they did not select; with respect to delivery medication, the discrepancy resulted from their not receiving what they wanted. With middle-class women, the greater discrepancy surrounding the use of a fetal monitor and transfer to the delivery room derived from the procedures being imposed against their wishes (like enemas for working-class women).

The data do not indicate that doctors impose their will on working-class clients more frequently than on middle-class clients; nor do the data indicate that working-class clients are less effective in stating what they want than are middle-class clients. Both working-class and middle-class models of birth conflict with hospital protocol. Women in neither group were entirely successful in getting their way (see Table 6.5).

Postpartum Attitudes

Working-class women and middle-class women had different ideas about what they wanted to happen during childbirth and different experiences during the birth. They learned different lessons from these experiences.

A series of open-ended questions was designed to obtain general information from the clients about their feelings after going through labor and delivery. These questions proved very useful because they did not presume anything about client knowledge of, or specific client attitudes toward, birth.

TABLE 6.5. Discrepancy between Choice and Event: Percentage of Clients Who Got What They Wanted*

Procedure	Working-Class		Middle-Class		% Difference: Working-Class versus Middle-Class
	%	No.	%	No.	
Shave	65	34	56	52	9
Enema	50	38	65	51	−15
Labor medication	59	37	59	37	0
Delivery medication	53	51	78	60	−15
Artificial rupture of membranes	50	20	38	13	12
Episiotomy	67	9	61	28	6
Fetal monitoring	87	23	58	31	29
Delivery site	86	66	70	60	16
Support person present during labor	86	85	98	87	−12
Support person present during delivery	79	84	95	87	−16
Watching the birth	48	84	44	73	4
Holding baby at birth	83	76	84	81	−1

*Based on the number of clients who made a choice—either positive or negative—with respect to the procedure.

The first of these questions was asked after a long series of detailed questions about what had happened during labor and delivery. Women were asked, "Is there anything else you would like to tell us about your labor and delivery?" In the majority of cases, the answer was a simple "No"—not a surprising response from women who had just finished answering approximately 100 questions eliciting both factual and attitudinal information.

The responses of those clients who did have more to say were informative. First, there were differences in the sheer quantity of responses: middle-class clients were more likely than working-class clients to have something that they wanted to add. Second, there were differences in the style of the responses: the middle-class women who responded did so at great length; the working-class women gave short answers. Third, there were differences in the content of the responses. The working-class women expressed either extremely positive or extremely negative attitudes toward the birth. Negative comments (of which there were more than positive comments) stressed pain and the length of labor. Many of the comments used a passive voice: "I was very pleased that it happened to me"; "I was made to get up too soon"; "Things were explained to me better than last time." Among the middle-class women, there were more responses containing both positive and negative factors. For instance, a middle-class woman might have responded that there were some rough moments but that the staff was reassuring, or, conversely, that the birth had gone well but that staff actions created problems. Middle-class women rarely mentioned discomfort and never spontaneously commented on the length of labor. Instead, they gave detailed criticisms of the staff and the procedures implemented. In so doing, they demonstrated their sophisticated knowledge. The passive voice was rarely if ever used: middle-class clients were actors during the birth, not the recipients of the actions of others. Finally, middle-class women frequently used the concept of experiencing a birth; working-class women almost never used this concept.

In response to a question asking the women what they would do differently if they were to have another baby at the same hospital, different themes predominated among working-class and middle-class women. Working-class women often referred to a detail of the experience over which they might have had control. They criticized themselves for not being adequately prepared for childbirth, for aspects of how they behaved during the birth, and for arriving at the hospital too late. In contrast, the middle-class women were basically self-congratulatory: they felt that they did their part right but that the staff should have done things differently or that hospital routines should be altered.

Studies demonstrating the effects of preparation for childbirth argue that prepared women are more likely to see themselves as the locus of control than are unprepared women (Felton and Segelman, 1978). The findings noted earlier support this conclusion only with respect to positive behaviors. Middle-class women, typically better "prepared," did speak in a more active way about their role in the birth and were rarely critical of this role; working-class women often used the passive voice when reporting events, but when they did speak in an active voice, they were more likely to be critical of their own activity. My interpretation of this finding relies on my earlier analysis of the differences between middle-class and working-class clients with respect to antepartum planning and draws on the concept of social distance. The interpretation enriches our understanding of what women learn during the process of childbirth.

Earlier I noted that middle-class women were more likely than working-class women to assume control over what was going to happen when they entered the hospital: they made more concrete choices. When the birth proceeded in the manner they had anticipated, they were pleased with themselves. The preparation had paid off. When the birth ran counter to their expectations, they blamed someone or something else. Because they were usually of a higher social status than the nurses and close in status to physicians, they could be critical of these individuals. The hospital itself is supported by their payments and contributions: it too is subject to evaluation.

For working-class women the situation is different. They enter the hospital less prepared to assume control and less interested in active participation. They learn that they have to participate and that their performance is subject to evaluation.

Ehrenreich and Ehrenreich (1978) refer to the patient-physician relationship as one that, because authority, intimacy, and social distance are combined, holds great potential for conveying nonrelevant messages. In the case of working-class women in labor, comments made by medical personnel may be internalized. Those women who are told that they are doing well, that they are being good patients, may learn to see themselves as such and assume pride in their own behavior. Those women who are told that they are acting poorly, not relaxed enough, pushing too soon, getting too hysterical, may learn to see their own behaviors as problematic. The social distance that inhibits their own criticism of the staff may ensure internalization of comments made by the staff.

Working-class women and middle-class women learned different lessons during childbirth. The middle-class women learned that what you want is not necessarily what you get; the working-class women learned that what you do or how you act will not necessarily meet the approval of those in authority. It is not surprising that the women walked away from birth with different impressions.

A final question concerned impressions of the experience: "If you were to tell a woman who had never given birth what it was like, what would you say?" Both working-class and middle-class women indicated that birth was worthwhile. But working-class women said that it was worthwhile despite the pain because there is a baby at the end: "I think it's worth it, a day of pain for all this." At the same time, many working-class women said that they forgot about the pain quickly. They said they wouldn't frighten other women, the way they had been frightened, with predictions of pain, and that women should not believe all the terrible things they heard about giving birth.

Middle-class women had a very different set of ideas about what it was appropriate to tell a woman who had never given birth. First, they said that they would focus on the process as an experience itself: "a high and painful experience"; "a fantastic experience." Second, they would talk about the work involved: "It's hard work; preparation is important"; and "Now I know why it is called labor. You really have to work." Third, they would be more likely to give details. Indirectly, they suggested that they had been told positive things about birth by their peers: "It's as good an experience as I had been told it was"; "It was even better than my friends said it would be."

These responses revealed a further basic difference between the two groups of women. The working-class women did not appear to value the process of birth itself. They focused, instead, on the product—the baby. Labor and delivery were something to be endured to get the product. Middle-class women valued the process as well as the product. They felt fortunate to be able to enjoy the experience of birth en route to motherhood.

DISCUSSION

I will briefly summarize my data analysis. From the material available about the antepartum attitudes of clients, we learned that middle-class and working-class women were involved in prenatal planning for birth in different proportions and that the members of each group who made choices worked toward different goals. Middle-class women wanted births in which they could actively participate while avoiding intervention; working-class women wanted quick and easy births with as much intervention as they perceived to be required to bring about this end. Neither of these models of birth was entirely congruent with that of the physicians who worked with them.

When the women entered the hospital, they had some, though not all, of their antepartum wishes respected. Middle-class women received more intervention than they wanted, but less than working-class women; working-class women got less intervention than they wanted, but more than middle-class women. Women in each group were forced to modify their expectations in the face of hospital protocol.

Working-class women learned that birth can be survived. Because they valued the process primarily because of the product, they ultimately felt that it was worth it—it certainly wasn't fun but when all was said and done it could be forgotten. Some working-class women also were told by hospital staff that the manner in which they handled themselves during the birth was not appropriate; they may have left with diminished self-confidence. Middle-class women learned that birth was a powerful and important experience, even though the staff on occasion placed impediments to total enjoyment. Some of the middle-class women learned that next time they had better be prepared to fight harder for what they want.

How can we account for these different attitudes toward, and experiences during, the birth process? Two possible explanations have been implicit at various points in our analysis. I will consider them further here.

One possibility is that working-class women are simply more inhibited by the context in which birth occurs. They may not become interested in the birth process because they do not believe that they can determine what is going to happen to them. Caught between medical experts and nature, they see little room for individual initiative. This is clearly an element of working-class disaffection with birth. But working-class feelings of impotence cannot entirely explain the particular nature of the choices that some working-class women make, particularly because these choices are not entirely congruent with those of the professionals who manage their care.

A second possibility is that the greater interest of middle-class women in childbirth issues derives from greater knowledge. Not only are middle-class women more likely to prepare themselves for childbirth through reading and attending classes, but they also draw on different kinds of information.[6] But these facts also cannot entirely explain different attitudes: the middle-class women hold their attitudes regardless of whether they have educated themselves about childbirth. The same is not true among working-class women: those who are prepared frequently hold different attitudes from those who are not. In any case, the search for information is probably the result—not the cause—of interest in childbirth.

Why, then, are working-class women generally uninterested in learning about childbirth? Why do they reject the middle-

[6]Working-class women were far more likely than middle-class women to say that they relied on mothers and other relatives to provide them with information about childbirth. The apparent middle-class rejection of their mothers as a source of information about childbirth suggests that they were aware that the ideology about childbirth has changed since they were born and that their mothers' retelling of a painful—but ultimately anesthetized—birth offered little to them. Working-class women felt that more information could be obtained from their mothers, indicating that they had not recognized the changes that have occurred since the time when they were born.

class ideology that not only stresses the value of information but also holds as its goal a client-structured, "natural" childbirth? The answer lies in the contexts in which each group of women gives birth and in the fact that the movements that have created the middle-class model of the birth experience do not speak to both contexts equally.

As noted above, the working-class women in our study started their families at a younger age, and at every subsequent age level had more children living in the home than did the middle-class women. The working-class women were more likely to have accidental pregnancies. Furthermore, when they chose to become pregnant, relatively few factors were taken into account, and these factors concerned only the family structure. Middle-class women were more likely to plan their pregnancies and the total number of children they wanted to have. As with working-class women, the ideal family structure was central to their thinking, but this factor was diluted by self-concerns (work and career, child care facilities) and world concerns (overpopulation). Working-class women, then, had their children earlier, had more of them, and frequently had them without planning. They also had fewer material resources with which to raise these children.

The movements that created the middle-class model of birth experience do not clearly address the working-class context of childbirth. In the early 1960s, middle-class women were not very interested in childbirth; in the early 1970s only elite portions of the middle class took childbirth classes or attempted to define birth independent of the prevailing, high-technology, medical model. The change came with the convergence of (and occasional tension among) four social movements: 1) the natural childbirth movement; 2) feminism; 3) consumerism; and 4) "back to nature" romanticism.

Advocates of natural childbirth initially glorified it as a step toward motherhood. The movement appealed largely to middle-class women who were eager to be more active participants in this important event but who continued to accept professional (as distinct from technological) control over it. The feminist movement, however, told many of these same women that it was time to reject the authority of men in specifically female experiences in order to gain personal control over their lives and their bodies. Feminists also rejected the notion that childbirth was important primarily as a step toward motherhood. Consumerism advocated questioning attitudes toward any and all prevalent medical practices. And the back-to-nature movement advocated rejecting modern technology and returning to great-grandmother's way. None of these movements speaks to working-class women.

Natural childbirth preparation requires time, money, and a willing alliance with professionals. Within the feminist movement, the focus on middle-class concerns of access to professional jobs and consciousness-raising has alienated many working-class women who face employment problems of a very different cast and who are less able to live independent of their husbands' paycheck. Moreover, an "educated" contempt for professionals is easier for those who live among them that for those who may have to submit to experts in a wider range of life experiences. The failure of middle-class feminists to make contact with working-class concerns has been noted frequently: this analysis merely points to an additional consequence of this failure.

Consumerism depends on a steady income, mobility, and time. Middle-class women can afford to shop around for goods and services. But working-class women pay more out of necessity, not out of choice (Caplovitz, 1967); clinic clients see the doctor assigned to them. And a rejection of technology is the luxury of those who have already benefited from it. That class of women who have always had access to the most sophisticated medical technology may make the decision to reject some aspects of that class privilege; those women who have not yet consistently received those benefits may not be ready to abandon them.

In sum, the middle-class model of childbirth has its roots in social movements that do not have immediate relevance for working-class women. The model is also predicated on the idea of choice, the idea that one can take control of one's life and one's body (e.g., Boston Women's Health Book Collective, 1976). Working-class women have fewer opportunities for making choices; even pregnancy often appears to be outside their control.

The emerging model of hospital birth is, in fact, closer to the middle-class model than it is to the working-class model. Doctors have been greatly influenced by the criticisms of their most vocal clients and, in "progressive" hospitals, are making a conscious effort to "humanize" birth. Some of these changes may converge with working-class goals. But reducing the frequency with which medication is administered is foreign to working-class concerns and may seem like a threat to a woman (of any social class) who is unprepared to do without medication. In fact, physicians may use the middle-class model to force working-class compliance: one woman we interviewed said she was told by a doctor that if she "didn't stop yelling he would make [her] go natural."

Each of the two models of childbirth makes sense within its intended context. Each model confers benefits on the women who adhere to it. Each model also has its drawbacks. The middle-class model mystifies childbirth. Accepting the model can produce a sense of guilt and personal failure in women whose births fail to conform to its high standards. The working-class model engenders a dependence on potentially harmful medication and creates an anxiety that can prolong and complicate labor.

This kind of evaluation brings us back onto thin ice. My reading and research suggest that a single model of childbirth has too often been held up for all women. Initially, doctors defined the experience for all women. Then one group of women began speaking for all women. But women are not a single, undifferentiated category. Childbirth is a biological experience mediated by class position. We must learn more about what women at different locations in the social structure want for themselves rather than pass judgment on what they do. If changes are to come in either working-class or middle-class birth styles, they must come from the women themselves—not from one group of women speaking for another, or from physicians dictating to all of them.

REFERENCES

Boston Women's Health Book Collective. *Our Bodies, Ourselves.* New York: Simon and Schuster, 1976.

Brinley, Maryann B. "The First-time Mother: It's One Thing When You're 23, Quite Another When You're Approaching 40. Two Women Tell Their Stories." *Health* 13(October 1981):30–32.

Caplovitz, David. *The Poor Pay More.* New York: The Free Press, 1967.

Comaroff, Jean. "Conflicting Paradigms of Pregnancy: Managing Ambiguity in Antenatal Encounters." In *Medical Encounters: The Experience of Illness and Treatment*, edited by Alan Davis and Gordon Horobin. London: Croom, Helm, 1977.

Danziger, Sandra K. "The Uses of Expertise in Doctor-Patient Encounters During Pregnancy." *Social Science and Medicine* 12(1978): 359-367.

Doering, Susan G., and Entwisle, Doris R. "Preparation During Pregnancy and Ability to Cope with Labor and Delivery." *American Journal of Orthopsychiatry* 45(1975):825-837.

Doering, Susan G.; Entwisle, Doris R.; and Quinlan, Daniel. "Modeling the Quality of Women's Birth Experience." *Journal of Health and Social Behavior* 21(1980):12-21.

Ehrenreich, Barbara, and Ehrenreich, John. "Medicine and Social Control." In *The Cultural Crisis of Modern Medicine*, edited by John Ehrenreich. New York: The Monthly Review Press, 1978.

Ehrenreich, Barbara, and English, Deidre. *Witches, Midwives and Nurses*. Old Westbury, N.Y.: The Feminist Press, 1973.

Enkin, N. W.; Smith, S. L.; Dermer, S. W.; and Emmett, J. D. "An Adequately Controlled Study of the Effectiveness of PPM Training." In *Psychosomatic.Medicine in Obstetrics and Gynecology*, edited by Norman Morris. New York: S. Karger, 1972.

Felton, G. S., and Segelman, F. B. "Lamaze Childbirth Training and Changes in Belief About Personal Control." *Birth and the Family Journal* 5(Fall 1978):141-148.

Gaziano, Emmanuel P.; Garvis, Marlene; and Levine, Elaine. "An Evaluation of Childbirth Education for the Clinic Patient." *Birth and the Family Journal* 6(Summer 1979):89-94.

Greenfield, Debra S., and Tepper, Shelley L. "Childbirth Preparation and Urban Clinics." *Journal of the American Medical Women's Association* 36(December 1981):370-376.

Haire, Doris. "The Cultural Warping of Childbirth." In *The Cultural Crisis of Modern Medicine*, edited by John Ehrenreich. New York: The Monthly Review Press, 1978.

Hart, Nicky. "Parenthood and Patienthood." In *Medical Encounters: The Experience of Illness and Treatment*, edited by Alan Davis and Gordon Horobin. London: Croom, Helm Ltd., 1977.

Hubert, Jane. "Beliefs and Reality: Social Factors in Pregnancy and Childbirth." In *The Integration of a Child Into a Social World*, edited by Martin Richards. New York: Cambridge University Press, 1974.

Huttel, F. A.; Mitchell, I.; Fischer, W. M.; and Meyer, A. E. "A Quantitative Evaluation of Psychoprophylaxis in Childbirth." *Journal of Psychosomatic Research* 16(1972):81-92.

Kobrin, Frances E. "The American Midwife Controversy: A Crisis in

Professionalization." *Bulletin of the History of Medicine* 40(1966):350-363.

McGough, Helen, and Nelson, Margaret K. "An Evaluation of Obstetric Services at Medical Center Hospital of Vermont." Unpublished report, Department of Obstetrics and Gynecology, Medical Center Hospital of Vermont, Burlington.

Nash, Anedith, and Nash, Jeffrey E. "Conflicting Interpretations of Childbirth: The Medical and Natural Perspectives." *Urban Life* 7(1979):493-511.

Nelson, Margaret K. "The Impact of Childbirth Classes on Women of Different Social Classes." *Journal of Health and Social Behavior* 23(1982):339-352.

Norr, Kathleen L.; Block, Carolyn R.; Charles, Allan; Meyering, Suzanne; and Meyers, Ellen. "Explaining Pain and Enjoyment in Childbirth." *Journal of Health and Social Behavior* 18(September 1977):260-275.

Oakley, Ann. "A Case of Maternity: Paradigms of Women as Maternity Cases." *Signs: A Journal of Women in Culture and Society* 4(1979):607-631.

Romalis, Shelly. "An Overview." In *Childbirth: Alternatives to Medical Control*, edited by Shelly Romalis. Austin: University of Texas Press, 1981.

Rothman, Barbara Katz. *In Labor: Woman and Power in the Birthplace.* New York: W. W. Norton, 1982.

Shaw, Nancy Stoller. *Forced Labor: Maternity Care in the United States.* New York: Permagon Press, 1974.

Stewart, Mary, and Erickson, Pat. "The Sociology of Birth: A Critical Assessment of Theory and Research." *Social Sciences Journal* 14 (April 1977):33-47.

Wertz, Richard W., and Wertz, Dorothy C. *Lying-In: A History of Childbirth in America.* New York: Schocken, 1977.

Zax, Melvin; Sameroff, Arnold J.; and Farnum, Janet E. "Childbirth Education, Maternal Attitudes and Delivery." *American Journal of Obstetrics and Gynecology* 123(1975):185-190.

Zimmerman-Tansella, C.; Dolcetta, G.; Assini, V.; Zacche, G.; Bertagni, P.; Siani, R.; and Tansella, M. "Preparation Courses for Childbirth in Primipara: A Comparison." *Journal of Psychosomatic Research* 23(1979):227-233.

7

Cesarean Birth

PAMELA S. SUMMEY

At the foot of the bed, in Lizaveta Petrovna's skilful hands flickered the life of a human being, like the small uncertain flame of a night-light—a human being who had not existed a moment ago but who, with the same rights and importance to itself as the rest of humanity, would live and create others in its own image.

"Alive, alive! And a boy too! Set your mind at rest!" Levin heard the midwife say as she slapped the baby's back with a shaking hand.

"Mama, is it true?" asked Kitty.

The princess's only reply was a sob.

And in the silence there came, in unmistakable answer to the mother's question, a voice quite unlike the subdued voices that had been speaking in the room: a bold, insistent, self-assertive cry of the new human being who had so incomprehensibly appeared from some unknown realm.—L. N. Tolstoy, *Anna Karenin* (tr. Rosemary Edmonds).

The miracle of birth ties us to generations past and future. As we bring forth new life, we unite our families in the present and affirm our collective hopes for the future. Women's unique ability to give birth has always shaped their lives and given them meaning. A good part of a woman's adult life historically has been consumed by pregnancy and the bearing of children, attended by a constant fear of death in childbed (Rosaldo, 1974; Leavitt and Walton, 1984). Today, even with the twin burdens of continual pregnancy and risk of death lifted from the lives of most modern women, the importance of bearing children continues: women divide their lives into before- and after-children segments and define themselves at least in part as mothers of their children.

Childbirth itself is an important life event: reconstructed, retold, and relived in memory over and over again. The progression of labor to delivery, the physical sensation of birth itself, the first cry of the newborn infant, and the first moments with that infant are long remembered by mothers. As Nabokov reminds us, "Our existence is but a brief crack of light between two eternities of darkness" (1947:1). The welcome we give new beings can be compared in meaning only with our farewells to those leaving life.

To doctors, childbirth is seen as the work needed to deliver a healthy mother and baby from a potentially endangering situation. The mystery of birth is translated into an uncertainty in need of control. Even though the work is usually routine, the view persists that danger is always lurking. And the raison d'être of the medical profession rests, as Light put it, "on the claim that it can handle other people's emergencies with routine control" (1980:282).

We are thus left with two competing visions of modern childbirth—two players who do not agree on the scenario they are enacting. We have, on the one hand, the birthing woman, embarking on one of life's most significant and meaningful experiences, apprehensive of its possible dangers, trying to face her pain and fear with dignity and courage. On the other hand, we have doctors who see childbirth as both part of a routine day's work and a potentially dangerous situation to be controlled. Conflict in the situation is structured.

This chapter will focus on the doctor's view of childbirth vis-à-vis Cesarean delivery. I will argue that doctors present birth as a situation of uncertainty. Emphasis on the uncertain aspects of childbirth rather than its lawful and routine

aspects allows doctors considerable autonomy in their decision making and reinforces their dominance over both other
practitioners and birthing women. Cesarean delivery is used
as an example in which the uncertainty of outcome and the
dangers of birth are invoked to control birth and leave women
powerless.

THEORETICAL PERSPECTIVE

In his ideal type of the physician, Parsons stated that
physicians are expected to act for the welfare of the patient,
be guided by the rules of professional behavior, apply a high
degree of skill and knowledge to problems of illness, and be
objective and emotionally detached. In exchange for these
obligations, the physician is granted the "privileges" of
autonomy and dominance (Parsons, 1951). Freidson argued
that the most important characteristic of a profession is
autonomy over the content of work (1970a). Autonomy is
granted because of a profession's claims to expert skills or
knowledge and its guarantee of self-supervision and -regula-
tion. The dominance of a profession derives from the institutionalization of power in which other competing practitioners are controlled and both access to information and to
other alternatives for care are closed to the laity (Freidson,
1970b). The profession has the ongoing problem of protecting
its institutionalized authority from outside regulation and
challenges to its power and expertise.

The practitioner benefits from this institutionalization of
authority but has the daily problem of reaffirming his or her
dominance over both patients and colleagues. This problem
presents itself early in medical training when medical students, seriously lacking in both knowledge and skills, must
nevertheless begin treating patients and working with more
experienced medical staff. Medical students "train for uncertainty" and develop a "manner of certitude" in order to
manage this uncertainty and assert their position of dominance in the medical hierarchy (Fox, 1957).

The kind of uncertainty addressed by Fox was that of knowledge—either incomplete mastery of existing knowledge or
a limitation in the actual body of medical knowledge. In his
study of psychiatry training, Light expanded upon Fox's con-

cept by elaborating areas other than knowledge in which uncertainty exhibits itself and by examining how it is managed in medical practice. As Light wrote, "Training for uncertainty means learning techniques of control. . . . *Technically*, a profession's greatest need is for a better expertise in the form of knowledge and skills, but *sociologically*, a profession's greatest need is for control" (1980:282). Areas of uncertainty defined by Light include: professional knowledge, diagnosis, procedure, collegial relations, and client response. Using these categories, and some of Light's techniques for control, I will elaborate how medicine in general and obstetrics in particular have managed to institutionalize and maintain control on both the level of the profession and the level of the individual physician.

The first of Light's areas of uncertainty is that of professional knowledge; a profession must claim a body of knowledge as its own, and a practitioner must master this knowledge. Medicine has been successful in claiming its body of knowledge and in involving the state in the ongoing support of this claim. Obstetrics as a profession claimed the "diseases of women" as its body of knowledge in establishing itself as the first major specialty in medicine in 1930 (Dannreuther, 1931). Professional organizations, closed to all but "board certified" obstetrician-gynecologists, as well as three subspecialty boards set up in 1974, continue to assert the profession's claim to a specific body of knowledge and expertise.

Practitioners approach this constantly changing and expanding body of knowledge with a realization that they will never master it all. There are several techniques of controlling the uncertainty related to a vast and unlearnable body of knowledge. One is to limit oneself to a small area of expertise. Obstetrician-gynecologists often specialize in gynecologic cancer, infertility problems, or high-risk pregnancy and limit their practices accordingly. A second technique is to adopt a "school or philosophy of practice" (Light, 1980). The belief that there is no one right way in medicine often leads a physician to develop an "aggressive" or a "conservative" approach to medical management. Yet a third method is to project the "manner of certitude" described by Fox, thus covering up for a lack of mastery of knowledge.

The second area of control is that of problem definition or

diagnosis. On a professional level, this is intimately related to the establishment of the specialty itself and the institutionalization of its authority. Freidson argued that one of the major powers of a profession as the ability to define its work: "In developing its own 'professional' approach, the profession changes the definition and the shape of problems as experienced and interpreted by the layman. The layman's problem is recreated as it is managed—a new social reality is created by the profession" (1970a:xvii). This definition of the situation provides the underlying philosophy or ideology upon which a profession's work is based.

As discussed in Chapter 1, Joseph DeLee espoused the classic view of the "abnormality" of childbirth. He maintained that birth was innately a pathogenic situation, a perspective that provided the obstetrical profession with a basic interventionist philosophy (1920:39–40). This philosophy is echoed throughout the history of modern obstetrics, as illustrated by a classic exposition in 1932:

The most marked feature of present-day obstetrics, is the fact that there is a distinct spirit of activity, of being ever alert to do something to relieve the patient and to safeguard her and her baby from the dangers which are ever associated with labor, as against the older policy so often expressed of letting nature take its course (Bill, 1932:156).

And yet another in 1979: "You know that the trip through the birth canal is the most dangerous trip we ever take with the greatest chance of our dying of any one day in our lives" (Stone, 1979:2). The image of birth as a dangerous event from which only obstetricians can safely deliver women and their babies reasserts the importance of the profession.

The individual practitioner's definition of specific problems is based on this general philosophy of being constantly alert to danger, even in seemingly innocuous situations. There is a bias toward diagnosing illness (Freidson, 1970a) and the notion that it is better to impute disease where there is none than to overlook it where it truly exists (Scheff, 1963). In obstetrics, this translates into a tendency to see pathology even in normal labor and to view any deviation from a normal pattern as a serious problem requiring action.

After a problem is defined or diagnosed, then the procedures or treatments needed to manage it must be found. Having defined childbirth as pathologic, the obstetrical profession has developed an interventionist ideology of birth as well as a vast array of techniques and technologies to manage it.

In the case of the individual doctor, this translates into the availability of a battery of interventions and a bias toward action. "Successful action is preferred," wrote Freidson, "but action with little chance for success is to be preferred over no action at all" (1970a:168). The relation between action and its result is frequently overlooked in medicine. As Light noted, "A major way in which professionals learn to control the uncertainties of treatment lies in the subtle shift from considering technique as a means to considering it an end" (1980:287).

Problems of diagnosis and treatment depend on the constant invoking of the concept of uncertainty—that all labors are different and there is no right way to manage all of them. Doctors can thus choose their preferred method of delivery, invoking clinical experience as their guide, and remain answerable to no one.

Collegial relations is an area in which the medical profession has been very successful at gaining and retaining control. Historically, direct competitors were driven out of practice by medicine's strong and cultivated relationship with the state. Other less threatening occupations were controlled simply, as Freidson put it, "by gaining from the state control over those occupations' activities so as to limit what they could do and to supervise or direct their activities" (1970a:47). Thus, the obstetric profession's long-standing concern with the "midwife problem" (Williams, 1912; Kobrin, 1966) has been a central aspect in the maintenance of professional dominance over colleagues.

Individual doctors are protected in their collegial relations by the institutionalized dominance of the profession. Nevertheless, the need for control over others is evidenced in the tendency to work alone, the reluctance to call in consultants, the hesitancy in delegating any but the most demeaning work, and the tendency to keep much of their work "invisible" and thus not subject to review or criticism (Freidson, 1970a).

Client response is the last area over which a profession must retain control. The medical profession controls this sphere by closing off alternative sources of care and by maintaining a dominant class position vis-à-vis the patient. Because physicians are of a higher social class than most of their patients, class dominance is inherent in the doctor-patient relationship (Freidson, 1970b).

Individual physicians begin with this position of class dominance over their patients. In obstetrics, this dominance is reinforced because most doctors are men and all patients are women. Doctors also maintain their position of superiority by keeping patients ignorant (Waitzkin and Waterman, 1974) and by invoking ideologies and rituals of medicine that command the patient's submission. In obstetrics, for example, many birth rituals serve to keep the patient in her place and the doctor in control (Haire, 1972; Eakins, 1982). In addition, when a birthing woman is presented with the possibility of a damaged baby, she will do whatever her doctor advises in the situation.

With this theoretical perspective, I will now argue that the use of Cesarean delivery in obstetrics can be a powerful technique of control. For the profession, it reinforces the ideology of birth as a dangerous event and the importance of interventions to save women and infants from these dangers. The surgical skills required enhance the profession's prestige and ensure its dominance over others who deliver children (midwives, family practitioners) as well as over women who desire increased participation in childbirth. For the practitioner, Cesarean delivery is the culmination of an "aggressive" philosophy of childbirth in which the dangers to women and children are emphasized and modern technologies are the way to "better babies." Doing Cesareans helps physicians gain and maintain control over the uncertainties of diagnosis and treatment as well as over the more tangible aspects of their work, such as the long hours and fears of malpractice suits.

Because of the lack of agreement in both diagnosing problems of childbirth as well as the preferred manner of treating those problems, doctors have great freedom to use Cesarean delivery whenever they see fit. Doctors use Cesarean delivery in different ways depending on their practice situations, their perceived practice problems, and their view of the technique as a potential means of controlling these problems. Cesarean delivery, far from being simply an example of "the application of scientific knowledge to problems of illness and health" (Parsons's 1951 definition of modern medical practice), can be and often is used as a technique by which doctors control birth.

My focus in this chapter will be the work of individual practitioners. The arguments of how the obstetrical profession has gained and continues to maintain control have been discussed in depth elsewhere (Wertz and Wertz, 1977; Summey and Hurst, 1984).

CESAREAN DELIVERY AS A MEANS OF CONTROL

Cesarean delivery is the ultimate medical control over childbirth. It is the surgical delivery of a child by a doctor, with little or no participation of the birthing woman or her family. The decision to do a Cesarean is nearly always made by the physician alone, and the conditions under which it is performed are often totally controlled by the doctor and/or hospital policies and regulations. Today more than one out of every five babies born in the United States is born by Cesarean (Taffel, Placek, and Moien, 1985). The rate has more than tripled in the past decade.

A Cesarean is a dangerous procedure for women, with a four times greater risk of death and a ten times greater risk of infection than a vaginal delivery (Consensus Development Conference, 1981). Apart from the medical risks, Cesareans are also psychologically difficult for women, leading to feelings of failure and self-blame or depression over loss of control over the birth process. Although Cesareans are usually done for the benefit of the infant, the advantages to infants remain largely undocumented.

The subjectivity of indications, and wide variations in accepted use give physicians enormous choice in whether or not to do Cesareans. To explore this issue, I examined the practices of thirty-one obstetricians delivering at a New York City teaching hospital from 1978 to 1980 (see Table 7.1). These physicians all had their own private offices with full general ob-gyn practices during the period of my study. Twenty of the doctors were in group practices. Only one of them had what could be considered a high-risk practice. Areas of uncertainty were explored with these doctors, and ways in which they controlled this uncertainty were examined.

TABLE 7.1. Cesarean and Forceps Rates by Year, in Percent

Measurement	1978	1979	1980	Total
Average Cesarean rate	26.9	23.9	27.1	25.6
Range in individual rates	8–66	10–51	13–52	12–51
Year-to-year correlations of individual rates		r = .71 1978–79 r = .67 1978–80	r = .65 1979–80	
Average forceps rate	31.1	30.3	30.8	30.4
Range in individual rates	0–75	6–73	7–75	9–74
Year-to-year correlations of individual rates		r = .84 1978–79 r = .79 1978–80	r = .88 1979–80	

The Cesarean rates of these physicians were remarkably consistent year to year, as were their rates of forceps deliveries. This consistency indicates that physician practice is a highly stable characteristic, dependent less on the medical characteristics of patients than on the preferred practice style of the individual physician.

The data in Table 7.1 indicate that, on the average, these private physicians did 25.6 percent of their deliveries by Cesarean and used forceps in 30.4 percent of all deliveries over the three years studied. If we combine the two figures, we find an average intervention rate of 56 percent. When we examine individual rates, we see enormous variation: Cesarean rates range from 12 to 51 percent; forceps rates range from 9 to 54 percent. This translates into overall intervention rates ranging from 29 percent (9 percent forceps plus 20 percent Cesarean rate) to 95 percent (74 percent forceps rate plus 21 percent Cesarean rate)! That two doctors, practicing at the same hospital under similar conditions, differed so much in their propensity to intervene in the birthing process is astonishing. The fact that these were not extreme scores, but that the other twenty-nine physicians in my study were fairly evenly distributed between the two endpoints, illustrates the great divergence in obstetrical practice today. Incidentally, the one obstetrician with the high-risk practice fell well into the middle range, with a Cesarean rate of 32 percent and a forceps rate of 28 percent, for a total intervention rate of 60 percent.

How did doctors explain their generally high Cesarean rates, and what factors accounted for the enormous variations in rates in this study?

Professional Knowledge

The practice style of an individual physician reflected his[1] resolution of the problem of uncertainty in professional knowledge. Two physicians with very high Cesarean rates emphasized the many aspects that could go wrong in childbirth and the importance of intervening:

> We should be well aware of what comprises danger and what doesn't comprise danger or risk. I think there is a tendency in some quarters toward thinking there is no reason any child practically can't be delivered vaginally, even if it's molded into the shape of a banana, as long as the fetal monitor is okay. The fact of the matter is that we still must not lose sight of the fact that we are dealing with a physical system where injury can occur not only because of physiologic deprivation but also because of physical injury. An infant's skull can be rammed against a bony pelvis for only so long without causing rupture of blood vessels and bleeding on a traumatic basis.

> I wish that emergency situations like fetal distress and bleeding and cephalopelvic disproportion, and all of those things never occurred in obstetrics, because I would love to go to people's homes and sit around with them, open up a jug of wine, and deliver a baby and have their children come in and their neighbors and anybody else who wanted to. I wish that those things either never would happen or that I was ignorant to their possibility. But since I am neither ignorant and have seen too many things happen, and because I care a great deal about how a labor turns out, I am filled with much too much anxiety built in relative to

[1]The male pronoun will be used in this discussion of individual practitioners. Few women were involved, and use of the female pronoun could unnecessarily identify these women, thus breaching my promise of confidentiality.

the childbirthing process to be able to take any of those risks.

One of the foreign-trained doctors in my sample commented on the difference between his British medical colleagues and his newer American ones in terms of their attitudes toward birth: "Not everything is a life and death situation as American doctors would have us believe. Here, you can have a woman in normal labor and everyone treats her as if this is a disaster!"

More conservative physicians with lower Cesarean rates expressed fewer fears of danger in childbirth and more trust of the natural process. Several times in my interviews I heard the "cigar story," that classic of conservative philosophy in obstetrics:

I had a professor of obstetrics who had a great axiom: "When you run into trouble, go into the waiting room and smoke a long cigar. By the time you finish, your problem will probably have resolved itself." Much more damage, especially in obstetrics, comes from doing too much too soon than too little too late.

Professional ideology does not exist in a vacuum. It is continually influenced by the social climate and external events. In the case of obstetrics, the recent fall in the birth rate, combined with an increase in the number of obstetricians, has affected the general outlook of the profession. Most obstetricians agree that there is more than enough work for everyone but make one remarkable shift in attitude to accommodate the change:

I think there has been a very marked shift in emphasis from what used to be called quantity to quality. Most obstetricians are delivering significantly fewer patients in a month or a year than they used to, and, simultaneously, there have been a number of advances in obstetrics that have made it possible to assess the well-being of the baby much more carefully than in the decade before.

And the concept came about that every baby was a quality baby and that no risks should be taken at all. This gave us the opportunity to devote significantly more time to each woman in labor. Every patient was then monitored, watched carefully for signs of difficulty, and the pattern that we have today of rigorous monitoring of every facet of pregnancy, labor, and delivery came about.

Professional ideology not only allows physicians to control the problem of uncertainty in their knowledge but it also fosters a certain approach to diagnosis and treatment. Focus on the dangers of birth and the importance of "quality" babies provides the groundwork for increased interventions, particularly Cesarean delivery.

Diagnosis and Treatment

To solve uncertainties of diagnosis and treatment, doctors fall back on their training and clinical experience and tend to focus on technique as an end in itself. Many of the doctors I interviewed underlined the uncertainty of when to do a Cesarean and the aspect of choice on the part of the doctor:

There are some people who say that all breeches should be sectioned; some people who say that none of the breeches should be sectioned; and there are the middle-of-the-road people who say you should check through pelvimetry, check how big the pelvis is, and then, above a certain diameter, certain parameters, the baby should be delivered from below. You get ten different opinions on the way to properly deliver a premature vertex, a premature breech, whatever.

It's highly individual. I think anyone who reads statistics on primigravida breech deliveries, with their wife or sister in labor, they would inevitably section that patient. But that's my own personal belief.

The delivery techniques learned in training seemed to have a great influence of doctors' attitudes about delivery, but a lesser effect on their actual practices. Obstetrical training for older doctors meant delivering babies with "technical virtuosity": "We were trained more in the arts of obstetrics where manipulation was the mark of the really good obstetrician." More recent training in the words of a young obstetrician, emphasizes the attitude that Cesarean section is certainly not as dangerous as it used to be and that it is much better to perform a Cesarean section than some heroic gesture of delivering the baby vaginally. [We have come] from an attitude that Cesarean section was a defeat to the obstetrician to the feeling that, far from a defeat, it really is beneficial to a lot of babies that would have been harmed otherwise.

Despite disagreements on the relative merits of various interventions, in the end, one older doctor admitted: "You do things that you feel comfortable with. The younger people are not trained to do what I was trained to do. So they're better off doing a Cesarean section. Now whether my results would be different from theirs, I don't know."

Reliance on clinical experience is another way of resolving the dilemma of uncertainty. A bad experience seems to be the most effective teacher:

I've seen many instances myself where, for no good reason, because of a poor outcome in a previous delivery, a c-section is done with an indication that would not even toss a mosquito off balance. And yet a c-section is done, clearly because this time we're going to get a good baby, no matter what.

I don't want to risk doing an operation for an indication that I'm not comfortable with. And I think [that is because of] an experience I had as a resident. A woman almost died after a Cesarean. I mean, really almost died. I thought she was going to die. It was very touch and go. She was in a coma and everything. And the section was done for CPD [cephalopelvic disproportion, an often subjective estimate by the doctor that a baby is too large to be born vaginally]. Having seen this woman almost die very early on [in my training] impressed upon me that this is not nothing. A Cesarean is significant. And I just always want to feel comfortable that, God forbid something should happen, I can sleep easy and know that the operation had to be done.

Clearly, from the examples presented here, experience can lead a physician to do more or fewer Cesareans, depending on the circumstances.

Data from these physicians' practices do not show that earlier-trained doctors were necessarily less likely to do Cesareans than those more recently trained. In fact, the rates of the older doctors and the most recently trained doctors were quite similar and on the low end of the range. The highest Cesarean rates in my sample were among physicians trained in the late 1950s and 1960s.

Forceps use was tied much more to when a physician was trained. The correlation coefficient between years since medical school graduation and rate of forceps use was .49, indicating that more recently trained physicians were less likely to use forceps. The influence of time of training was even greater on midforceps use, a practice now considered outdated in obstetrical training. Only six physicians in my sample had midforceps rates higher than 2 percent. Of these six, the average number of years since their medical school graduation was thirty years, and the group included the two oldest doctors in my sample.

Doing Cesareans solves more than just problems of uncertainty. It allows doctors more control over their time. Clearly, delivering babies is an unpredictable business. This is especially problematic to doctors who must juggle deliveries with an office practice, surgery, hospital rounds, teaching, and, presumably, a private life as well. Deliveries, furthermore, take place in a hospital environment in which an "optimal tempo" of births must be maintained (Rosengren and DeVault, 1963).

Looking at when doctors were most likely to do primary Cesareans—that is, Cesareans that are emergency in nature—I found that the doctors in my study were more likely to do primary Cesareans on weekdays than on weekends or holidays. This finding has been reported by others as well (Fleck, 1980; Phillips et al., 1982). Further, these doctors were more likely to do primary Cesareans at nine o'clock in the morning than at any other time of the day. At least 10 percent of the primary Cesareans took place around 9 A.M.

Two doctors predicted that common time, stating: "I can explain that by the fact that they were up all night long, they had reached a point of disgust, and they wanted to get [the delivery] done before they then had to start their scheduled day's activities." And again: "Physicians do sections before office hours. They 'pit' women [give pitocin to speed up labor] at night, then do the sections early in the morning to get to the office on time."

In his study of upstate New York hospitals, Fleck (1980) found that doctors were much more likely to do primary Cesareans during the day, concluding, "Primary Cesarean births do not have the attributes of emergency procedures and resemble much more closely the kinds of things you would expect for a tonsillectomy, herniorrhaphy, and other elective surgical procedures."

Some of the interviewed doctors admitted that doing Cesareans not only helped them control their time but actually saved time:

If it looks like someone's going to have a Cesarean section, rather than wait the two or three hours to see if they can push it out, they go ahead and do the Cesarean section rather than wait it out. To deliver repeats or breeches from below certainly is much more time consuming. That's the reason I'm in a group so that we can have the time to spend—we know that despite the time we spend up with the patient, we'll have the next few nights off.

The doctors in my study who were in group practice did fewer Cesareans than did doctors in solo practice, reinforcing the statement that doctors can wait out a long delivery if others can cover other obligations for them. Nevertheless, the doctors in my study with the largest practices tended to have the lowest Cesarean rates, thus arguing against the use of Cesarean delivery as a means of controlling time.

Like Mizrahi's interns, whose orientation was to "Get Rid of Patients" (GROP) in order to avoid work and avoid the possibility of a problem (1983), the doctors I interviewed were generally motivated to get deliveries over with to save both time and worry:

I don't really think that Cesareans are done for money reasons. They might be done for other reasons: to get you out of trouble without having to put so much sweat in, or to avoid sitting there doing a real test of labor by doing a Cesarean section a little bit earlier.

Many times when I've been slow I was sorry. Not that the outcome was bad, but, three things: 1) it's rough on the baby: long, hard labor; 2) rough on the mother, and 3) it's rough on the obstetrician's coronaries. You sit up all night and you worry, should I do it now? And you wait and she's making a little progress. You go another hour or two, and you end up doing a section anyway. You say, why didn't I do it ten hours ago?

These last two comments were made by two of the older and more conservative doctors in my study, who leaned heavily toward what they considered to be the more problematical school of "watchful waiting."

Collegial Relations

The struggle for monopoly over others who deliver babies has been a persistent theme in the history of the obstetrical profession. Continued dominance over family practitioners and midwives is essential to the profession both for economic reasons and for prestige. One doctor in my sample practiced with a midwife and discussed his colleagues' reactions to the situation:

There were some people on the staff at this hospital who, when I tried to bring a midwife into my office initially, said that I was killing the goose that laid the golden egg. Board-certified obstetricians who've had four or five years of postgraduate medical training or more, should not be caring for normal, healthy women who don't need their expertise. I think that midwives could very well care for 50 to 60 percent of the private obstetrical population. The only problem is that New York obstetricians would have smaller incomes. I think it's a very simple economic issue.

The issue of dominance cannot be dismissed: maintaining control over other practitioners maintains professional prestige as well as income. One way in which this dominance is accomplished is by emphasizing the dangers of birth and the unpredictability of bad events:

Consumers are being pushed into alternate birth centers with nurse-midwives who deliver all the "uncomplicated, low risk" patients. The only problem is that most problems develop during labor, intrapartum. They are not predictable events. The patients that develop difficulties in labor, if they're in alternate birthing centers where they're an hour away from possible remedy to the medical problem, will wind up creating more obstetrical problems as a result.

Doing Cesareans helps maintain the focus on the danger of birth, the need for hospital delivery, and the imperative that highly trained specialists manage births.

Client Response

Uncertainty in their relations with patients has intensified for obstetricians during the past decade. The 1970s were years of defensiveness for the profession, which felt attacked from all sides: "We are under siege," said Stone in his 1979 presidential address to the American College of Obstetricians and Gynecologists (ACOG), "from the consumerists, environmentalists, women's liberationists, civil rightists, and other special interest activists yet to be organized" (1979:1).

Women's demands for a "perfect baby" were one of the major perceived pressures on the doctors in my study:

The majority of my patients don't have gigantic families. They have one or two kids, chosen exactly when they want them. And they're concerned about every aspect: what medicine to take, what not to take, what to do, whether to smoke, to drink, and they're very religious in their ways of making a perfect baby. And the medical-legal ramifications are such that whether the patients or whether the system puts a pressure on the physician, it's a very anxiety-producing situation.

A Cesarean provides a solution to that anxiety in two ways: 1) it hastens delivery, thus shortening the time an obstetrician must worry about the outcome, and 2) it protects the doctor from a legal challenge that he did not "do everything possible" to deliver a perfect baby. Consumer pressure in the form of malpractice suits has had an important impact on the practice of obstetrics. Marieskind found it to be the "most frequent reason for the increase in the Cesarean section rate given by physicians" in her interview study (1979:82). The two doctors in my sample with the highest Cesarean rates did expert-witness work on malpractice cases and were very in-volved in the legal aspects of obstetrical practice.

The recent ACOG study of malpractice (1983) showed that 60 percent of U.S. obstetricians have been sued at least once, and in New York, nearly 50 percent have been sued three times or more. Doctors in my study paid between $40,000 and $50,000 annually in malpractice insurance premiums, and nearly all agreed that this had an impact on their practice. Whether doctors who had been sued more had higher Cesarean rates could not be determined from my research, but those with the highest rates were also the most verbal in interviews about the malpractice situation and about their own lawsuits.

Because of the large number of publicized suits brought against obstetricians for failure to perform a Cesarean or for performing one too late, doing a Cesarean "in good time" is perceived as the safest path legally:

There is an inner fear in many practicing physicians about the legal aspects of what they're doing. If they wait another two hours and have the woman push, what happens if the baby is brain-damaged? Would it be better to do a Cesarean section and get it over with and get a good baby and not worry about it? We're talking about the prime baby—the one shot—the one-child or the two-child family, and there's a lot of pressure. I think that it's many times easier to take the pressure off and do a Cesarean section whenever there's a question of a problem rather than persist and possibly have a problem.

Obstetricians have two patients and thus are responsible for the health of both mother and child. A recent court decision upheld the duty of a doctor to do a Cesarean for the health of a child, despite the objections of the mother (Bowes and Selgestad, 1981). The fact that most women would prefer to avoid a Cesarean if possible often puts them in an adversary position vis-à-vis the physician. But playing on the shared desire for a healthy baby, obstetricians maintain control over the situation, even when it means an undesired Cesarean:

My final goal is a perfect, perfect baby. That's what I want to hand parents. Sometimes it's tough. They come to me expecting a vaginal delivery. Presenting them with a sec-tion sets me up as their enemy. Sometimes it's quite a wrestling match. I always win. Because the argument of a cerebral palsy baby, knocking off I.Q. points, continuing the labor with fetal distress, is too overwhelming in my experience to date for a patient to refuse a section. So we always win for obvious reasons.

Cesarean delivery is presented, by those with the highest rates, as the ultimate in a good doctor-patient relationship:

We do a lot of Cesareans because we really care about our patients and are involved in their deliveries. If you know a patient well, take care of her during her pregnancy, you are much more likely to do a Cesarean than for a patient whom you don't know and don't care much about.

Another physician gave an example of a Cesarean done recently with no apparent indication other than a bad outcome from a previous delivery:

My partner just sectioned a woman who two years ago I delivered an absolute monster for. Even though this time we had chromosomal evidence of total normality, the pressure was still tremendous because they were such wonderful people, both of them, and they had gone through this together with such strength. Even though we had pressed all the right diagnostic buttons and done all the right things, we still had tears in our eyes when a normal baby was born, because, God knows, they deserved it.

Once again, we see the importance of controlling the vast uncertainty of birth and the effectiveness of Cesarean delivery as a technique of control.

Childbirth remains a mystery, an uncertainty, to both women and their doctors. Women, fearing the uncertainty, often choose to deliver in hospitals with doctors as their assistants. Thus their uncertainty is reduced as they relinquish some of the control to doctors. Doctors see the uncertainty of birth as problematic, yet use the concept of uncertainty to ensure their autonomy and dominance. Uncertainties about professional knowledge, diagnosis, and treatment are translated into powerful ideologies of childbirth that define it as dangerous and in need of expert control. Uncertainties of collegial relations and client control are translated into the closing off of alternative sources of care and again the invoking of an ideology relating expert medical intervention with improved outcomes for babies. Cesarean delivery represents the triumph of this medical control. The ideology linking Cesareans to "better babies" continues to guarantee the autonomy of obstetricians and their dominance over birth.

REFERENCES

American College of Obstetricians and Gynecologists. "ACOG Committee Statement on Dystocia." Washington, D.C.: American College of Obstetricians and Gynecologists, 1982.

———. *Professional Liability Insurance and its Effects: Report of a Survey of ACOG's Membership.* Washington, D.C.: American College of Obstetricians and Gynecologists, 1983.

Bill, Arthur H. "The Newer Obstetrics." *American Journal of Obstetrics and Gynecology* 23(1932):155–164.

Bowes, Watson A., Jr., and Selgestad, Brad. "Fetal Versus Maternal Rights: Medical and Legal Perspectives." *Obstetrics and Gynecology* 58(1981):209–214.

Consensus Development Conference. *Cesarean Childbirth.* Bethesda, Md.: National Institutes of Health, 1981.

Dannreuther, Walter T. "The American Board of Obstetrics and Gynecology: Its Organization, Function, and Objectives." *Journal of the American Medical Association* 96(1931):797–798.

DeLee, Joseph B. "The Prophylactic Forceps Operation." *American Journal of Obstetrics and Gynecology* 1(1920):34–44.

Eakins, Pamela S. "Fundamental Complications of the Contemporary Medical-Obstetrical Paradigm." Paper presented at Society for the Study of Social Problems Meetings, San Francisco, September 1982.

Fleck, Andrew C., Jr. Data cited in letter to Marsha Hurst, March 20, 1980.

Fox, Renée C. "Training for Uncertainty." In *The Student-Physician,* edited by Robert K. Merton, George G. Reader, and Patricia L. Kendall. Cambridge, Mass.: Harvard University Press, 1957.

Freidson, Eliot. *The Profession of Medicine.* New York: Dodd, Mead, 1970a.

———. *Professional Dominance.* New York: Atherton Press, 1970b.

Haire, Doris. *The Cultural Warping of Childbirth.* Milwaukee: International Childbirth Education Association, 1972.

Kobrin, Frances. "The American Midwife Controversy: A Crisis of Professionalization." *Bulletin of the History of Medicine* 40(1966): 350–363.

Leavitt, Judith Walzer, and Walton, Whitney. "Down to Death's

Door: Woman's Perceptions of Childbirth in America." In *Women and Health in America*, edited by Judith Walzer Leavitt. Madison: University of Wisconsin Press, 1984.

Light, Donald. *Becoming Psychiatrists*. New York: W. W. Norton, 1980.

Marieskind, Helen I. *An Evaluation of Caesarean Section in the United States*. Washington, D.C.: Department of Health, Education, and Welfare, 1979.

Mizrahi, Terry. "The Impact of Graduate Medical Socialization of Internists on the Doctor-Patient Relationship." PhD diss., University of Virginia, 1983.

Nabokov, Vladimir. *Speak, Memory*. New York: G. P. Putnam's Sons, 1947.

Parsons, Talcott. *The Social System*. Glencoe, Ill.: The Free Press, 1951.

Phillips, Robin N.; Thornton, John; and Gleicher, Norbert. "Physicians Bias in Cesarean Sections." *Journal of the American Medical Association* 248(1982):1082–1084.

Rosaldo, Michelle Zimbalist. "Woman, Culture, and Society: A Theoretical Overview." In *Woman, Culture, and Society*, edited by Michelle Zimbalist Rosaldo and Louise Lamphere. Stanford: Stanford University Press, 1974.

Rosengren, William R., and DeVault, Spencer. "The Sociology of Time and Space in an Obstetrical Hospital." In *The Hospital in Modern Society*, edited by Eliot Freidson. New York: The Free Press, 1963.

Scheff, Thomas J. "Decision Rules, Types of Error, and Their Consequences in Medical Diagnosis." *Behavioral Science* 8(1963):97–107.

Stone, Martin L. Presidential Address to the American College of Obstetricians and Gynecologists. *ACOG Newsletter,* 1979, 1-passim.

Summey, Pamela S., and Hurst, Marsha. "OB/GYN on the Rise: The Evolution of Professional Ideology in the Twentieth Century." Paper presented at the Sixth Berkshire Conference on the History of Women, June 2, 1984.

Taffel, Selma M.; Placek, Paul J.; and Moien, Mary. "One-fifth of 1983 U.S. Births by Cesarean Section." *American Journal of Public Health* 75(1985):190.

Tolstoy, Leo N. *Anna Karenin* (tr. Rosemary Edmonds). New York: Penguin, 1976.

Waitzkin, Howard B., and Waterman, Barbara. *The Exploitation of Illness in Capitalist Society*. Indianapolis: Bobbs-Merrill, 1974.

Wertz, Richard W., and Wertz, Dorothy C. *Lying-In: A History of Childbirth in America*. New York: The Free Press, 1977.

Williams, J. Whitridge. "Medical Education and the Midwife Problem in the United States." *The Journal of the American Medical Association* 58(1912):1–7.

8

Childbirth and the Malpractice Insurance Industry

WENDA BREWSTER O'REILLY
PAMELA S. EAKINS
MYRA GERSON GILFIX
GARY A. RICHWALD

Anne Robison's doctor decides that her labor is moving along too slowly. "We are going to make your contractions more effective," he tells her. He orders the nurse to give her pitocin. The pitocin-induced contractions are not only stronger but more frequent. They do not build gradually and fade as natural contractions do; they come on suddenly with almost full force. The doctor orders an epidural to relieve Anne of the much less manageable pain of pitocin-induced contractions. The doctor also decides to use an internal electronic fetal heart monitor to assess the effects of these interventions on the baby. To do so, he artificially ruptures her membranes to attach an electrode to the baby's skull.

Each intervention has led to another as Anne Robison finds herself involved in a cascade of medical technology. With each intervention, the risk of complications increases. The scenarios of complications are numerous. Here are just a few:

1. Because the pitocin-induced contractions are strong and frequent, each contraction cuts off the baby's oxygen supply, leaving little time between contractions for the baby to fully recover. Fetal distress results, an indication for Cesarean section.
2. Being wired to the electronic fetal monitor makes it difficult for a laboring woman to walk or even readily change positions. She spends a lot of time nearly flat on her back in deference to the machine's needs. In that position, less blood and oxygen reach the fetus, whose heart rate and blood pressure drop. The result: a diagnosis of fetal distress followed by a Cesarean section.
3. Many people experience adverse reactions to anesthetics. It is not uncommon for anesthetics to slow labor, leading to an eventual diagnosis of "failure to progress." One possible result: Cesarean section. Other women find it impossible to push effectively during the later stage of labor since they cannot fully feel the contractions while anesthetized. One possible result: a forceps delivery.

As minor interventions lead to major ones, the risk of severe complications increases. Nearly 100 percent of Cesarean sections involve minor complications; approximately 50 percent result in more than minor complications, including infections, hemorrhage, surgically related problems that may compromise future childbearing, and, in rare instances, death. The risk of death, while small, is nonetheless twenty-six times greater with Cesarean section than with vaginal delivery (Cohen and Estner, 1983:26–33). Complications from such procedures as Cesarean section represent a large portion of the lawsuits against obstetrician-gynecologists.

Many procedures—diagnostic or therapeutic—developed for use in the intrapartum period may be beneficial when appropriately and discriminately used. However, it has become increasingly evident that when routinely used these same procedures may induce complications, some being the very ones sought to be prevented in the first place. Virtually no medical procedure or treatment is risk-free: each has its inherent risks. In addition, there is always the risk of faulty human performance in instituting them (e.g., inadequate sterilization, improper placement of a fetal scalp electrode, substandard care in performing surgery).

Ironically, the fear of being sued is leading doctors to perform more tests and diagnostic procedures than ever before. A major survey of the American College of Obstetricians and Gynecologists stated that obstetricians increased prenatal testing by as much as 76.2 percent and electronic fetal heart monitoring by 72.3 percent directly because of the fear of a lawsuit (American College of Obstetricians and Gynecologists, 1983). Yet the cascade of interventions that follows overtesting increases the incidence of medical complications, a certain percentage of which end up in court.

Medical practitioners find themselves in a vicious cycle involving fear of a lawsuit, increased rates of medical intervention, and increased complications that in turn increase the risk of lawsuit (see Figure 8.1).

DEFENSIVE MEDICINE

Defensive medicine is the practice of ordering a particular test or procedure to be performed not because it is medically necessary, but because the physician fears he or she may be liable to lawsuit unless such procedures or tests are done (Gilfix, 1984; Keeton, 1979). Keeton describes defensive medicine as departures by physicians from their usual practice or from following their best judgment in order to avoid the possibility

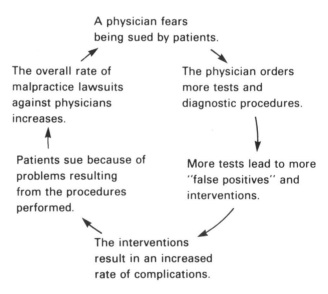

FIGURE 8.1.   The Vicious Cycle of Medical Malpractice and
Defensive Medicine

of a lawsuit and to provide what the physician believes will be a good legal defense if sued.

Ironically, departures from usual practice—such as ordering an unnecessary test or a test that cannot lead to a possible therapeutic benefit—may themselves be considered malpractice (Gilfix, 1984). At best, the patient is exposed to an unnecessary intrusion and at worst to risks that may cause injury. Fears of malpractice liability are real. However, the practice of defensive medicine is in most cases an irrational and destructive response to such fears.

As stated in Chapter 7, Marieskind reported that the threat of a malpractice suit if a Cesarean were not performed and the outcome was less than a perfect infant was the most frequent reason that physicians gave for the increase in their Cesarean section rate (Marieskind, 1979). The fear of liability was also one of the most frequently mentioned reasons for performing Cesareans in a survey of fifty prominent U.S. obstetricians done by O. Hunter Jones: "Almost all replies to the questionnaire mentioned malpractice suits. Undoubtedly this is a factor in the increased Cesarean section rate everywhere. In 1983 . . . no one would have ever thought the malpractice threat would become an indication for Cesarean section" (Gilfix, 1984).

In her study of Cesarean sections in the United States, Marieskind wrote: "When questioned, physicians freely agreed 'off the record' that fear of a suit prompted Cesareans and that this was commonly discussed among colleagues." Further, she cited a Chicago obstetrician who stated that the fear of malpractice suits rather than solid medical criteria is the reason for the rise in Cesarean sections. When contacted by Marieskind, the obstetrician agreed that he did not know of anyone who had been sued but that it was a commonly expressed concern. "Physicians said that a Cesarean is 'defensive medicine' and that even if the baby was 'less than perfect,' if a Cesarean had been done they were covered."

However, even in cases in which Cesarean section is considered the most that could be done, a physician will not necessarily be shielded from liability for a problematic outcome. Data suggest that malpractice claims are associated with the Cesarean surgery itself, rather than with failure to perform a Cesarean where it was believed that such intervention would improve the outcome. Reviews of some Cesarean-related lawsuits decided between 1970 and 1976 indicate that most of the suits were for malpractice associated with Cesarean surgery, rather than for failure to perform the procedure. Thus, physicians may not only not avoid liability simply because they performed a Cesarean section, they may actually risk liability.

This point is well illustrated by the findings of a National Association of Insurance Commissioners study of closed malpractice insurance claims from July 1975 to June 1976. Of the claims studied, 637 were against obstetrician-gynecologists, 61 of which (9.5 percent) were related to Cesarean section. The total indemnity paid for these suits was $2,596,564. In comparison, 50 claims (7.8 percent) were related to vaginal deliveries, with a total indemnity of $798,138—less than one-third the amount paid for Cesarean-related suits. A further 25 claims were related to newborn injuries, with a total indemnity of $1,700,001 (Marieskind, 1979:83–87).

WHAT IS MEDICAL MALPRACTICE?

In general, whether conduct is negligent is determined by whether it "falls below the standard established by law for the protection of others against unreasonable risk of harm" (Gilfix, 1984). The conduct of a defendant in an ordinary (i.e., not medical malpractice) negligence case is compared with that expected of a reasonable and prudent person under the same or similar circumstances. Evidence that the defendant acted in accordance with or failed to conform to a customary or fairly well-defined and regular practice among those in the same industry, profession, or craft is considered relevant but not definitive in establishing the standard of behavior under the circumstances (Gilfix, 1984). In other words, it has been recognized that an entire business or industry could be operating in an unnecessarily dangerous manner. A customary practice, then, may be judged by the courts to be unreasonable or negligent.

Unlike ordinary negligence standards, what is customarily done in a particular circumstance usually determines the standard of care regarding what constitutes medical negligence or malpractice. A medical professional is said by tort law to be obligated to possess that degree of learning and skill ordinarily possessed by reputable medical professionals in the same category, who practice in the same or similar locality and under the same or similar conditions or circumstances. The medical professional must, of course, not only possess but actually use that degree of skill and learning. This is usually referred to as practicing in accordance with the customary or community standard of care.

Similarly, the standard of care required on the part of a health care institution is generally the same care, skill, and diligence ordinarily used by similar health care institutions operating in the same or a similar locality and under similar circumstances. Note, however, that for most purposes, there is a national (rather than local) standard of care for specialists in medicine.

The judge or jury, then, generally needs to decide only whether the physician (or health care facility) conformed to that community or customary practice, not whether the practice itself was reasonable in light of an independent analysis of the risks and benefits. Thus, the medical profession basically sets its own standard of care.

In a medical malpractice suit, the plaintiff usually must prove all three of the following:

1. The medical professional accepted the plaintiff as a patient. The resulting relationship evokes the duty owed to the patient.
2. The medical professional breached his or her duty by way of substandard conduct—conduct that did not meet the medical malpractice standard of care, which, as described earlier, is generally established by what is customarily done. It is important to point out, however, that courts have sometimes departed from the rule; some have applied ordinary negligence "reasonableness" standards, and some have invoked duties on the part of the medical professional a) to keep abreast of new information and b) to use his or her best judgment (Gilfix, 1985).
3. The medical professional caused, by such conduct, harm and damage to the patient.

Thus, duty, breach of duty, causation, and actual damages must be established for the plaintiff to prevail in a medical malpractice lawsuit. Courts typically rely on evidence of what is commonly done in medicine. Therefore, since certain obstetrical procedures are now routine, hospitals and practitioners believe that they must conform to them. They believe this despite the fact that many of these procedures are not necessarily efficacious, nor have they been proved to be of benefit in many circumstances. Some may even prove harmful.

Although there are certain reasons why the medical community's typical behavior should set the standard of care, there are problems with the "customary practice" rule in medicine. One of the problems is that "medicine has an antiquated, largely unstructured, and inadequate system for evaluating the flood of new approaches that are fast being introduced" (Robin, 1984:86). Many of these become customary practice before such evaluation can be done.

Medical history unfortunately includes many examples of unreasonable customary practices. Among them is the well-known use of DES to prevent spontaneous abortion, which exposed the children of the treated women to the development of genital cancer at relatively early ages (Gilfix, 1985; Robin, 1984). Another customary practice, now discredited, has been the administration of high oxygen concentrations to premature infants without adequate precautions—which, in the 1950s, was the leading cause of blindness in children. A third example is radiation to the neck for "status thymaticus," in which normal infants who were considered to be at risk from an enlarged thymus gland were treated prophylactically with X-rays. Now it is known that the disease never existed, but "an unknown number developed cancer of the thyroid gland" (Robin, 1984:77).

The law generally deals inadequately with treatments and technologies in medicine that have become customary practice while effectively still experimental. Further testing and long-term use may later indicate their drawbacks, yet many such treatments or procedures continue unchecked, sometimes for a very long time.

In recent years, however, some courts have deviated from looking just at customary practice as a determinant of medical negligence. Their approaches have included applying ordinary negligence criteria. This involves 1) looking at the reasonableness of the conduct, with custom being only one factor in the possible determination of negligence; 2) applying the specific duty to keep abreast of new developments; and 3) the duty to use one's "best judgment."

THE MEDICAL MALPRACTICE INSURANCE
CRISIS OF THE MID-1980S

As a result of the medical liability crisis of the mid-1980s, medical centers and practitioners throughout the country have experienced skyrocketing insurance premiums and cancellation of policies. The crisis has not been limited to the field of medicine. It has also affected public transportation systems, bankers, fishermen, firefighters, architects, civil engineers, car dealers, child care providers, lawyers, and numerous other groups. The medical field, however, has been one of the hardest hit, both in terms of increases in the rate and size of suits brought and in terms of malpractice insurance premium increases. In 1975, 14,074 claims were brought against physicians for malpractice; by 1983 there were close to 40,000. In 1978 3.3 claims were brought against every 100 physicians, but by 1983 the rate had more than doubled, to 8 claims (American Medical Association, 1984).

By the mid-1980s, the insurance industry had responded with soaring premiums and canceled policies. Insurance companies claimed that these changes directly reflected their financial losses in the areas of medical malpractice. Between 1979 and 1983, insurance company losses climbed from $817 million to $2 billion (Koch, 1985). In general, the amount of claims paid rose 143 percent in the West and 142 percent in the Northeast from 1979 to 1983. In Florida during that period, the average claim payment by physician-owned insurance companies rose 712 percent to $106,712 (Cuniberti, 1983).

The actions taken by the St. Paul insurance company typify the insurance industry's reaction. In 1984 the company carried more medical malpractice policies than any other insurance company in the nation. It insured 57,000 physicians, 100,000 nurses, and 1,500 hospitals in forty-four states, accounting for a 15 percent share of the $2 billion in malpractice insurance premiums paid annually. As a result of the skyrocketing number of claims made, the company raised its rates 25 to 30 percent in 1984 alone. Further, it changed its system from "occurrence policies" to "claims made policies"—meaning that medical professionals had coverage only for medical occurrences during the period they paid premiums to a given company, rather than coverage for any claims brought during the premium period (including claims related to occurrences before the premium period).

Among medical specialties, obstetrics and neurosurgery have probably had the greatest malpractice problems. Obstetrician-gynecologists are sued twice as often as other doctors (Cuniberti, 1983). A report from the American College of Obstetricians and Gynecologists stated that as of 1983, two-thirds of its members had been sued for medical malpractice and one in five had been sued three or more times (American College of Obstetricians and Gynecologists, 1983).

For ob-gyns in California, annual premium rates in 1985 ranged from $25,000 to $80,000 (California Medical Association, 1985a). In a *San Francisco Chronicle* interview, Dr. Clarence S. Avery, president of the California Medical Association, stated, "A typical obstetrician delivers 110 babies a year, and a professional liability insurance premium of $33,000 a year costs that doctor $300 per baby" (*San Francisco Chronicle*, June 7, 1985).

Soaring malpractice premiums have affected midwives as well. In June 1985, the Philadelphia-based Mutual Fire, Marine and Inland Insurance Company, which provided malpractice policies for more than 1,400 of the 3,000 licensed midwives in the country, announced that it would not renew the policies. It had been providing each of these midwives with $1 million in coverage for less than $1,000 annually. The president of the company, Richard Guilfoyle, acknowledged that the decision not to renew the policies had nothing to do with the record of the midwives (Fresco, 1985). In fact, only 6 percent of midwives had ever been sued (American College of Nurse Midwives, 1985). A memo to its membership from the National Association of Childbearing Centers, concerning the problem with Mutual Fire, Marine and Inland Insurance Company, stated that the policies would not be renewed because of 1) rising claims in obstetrics, 2) higher awards, especially in obstetrics, 3) a lack of actuarial information, making it difficult to determine risk (especially since parents can sue up to ten to twenty-one years after a birth), and 4) a changing and unclear definition of negligence in a rapidly changing health care delivery system.

Since the cancellation of Mutual Fire, Marine and Inland's underwriting, the American College of Nurse Midwives tried to obtain malpractice coverage for the 1,400 members left without coverage. The organization's insurance broker was "turned down by every insurance company now writing insurance," reported Karen Ehrnman, the college coordinator. Because of the insurance industry's record losses of $4 billion in 1984, insurers and reinsurers had fled the market.

The New York Medical Malpractice Insurance Association responded by offering premiums for midwives practicing in New York that ranged from $24,000 to $72,000 per year depending on the circumstances of the midwife's practice (Fresco, 1985). Such a policy decision clearly ignored the fact that licensed midwives make an average of $22,000 to $25,000 a year. The association argued that midwives represent a very small premium pool, that it is hard to establish a valid claims record for midwives because some of them work at hospitals, some work at free-standing birth centers (FSBCs), and some work in private homes, and that the liability faced by midwives is potentially as costly as that faced by obstetricians (Fresco, 1985).

Such a decision reflects the insurance industry's general fear of anything related to obstetrics, and also a fear that in the future the rate of suits for less-than-perfect birth outcomes will continue to climb, affecting doctors, midwives, and birth centers alike.

THE EFFECT OF THE INSURANCE CRISIS ON CHILDBIRTH SERVICES

The malpractice insurance crisis has significantly altered the nature and availability of obstetrical care by physicians, midwives, and FSBCs.

Physicians

As a result of the malpractice crisis, obstetrician-gynecologists have raised their professional fees and stopped delivering babies. A 1985 survey by the American College of Obstetricians and Gynecologists found that by 1985, 12 percent of its fellows had given up obstetrics because of liability insurance problems, an additional 14 percent had decreased their deliveries, and 23 percent had decreased high-risk medical care (American College of Obstetricians and Gynecologists, 1985). An American Medical Association survey also found that 10 to 35 percent of obstetrician-gynecologists had discontinued their obstetrical practice (Koch, 1985). More than four out of five obstetricians (83 percent) indicated that they had raised their fees as a direct result of increased insurance premiums (American College of Obstetricians and Gynecologists, 1985).

The California Medical Association also surveyed its members in 1985: 29 percent of California obstetricians-gynecologists said that they had eliminated or curtailed the number of deliveries performed—16 percent had eliminated deliveries entirely, while an additional 13 percent had reduced the number. The situation for family physicians in California was even worse: Almost three out of five (58 percent) had either eliminated deliveries, reduced the number, or were thinking about doing so. Nearly one-third (32 percent) had already stopped delivering babies (California Medical Association, 1985d).

Midwives

The availability of obstetrical care by nurse midwives has also been threatened by the insurance crisis. Between July 1984 and July 1985, approximately 1,400 of the nation's 3,000 nurse midwives had their malpractice insurance coverage canceled, as stated before. As a result, up to 800 nurse midwives faced immediate closure of their practices. Although other insurance was available, there was a crisis in affordability. During the seventies, midwives paid $38 per year in malpractice premiums. By 1985 this had risen to an average of $1,000 per year (American College of Nurse Midwives, 1985). By 1986, when insurance was no longer widely available, the cost had skyrocketed in the aforementioned New York case. Essentially, this meant that midwives could no longer afford insurance.

Even though nurse midwives deliver only 2 percent of the nation's obstetrical care, 50 percent of their services go to the poor (Koch, 1985). Between rising fees (to compensate for increased premiums) and closing practices, the poor once again are the ones who have lost the most, in terms of their access to medical care.

Free-Standing Birth Centers

The withdrawal of Mutual Fire, Marine and Inland's coverage also affected FSBCs. In 1985 the company underwrote medical malpractice insurance for at least one-third of the FSBCs in the United States. As a result of the cancellation of malpractice policies, seven birth centers immediately closed their doors (Wells, 1985). Countless others faced eventual closure.

FSBCs traditionally have charged less than half what acute-care hospitals charge for labor and delivery services (Ernst, 1985). They have been affected in several ways. For example, the malpractice crisis has crippled volunteerism, especially by discouraging people from serving on boards of directors where, without malpractice insurance, they feel legally exposed. Birth centers are also adversely affected by the insurance crisis in that it promotes the practice of defensive medicine, even in low-risk cases. Such a practice means that a certain percentage of women unnecessarily are excluded from low-risk birth settings.

Finally, FSBCs, like physicians and nurse midwives, have been forced to increase their fees. When insurance is available, it is more expensive. For an increasing number of FSBCs, however, insurance is no longer available at any price. These centers have had to make the painful choice either to practice without insurance or to close.

Although FSBCs serve fewer than one-half of 1 percent of American women annually (National Association of Childbearing Centers, 1985), they represent an important trend in obstetrical care—a trend toward the appropriate use of technology in childbirth and toward women and their families having a voice in the medical management of the birth of their children. FSBCs are a rapidly growing alternative in the United States. Yet at the very time this alternative is solidifying, it is being threatened by the insurance industry crisis.

Summary

In summary, family physicians, obstetrician-gynecologists, midwives, and FSBCs—in short, nearly all childbirth services—have been crippled by the malpractice insurance crisis. Family physicians, nurse midwives, and birth centers traditionally have offered high-quality obstetrical care at affordable prices to women with low-risk pregnancies from all socioeconomic groups. Ironically, family physicians, nurse-midwives, and FSBCs—the groups with the lowest rate of obstetrical claims and suits brought against them—run the highest risk of having to close their practices because they are least able to afford the increased costs. As they are forced to go out of business, women will lose not only cost-effective health care delivery systems but important childbirth options as well.

Various factors have contributed to the liability insurance crisis of the mid-1980s. The insurance industry has cried out for tort reform—that is, major revisions in the laws that dictate who can sue, for how much money, and during what period of time following a medical incident. Lawyers who prosecute malpractice cases, however, claim that only a small percentage of people injured by medical malpractice actually sue their doctors. Their assertion has been that impaired doctors and those whose procedures repeatedly result in serious complications are too readily allowed to continue to practice medicine.

A third factor involves the expectations of patients regarding medical care. A task force of the American Medical Association found that a contributing factor to the malpractice insurance crisis is the public's unrealistic expectation of a perfect medical outcome 100 percent of the time (American Medical Association, 1985). The International Childbirth Education Association also stated that the problem has been exacerbated by the public's expectation of a perfect baby and a perfect outcome—an expectation that the association maintains is encouraged by the medical profession (International Childbirth Education Association, 1984).

Yet another factor is the current practice within the insurance industry to settle cases out of court that involve no fault of the doctor but that involve a particularly sad outcome. Insurance company lawyers may be afraid of judges or juries who might base their decisions on sympathy for the plaintiffs, or they may view a case as more expensive to fight than to settle. The result, however, is an increase in the number of suits brought that involve maloccurrence but not malpractice. In addition, medical care providers are increasingly frustrated that they are being forced by insurance companies to settle out of court for cases they feel involve no real medical malpractice. For their reputation's sake, they want their day in court.

Certainly, one of the major factors contributing to the malpractice insurance crisis is that there is currently no other means by which people who have experienced an unfortunate medical outcome can receive any kind of financial assistance for further medical expenses. The only way to receive assistance is to prove the doctor wrong in court. Such a system is so expensive that only twenty-eight cents of every insurance premium dollar is paid to the injured patient (*New York Times*, February 4, 1985).

In summary, the current medical malpractice insurance crisis is a manifestation of the fact that our medical, legal, and insurance systems no longer work well together. The existing set of systems encourages the practice of defensive medicine. Not only is this hazardous to the patients involved, but it is also exacerbating the insurance problem rather than reducing it. Furthermore, defensive medicine substantially increases the general cost of medical care. As nervous physicians turn away high-risk patients and order more tests than are medically necessary just to ward off a charge of negligence, patients not only experience less access to quality medical care and the discomfort and hazards of extra procedures; they also face inflated medical bills.

The American Medical Association's Committee on Professional Liability estimated that defensive medicine may increase the nation's medical bill by $15.1 billion per year. But a recent Harvard University study estimated that such defensive practices could add up to $42 billion per year to America's health care costs (Marchasin, 1985). Marchasin commented, "Unfortunately, it is the patients, the government and the local businesses that purchase insurance for their employees that ultimately foot the bill for [defensive medicine], and it is all for naught—an expense that has nothing to do with medical care."

Finally, sociological studies of who sues and who does not touch repeatedly on the theme of good doctor-patient relations. As our medical system becomes larger and more technologically complex, it is easy (especially for large medical institutions) to lose sight of the person who is the patient. One reason that lawsuits against birth centers and midwives are so few and so small in amount may be because birth centers and midwives provide high-quality, one-to-one medical care, in which the patient has a great deal of control over the medical management of her labor and delivery. She and her care provider thoroughly discuss medical options as labor progresses. Ironically, the current malpractice insurance crisis is having its strongest negative impact on the very care providers and services demonstrating the least real vulnerability to large lawsuits and who are offering some of the best care to low-risk patients, at a low cost.

RECOMMENDATIONS

The liability insurance crisis essentially is a manifestation of a much broader set of problems involving 1) the modern American legal system, 2) our predominant philosophy and practice with regard to health care delivery and the role of doctor, patient, and medical institution, and 3) the manner in which the insurance industry sets policies that dramatically affect the ability of large segments of society to offer valued social services. Any real solution to the crisis will be one that addresses all of these issues in depth.

The solution also must place women at the center of their own childbirth experience. Given that the care providers who are the least sued are those who act as women's partners in the decision-making process, it is logical to assume that the policies and practices that will have the greatest impact on reducing lawsuits will be those that increase women's voice.

We are now experiencing a vicious cycle of fear of lawsuit, defensive medicine, increased complications, and increased lawsuit rates. To transform this negative cycle into an upward spiral of fewer suits and greater satisfaction with obstetrical care requires, first, that women be given the primary voice in decisions regarding the birth of their children. We cannot underestimate the radical departure that this represents from trends in current obstetrical practice. We are advocating that women be the decision makers, fully informed by their care providers, rather than having doctors make decisions for them and about them and their children.

Why should this be the case? At present, a powerful group (the obstetrical establishment)—in direct response to the threat to their livelihood, their reputation, and their sense of self-esteem—is acting to maintain control as a matter of self-preservation. The real solution requires just the reverse: rather than holding onto power, that power must be freely shared with patients. With shared power comes shared responsibility; with shared responsibility comes a reduced impetus to sue. As we have seen, one reason that people turn to the legal system is because they have no voice elsewhere. We are not suggesting that this is the only step needed in order to reach a solution, but it is a necessary first step, without which any other solution will not be fully effective.

It is also necessary that any solution address the differences existing between malpractice cases and cases of medical maloccurrence. To solve the problem of a negative medical outcome in which no one is at fault, we need an insurance system similar, for example, to worker's compensation. Such a system would enable people who have experienced a medical maloccurrence involving thousands (or hundreds of thousands) of dollars to receive assistance. With the current system, the only way to receive such assistance is to prosecute one's doctor in court.

Finally, true reform will require replacing a power dynamic that incorporates aspects of fear and distrust with a new dynamic involving trust and shared power. Such a basic paradigmatic shift will make it possible for other reforms to be negotiated.

REFERENCES

American College of Nurse Midwives. *Nurse-Midwives and the Malpractice Crisis*, Fact Sheet. Washington, D.C.: ACNM, October 1, 1985.

American College of Obstetricians and Gynecologists. *Professional Liability Insurance and Its Effect: Report of a Survey of ACOG's Membership*. Prepared by Needham, Porter, Novelli, Washington, D.C.: ACOG, November 1985.

_____. *Professional Liability Insurance and Its Effects: Report of a Survey of ACOG's Membership*. Prepared by Porter, Novelli, and Associates, Washington, D.C.: ACOG, August 31, 1983.

American Medical Association. *Professional Liability in the 80's, Report 1*. AMA Special Task Force Report on Professional Liability and Insurance. Chicago: AMA, October 1984.

_____. *Professional Liability in the 80's, Report 3*. Special Task Force Report on Professional Liability and Insurance. Chicago: AMA, March 1985.

California Medical Association. *Professional Liability Coverage Program for Physicians in California*, San Francisco: CMA, first quarter 1985.

———. "Arbitration in Medical Professional Liability." *Socioeconomic Report* 25 (January/February 1985).

———. "Professional Liability Issues in Obstetrical Practice," *Socioeconomic Report* 25 (July/August 1985).

———. "Professional Liability Issues in Obstetrical Practice, Part 2." *Socioeconomic Report* 25 (October/November 1985).

Cohen, N. W., and Estner, L. J. *Silent Knife: Caesarean Prevention and Vaginal Birth after Caesarean*. South Hadley, Mass.: Bergin and Garvey, 1983.

Cuniberti, B. "Doctors Reel under Lawsuit Threat." *Los Angeles Times*, September 13, 1983.

Ernst, E. K. M. "Alternative Birth Centers: The National Perspective." Paper presented to The National Perinatal Association, Orlando, Florida, November 1985.

Fresco, R. "Midwives Face Insurance Crunch." *Newsday*, August 19, 1985.

Gilfix, Myra Gerson. "EFM, Informed Consent and Malpractice." *ICEA News* (August 1985).

———. "Electronic Fetal Monitoring: Physician Liability and Informed Consent." *American Journal of Law and Medicine* 10 (Spring 1984).

International Childbirth Education Association. "Malpractice Issues in Obstetrics." Minneapolis: ICEA, August 15, 1984.

Keeton, M. "Medical Negligence—The Standard of Care." *Texas Tech Law Review* 10 (1979).

Koch, S. "Malpractice Situation Once Again at Crisis Proportions." *OB.Gyn. News* (March 1-14, 1985).

Marchasin, S. "The New Crisis in Malpractice—If You Liked It in 1975, You'll Love It Now." *Sacramento Bee*, February 3, 1985.

Marieskind, Helen I. *An Evaluation of Cesarean Section in the United States*. Washington, D.C.: U.S. Department of Health, Education and Welfare, 1979.

National Association of Childbearing Centers. *NACC News* (Fall 1985).

New York Times. "Again, the Malpractice Crunch." February 4, 1985.

Robin, E. "Matters of Life and Death: Risks vs. Benefits of Medical Care." *The Portable Stanford*. Stanford, Calif.: Stanford Alumni Association, 1984.

San Francisco Chronicle. "Fewer Doctors Are Willing to Deliver Babies." June 7, 1985.

Wells, P. "National Malpractice Crisis Threatens Birth Alternatives." *Special Delivery* 2 (Fall 1985).

PART III
Woman-Centered Birth

Has the American medical system failed women? Failed would be too strong a word. Nevertheless, for thousands of years childbirth—an experience that resonates deeply in female culture and the female psyche—was woman centered. Only within the last seven decades has birth been redefined, relocated, and placed within a medical model, a professional paradigm that dictates specific routines and rules for participation. Many women can still remember when childbirth was a woman-centered event.

The medicalized birth—as a cultural production—is still in its infancy. It is swayed by external pressures: legal, political, and cultural. It has undergone, and is undergoing, many changes. Since the early congealing of the medical model, women have fought for reforms ranging from the right to have access to anesthesia in the early 1900s to the right to unmedicated birth in the 1960s. The natural childbirth movement, which emerged in the 1950s, struggled for the right to nonroutine, drug-free birth, freedom of birth position, husbands in the delivery room, along with the mother's right to keep the baby with her after the birth.

Two distinct and contradictory streams in the cultural production of American birth emerged: 1) the extreme

213

mechanization of birth by the scientific medical profession and 2) the consumer movement for the humanization of birth, which in practice typically involves "low technology" approaches as well as greater consumer control.

In 1964 the medical profession made its first "compromise" with the advent of an in-hospital "alternative birth center" (ABC) in Connecticut. While providing emergency equipment and requiring strictly enforced eligibility for use, this ABC offered women homelike furnishings; labor, birth, and recovery in the same room; and one-to-one nursing care. Relatives and friends could be present, and parents were not separated from their infants. Women and their babies were eligible for early discharge.

In 1968 the American College of Obstetricians and Gynecologists (ACOG), the Nurses Association of ACOG, the American Association of Pediatricians, and the American Nurses Association all made public statements endorsing ABCs. Since then, the growth of these "more humane" units has been rapid. In 1975 three of these units existed in California. There were seventy in 1979, and, at present, the number is still growing (May and DiTolla, 1982).

Another, more radical, component of this movement to humanize birth practices has been the advent of the free-standing birth center (FSBC). In 1975 there were four in the United States. By 1981 there were more than 150 in twenty-eight states (Eakins, 1984). Although FSBCs currently do fewer than one-half of 1 percent of American births, they represent an important philosophical trend and their numbers are increasing dramatically. These centers exist outside hospitals and are generally midwife or consumer owned and operated. The philosophy they espouse involves offering women control over their birth experiences in a medically safe environment. During a tour of fourteen FSBCs in 1979, Ruth Watson Lubic, president of the National Association of Childbearing Centers, found that the work of each center represented a total commitment by the pioneers who struggled to serve the childbearing parents making the decision not to give birth in the acute care setting of the hospital.

The primary thrust of these centers is toward placing decision-making power in the hands of the birthing woman. She is conceptualized not as sick, but rather as capable of making decisions. Medical specialists and equipment are reconceptualized as resources rather than as main actors or central components in the birth room. The birth room itself is arranged to meet women's needs. FSBCs allow for the introduction of ritual—other than the ritual of hospital routines—into birth, while downplaying the presence of technical devices. The key element in this movement is that in taking birth out of the standard medical system, birth is redefined as natural and normal. The movement toward FSBC birth is directed toward allowing women to fully experience the birth of their children as the desired rite of passage in a place in which emergency care is available. Thus, proponents of FSBCs claim that they represent the best of both worlds: they are woman centered and medically safe.

Nevertheless, FSBCs refer all high-risk births to hospitals, and very strict screening procedures are used. If complications arise, the woman will be transferred out. Some social commentators claim the ABCs and FSBCs, while they are more woman centered than the hospital delivery room, still leave ultimate decision-making power in the hands of medical professionals. Even in FSBCs, it is argued, women still deliver on foreign ground. They are still at the mercy of medical professionals who remain in control of the situation. Birth, even in a normal situation, is still defined as pathogenic. The balance of power, these critics would say, has not changed. ABCs and FSBCs have been criticized as coopting the alternative birth movement without addressing the deeper problem of medicalized birth—the question of power (Rothman, 1981; May and DiTolla, 1982). Nonetheless, through espousing a philosophy that places women more toward the center of their own experience, these units have significantly influenced consumers who have then demanded a more "humane" experience in the hospital.

Home birth is, by definition, woman-centered birth. It takes place on the woman's own territory, and she makes the decisions about who will attend her, what she will eat, what she will wear, and so on. There has been a small but significant increase in the number of home births in the past decade, though only about 2 percent of the nation's births currently occur in the home.

In Chapter 9, Pamela S. Eakins shows how out-of-hospital

birth decreased from 1940 to 1970 and then began to increase. In asking why, she finds that women choosing to deliver outside the hospital are indeed reacting negatively to medicalized birth. These women want to avoid the visual, technical, and philosophical environment of the hospital, as well as the cost. They define pregnancy as "a part of everyday life" and they do not want to become patients—"pawns in the medical system."

In Chapter 10, Regi L. Teasley examines contemporary midwifery. She contrasts professional and lay midwives and outlines their struggle to attain an occupational niche that challenges physicians' claims to a monopoly over expectations. In order to compete, they, like obstetricians in the nineteenth century, have taken up a strategy of professionalization: producing and articulating new ideologies and tailoring them to fit social circumstances. Teasley examines how the new world view of contemporary midwives—based on an ideology of informed choice, personal autonomy, and responsibility for parturient women—has been culturally produced in Vermont.

The ancient art of midwifery is more easily observable in the traditional black lay midwives of the Southern United States. In Chapter 11, Linda Janet Holmes shows how these midwives have been revered as key community members, responsible for sustaining tradition and cultural continuity within the childbirth experience. In Southern lay midwifery, traditional customs, such as sprinkling the placenta with a handful of salt and guarding the birth fire, are preserved. These rituals are followed to elevate the birth experience and preserve the spiritual nature of birth. Such midwifery is woman centered, emphasizing the supporting role of the midwife.

But lay midwives, unlike the midwives of Vermont, are disappearing. They face a formidable medical superstructure, and, since they lack formal organization, legal protection, and leverage, they cannot counter the high-powered antimidwife campaigns of the medical profession.

In Chapter 12, Deborah LeVeen states that the readmission, albeit cautious, of midwives into medicalized birth can be viewed as a major victory by feminists, childbirth advocates and other childbirth reformers. Yet, she states, institutionalizing the new nurse midwifery is problematic at best. What "excites" nurse midwives is supporting and empowering women by providing a better understanding of health needs and the birth process. But, while midwifery care centers around women's needs and is safe and humane, it is time-intensive and therefore costly from the point of view of hospitals, requiring more staff time per patient, more costs per unit of service, and more costs relative to revenue generated.

Midwives, states LeVeen, have been readmitted to the hospital system, but on terms that are not wholly compatible with the needs of midwifery care. How have midwives responded to this dilemma? In California, one group of midwives—those practicing at Highland General Hospital—unionized. This allowed midwives to claim, rather than be allowed, certain rights. It increased the midwives' power. But it did not eliminate the need for cooperation. Nonetheless, the experience of unionization at Highland, while unsuccessful on some levels, demonstrates the potential impact of a direct conflict strategy.

Part III outlines several strategies toward organizing childbirth around women. Some consumers have chosen to give birth at home and in FSBCs. Midwives have professionalized, striven to maintain traditional practices and customs, and unionized. In all of these areas, organization, on the part of consumers and providers, is the key to preserving and solidifying alternative choices.

REFERENCES

Eakins, Pamela S. "The Rise of the Free Standing Birth Center: Principles and Practice." *Women and Health* 9(1984):49-64.
May, K., and DiTolla, K. "Alternative Birthing Centers: Here Today, Where Tomorrow?" Paper presented at the UCSF Founders Day of the 2nd Century Conference, San Francisco, January 1982.
Rothman, Barbara Katz. "Awake and Aware, or False Consciousness: The Cooptation of Childbirth Reform in America." In *Childbirth: Alternatives to Medical Control*, edited by Shelly Romalis. Austin: University of Texas Press, 1981.

9

Out-of-Hospital Birth

PAMELA S. EAKINS

In 1940 a small majority of births in the United States occurred in hospitals, but by 1970 virtually all deliveries took
place in hospitals. Nonetheless, by 1975 out-of-hospital birth
was on the increase, and such deliveries had risen to a level of
about 1 percent of all births (Pearse, 1982). Alabama, Alaska,
California, Idaho, New Mexico, Oregon, Texas, and Washington state all had 2 percent or greater out-of-hospital births in
1977, 1978, or 1979.

In the late 1970s, the Department of Vital Statistics at the
National Center for Health Statistics noted that births attended by midwives—the bulk of out-of-hospital births—were
becoming prevalent enough to record. During the first year the
midwife-attended births were officially counted (1979), they
constituted .3 percent of the total number of U.S. births. By
1981, the latest year for which national statistics were available at the time of this writing, midwife-attended births had
increased to .35 percent.

In Oregon, for example, the out-of-hospital birth rate
doubled between 1970 and 1975, doubled again by 1977, and
by 1981 had increased another 16 percent. By 1982 the out-of-

hospital birth rate in Oregon was approximately 4.5 percent, the highest rate in the United States (Clarke and Bennetts, 1983). In California, where the total number of births remained fairly stable throughout the 1970s, increasing only 1 percent from 1970 to 1977, the number of births that occurred outside hospitals jumped threefold (see Table 9.1). These figures suggest that, at least in some states, out-of-hospital birth is a growing and complex phenomenon.

Also in the 1970s, out-of-hospital birth centers were mushrooming throughout the United States. An example is the free-standing birth center (FSBC), also called a birth center or birth home, which is a home environment adapted to a short-stay, ambulatory facility for childbirth (Cooperative Birth Center Network News, 1981). Midwife or consumer owned, the FSBC is seen as an alternative to both the home and the hospital, particularly in that it operates independently of the hospital in the official, financial, and physical sense and that it promotes "natural" childbirth, although all births at FSBCs are attended by physicians or nurse-midwives and operate with hospital backup for emergency situations (see Bean, 1975; Bennetts and Lubic, 1982; DeJong, et al., 1979; Eakins, 1984; Faison et al., 1979; Lubic, 1975 and 1982; Reinke, 1982; Shy et al., 1980). In 1972, Texas had the only FSBC known to

TABLE 9.1. Out-of-Hospital Births in California, 1970–1981

Year	Total	Out-of-Hospital	
		No.	*%*
1970	360,797	1,802	.50
1971	329,819	2,038	.62
1972	306,561	2,192	.72
1973	298,079	2,304	.77
1974	312,022	2,847	.91
1975	317,599	3,516	1.11
1976	332,232	4,628	1.39
1977	347,431	4,974	1.43
1978	356,203	5,625	1.58
1979	379,232	5,366	1.41
1980	403,007	5,175	1.28
1981	420,907	5,321	1.26

be operating in the United States. By 1975 there were four more, in California, New Mexico, New York, and Oregon, and at present there are well more than 100 operating in the country (Eakins, 1984). In California alone, there are at least twenty such centers.[1]

Although out-of-hospital births still represent only a small portion of American births, their rapid increase in both numbers and form is significant. The resurgence of out-of-hospital birth raises several questions:

1. Who is most likely to give birth out of the hospital?
2. What is the impetus behind out-of-hospital delivery?
3. What is the comparative outcome of in- and out-of-hospital births?

This chapter examines these questions in detail by providing a case study of out-of-hospital births in two adjacent counties in the San Francisco Bay Area, where the trends paralleled those in California at large (see Table 9.2).

METHODS

Over a three-year period in the early 1980s, seventy-six women in a two-county area south of San Francisco—Santa Clara and San Mateo counties—were interviewed retrospectively about their out-of-hospital births, which had taken place anywhere from four days to two years before the interview. They were asked about how they had selected their birth site and birth attendants, their obstetrical history, their birth experience, and the outcome of the delivery.

Thirty-eight of these women had planned a home delivery. The remaining half had intended to deliver in an FSBC. The birth center mothers were selected at random by means of the birth log (the central listing of cases) of one of the FSBCs. Only one woman who was contacted through the FSBC declined to participate, stating that she was too busy with her four-week-old baby.

The women who gave birth at home were more difficult to find. Two midwives supplied complete lists of all the women

---

[1]For more information on FSBCs in California, write to Project on Free Standing Birth Centers, School of Public Health, UCLA, Los Angeles, CA 90024.

TABLE 9.2. Out-of-Hospital Births in the San Francisco Bay Area, 1974–1981

Year	Total	Out-of-Hospital	
		No.	%
1974	62,696	485	.77
1975	58,079	557	.96
1976	65,333	828	1.27
1977	68,038	927	1.36
1978	69,664	1,052	1.51
1979	73,359	1,057	1.44
1980	77,176	991	1.28
1981	76,183	1,212	1.59

they had assisted in childbirth, from which a random sample of recent births was extracted. Other midwives provided partial lists of clients they had served. A total of forty home-birth mothers initially were contacted. One woman declined to participate because of lack of time, another because her husband disapproved. Overall, the women demonstrated a great willingness to share their experiences.

In all, the home-birth mothers had been attended by fourteen different midwives, both certified and lay, and two physicians. Thus, the women reflected a diversity of personal birth experiences, both positive and negative, and numerous styles of medical practice.

THE DATA

The Sample

What kind of woman chooses to deliver away from the security of the hospital? Abby Michaelson[2] is one example: age twenty-three, part-time electrical engineer, married to Jim, a project manager for an electronics company. Cassandra Hopkins, at age thirty-four a temporarily unemployed mental health worker, is another example and yet another is Libby Barnes, a twenty-four-year-old secretary married to Henry, a supervisor.

[2]All names have been changed to protect confidentiality.

Seventy-one (93 percent) of the women were legally married, four had permanent live-in relationships, and one had been separated from her husband since the birth of her baby. They ranged in age from nineteen to forty-two with an average age of thirty-one. Forty-one women (54 percent) had given birth to their first baby. Women selecting the birth center, with an average age of thirty, were somewhat older than the home-birth mothers, who had an average age of twenty-eight (see Table 9.3). Thirty-nine of the birth center mothers were Caucasian, and one was Hispanic. Thirty-four of the home-birth mothers were Caucasian, four were Hispanic, and one was black.

Twenty-one (28 percent) of the mothers identified themselves as homemakers. The remaining fifty-five (72 percent) held jobs outside the home. Their occupations varied from secretary to restaurant owner to dressmaker to assembler. The most striking occupational category, however, was health worker. Of the seventy-six women in the study, thirteen (17 percent) were employed in the health industry as nurses and other hospital workers, where they came into direct contact with patients. About 8 percent of the total work force of women is employed in the health field. Therefore, the number of women in this study who worked in health care was remarkably high, more than twice as high as in the general population.

Home-birth mothers had completed an average of fifteen years of education, just under a four-year college degree, and had an average annual family income of $20,000–24,999. Birth center mothers had an average of more than sixteen years of schooling, which meant, in general, a master's degree. Their average annual family income was $35,000–39,999. Clearly, there was a socioeconomic gap between the two groups.

TABLE 9.3. Some Characteristics of Home-Birth and Birth Center Mothers

	Age		Years of School		Annual Income	
Mothers	*Average*	*Range*	*Average*	*Range*	*Average*	*Range*
Home-birth mothers	28.7	19–41	15	10–20	$20–24,999	<$10–>$50,000
Birth center mothers	31.1	23–42	16.3	11–20	$35–39,999	<$10–>$50,000

TABLE 9.4. Reasons for Selecting an Out-of-Hospital Birth Site

Primary Reason Given	Birth Center Mothers		Home-Birth Mothers		Total	
	No.	*%*	*No.*	*%*	*No.*	*%*
"Not a hospital"	25	66	25	66	50	66
"Seemed right"	7	18	7	18	14	18
"Better than home"	5	13	—*	—*	5	7
"Cost"	1	3	6	16	7	9

*Not applicable.

Initial Attraction to Out-of-Hospital Birth
Philosophical Preference

Women selecting to give birth outside a hospital were not as interested in maintaining the comforts of home as they were in avoiding the "stark and regimented" hospital environment.[3] Fully two-thirds of the women delivering at home and two-thirds of the women delivering at the FSBC chose to deliver outside a hospital primarily because the location "was not a hospital" (see Table 9.4).

Seventy of the women interviewed (92 percent) had been patients themselves or spent time in a hospital during the illness of an immediate family member. Of these, fifty-two (68 percent) came away from the hospital with a negative impression. The hospital was seen as "knife-happy, filling beds and quotas," "noisy," "rigid," "bureaucratic," "white, boring and unfeeling," "dirty," "dangerous," "full of microbes," "badly managed," and "associated with pain and death."

Many of these women had experienced previous births in hospitals. Two mentioned feeling as if they were "on an assembly line." One woman described her experience as like "a cow going to slaughter." Another felt like an "inmate."

Most of the women saw themselves as "at war" with hospital staff who "treat you like you're a nonresponsive thing" and who were perceived as "cold," "insensitive," "impersonal," "masked and gloved," "tired," "overworked," and "su-

---

[3]Anything appearing in quotes without a citation is a direct quote from the interviews.

perior acting" ("it's an upstream struggle if you don't agree"). Generally, hospitals were viewed as political institutions motived by profit and not for patients, institutions that "serve the purposes of those who created them," institutions in which "the human element is missing." Only eight women (11 percent) had had a positive experience in the hospital.

Overall, these mothers asserted that hospitals were unsafe and uncaring environments for newborn babies. They viewed the hospital atmosphere as unconducive to relaxation, and the medications, so heavily relied on in the hospital setting, as potentially harmful. The women worried about the increasing practice of defensive medicine, and the first major recurrent theme that emerged in their rationale for selecting an out-of-hospital birth site was "My baby may be hurt if I give birth in the hospital."

The second recurring theme was that pregnancy was not a disease. To these women, who were experiencing healthy, uncomplicated pregnancies, the hospital environment was the antithesis of what they had come to expect in their childbirth education classes. The women in this sample, all of whom had taken birth preparation classes, generally had internalized the idea that the pregnant state is not a disease requiring medical procedures or intervention on a routine basis. As might be expected, multiparas who had given birth in a hospital were particularly vocal about the negative aspects of institutional procedures and protocols. College-educated Jane Atherton, age twenty-nine and bearing her second child, typified the experience of many:

> I had one baby in the hospital and I paid them $200 a day to yell at me. [I received no] continuity of care in the hospital. You may have more than one nurse. Even if you're there only a short time you may have two or three different nurses checking on you. It really doesn't help you relax and feel more comfortable. More mistakes can happen if there are too many cooks stirring the soup. . . . You're more likely to have interference if you're in the hospital and pick up infection.

Julia Greene, age thirty-four, with a masters degree and a family income of over $50,000, said the following about her first birth in a hospital: "[The hospital] had 400 patients a month giving birth, so we were not pampered. [My roommate] turned on the television set.... The door was always open. There was no sleep to be had. The impression was noise and chaos."

The Problem with Hospitals

Jane Atherton and Julia Greene each knew at the outset of their second pregnancy that they would give birth in an "alternative" setting. Thirty-two of the women (42 percent), had initially assumed without question that their babies would be born in a hospital. Of these, twenty-three (72 percent) toured the labor and delivery section of a hospital. Fifteen (65 percent) came away from the introductory tour with a negative or extremely negative impression. Cited as sources of concern were: the visual environment ("fluorescent lighting, linoleum floors, the whole combination of white and metal and hard surfaces," "terrible colors," "dull and unimaginative"); the technical environment ("This is what bothered me most, that thing that you put up your uterus with that little—put in the top of the head—the fetal heart monitor—that was the main thing"); the hierarchical structure ("People, as patients, lose control over what's happening to them"); the philosophy ("My own personal beliefs about what sickness is—a lot of it is the mind, and, at some level, sickness is an effort of the body to heal itself—I would really feel uncomfortable with a person who felt like the body was something he needed to fix up. That didn't have anything to do with my birth"); and the cost.

Amy Blum, experiencing her first pregnancy, summarized her feelings this way:

There was a little film and introductory talk by the O.B. nurse. It was a most insensitive film, very bloody and not very gentle. It seemed like a business assembly line. The film also included devices which I didn't want to be involved with, the internal fetal monitor, forceps, all of the paraphernalia in the delivery room. And we went from that unsettling experience right out to the intensive care unit for the preemies which was psychologically just about the worst thing the tour could have done for me. I came away feeling that if I had a sick child, if I gave birth to a sick child, that would be the place I would want to be, the hospital, but if I didn't give birth to a sick child, if it was a normal pregnancy and normal delivery, that was the last place I wanted to be. Abnormality seemed to be the main course of their business rather than the normal.... It felt consistent with my idea that you go to the hospital when you're sick.

The Fear of Becoming a Patient

Being in the hospital implied becoming a patient. Becoming a patient meant taking on a dependent role wherein the ability to make decisions was turned over to someone else. Not being able to make decisions meant relinquishing control. (Said one woman: "I certainly didn't want to be like a pawn in the medical system. I didn't want to be a patient at a hospital.") It was feared that the loss of decision-making power, in tandem with the heightened sense of "having to monitor the situation" (because of its unfamiliarity), would result in a loss of intellectual, emotional, and physical control. Many of these women feared being "caged in." It was felt that distraction, ensuing from preoccupation with the hospital routine, might cause tension, which could, in turn, lead to unnecessary intervention. As attorney Alana Bernard, having her first baby at age thirty-five, stated:

Frankly, I was afraid I couldn't relax, that there would be too much going on, and that I would be so distracted that I would experience the pain more and therefore end up having a medicated birth. I wanted my birth experience to be positive and loving and I just didn't see how I could do that in a hospital setting.

The general consensus was that an uncomplicated pregnancy did not require hospitalization. The women saw little need for most of the paraphernalia they observed while touring the hospitals. For all practical purposes, most of these women rejected the institutionalized hospital system in favor of attaining personal control.

Financial Incentives

The women who chose to give birth at the FSBC did not, by and large, consider home birth. Only five of the FSBC mothers (13 percent) seriously considered home birth, but ultimately lacked either confidence, insurance, or both. These women worried that they would not have adequate medical backup at home. Further, none of the birth center mothers had insurance to cover a home birth. Thirty-one FSBC mothers (82 percent), however, were covered for birth at the birth center. Many women stated that even if their insurance had not covered it, they would have chosen the birth center anyway. As one remarked:

> At the time we decided to go with the birth center, we questioned my insurance company and they said they would not pay for it. So we had a choice of going ahead and choosing the kind of birth we were going to have and where we were going to have it or letting an outside agency, because of monetary reasons, choose for us what we could or could not do.

Only one woman chose the birth center primarily for financial reasons. This woman had insurance that would have covered a hospital birth, but the hospital required the money in advance, and she was unable to meet the expense. Use of the birth center facility for delivery cost about $900, excluding physician or midwife fees, which were $500 and $1,200 for prenatal care, delivery, and postnatal care. This compared with about $2,000 for use of local hospital facilities for delivery alone, with the physician's fees also paid separately. The cost of using the birth center was about half that of the hospital.

Thus, the ability to purchase the desired alternative was clearly not a problem for the birth center mothers, who were well above average in income and education. In an area of the country in which the average income is about $29,000 for a family of four, the FSBC mothers' incomes averaged $35,000–39,999. The FSBC mothers' selection of the birth center clearly represented a conscious choice.

In general, the women choosing home delivery cited the same reasons for choosing out-of-hospital birth as the birth center mothers, although twenty of the home-birth mothers (53 percent) also cited the cost of hospital birth as a critical variable in their decision to give birth at home.

With regard to ability to pay, the home-birth mothers can

be divided into three groups. The first group, consisting of nine women (24 percent), was completely covered by insurance for birth at home with a certified midwife or obstetrician and would have been completely covered for birth in the hospital. Thus, their selection of the home environment represented a preference as opposed to a necessity. The average family income of this group was $25,000–$30,000 annually. Their home births cost an average of $880, which included complete midwifery services (prenatal, delivery, and postnatal care).

The second group, consisting of fourteen women (37 percent of the home-birth mothers), had insurance that would have covered hospital but not home birth. Four of these mothers mentioned that paying for the home birth was a hardship, but that they would have done it at any cost in order to avoid the hospital. For the remaining ten in this group, cost was irrelevant. Both of these first two groups had hospital coverage and clear plans for hospital backup in the event of complications, and they were generally similar to the birth center mothers in demography and philosophy.

The third group, consisting of fifteen home-birth mothers, (39 percent), had no insurance at all. For twelve of these women, whose average family income was $15,000–$19,000 annually, paying for the home birth posed economic difficulties. Of these women, nine (24 percent of the total group of home-birth mothers) initially had wanted to give birth in a hospital, but had no insurance and could not afford it. For these women, the average cost of a home birth was $850 when paid in cash. Other arrangements were made when cash was not available. As one mother stated:

> Well, we still haven't paid. The last time I talked to the midwife, I asked her how much we owed her. Originally, I thought she said it was four hundred dollars, and then I asked her later what that covered. She was real vague about it and I said, let us know. She never sent us a bill. My husband welds.... She said she needed some welding work done, so we still might go ahead with that.

A Catalyst to Alternatives: Financial Straits

The home-birth mothers who were uninsured and unable to afford a hospital birth were effectively rejected by the medical system, regardless of how they subsequently viewed their decision. When asked if money had been a factor in the decision for a home birth, one woman answered:

Yeah, I think if I'd had insurance, I wouldn't have looked into birth alternatives. It was a good thing because I really am happy with the way I did it. I think I would have gone right to the hospital and had it in the hospital, not knowing there was any other way.... If I had a whole bunch of money, I would have gone to the hospital without thinking.

Another home-birth mother, poet and artist Laverne Campbell, said:

I saw the medical doctor and, of course, she said she would only deliver in a hospital and ... so I said, well let me investigate. [The hospital cost] $5,000 at least! I mean the first thing they do is talk about money and you start adding up your savings account ... so the first thought was a hospital and then my mind just kind of rejected it.... It was there because that's the information from our culture, but I could not picture going into labor, getting into a car, riding somewhere, having a strange staff take care of me and this doctor walk in to get the baby's head.

Still a third woman remarked: "I didn't relish the idea of paying the kid off for five years."

Hospital Backup Arrangements

Almost all of the practitioners at the FSBC had admitting privileges at a major tertiary medical center that was a six-minute drive, door to door, from the FSBC. The few licensed midwives at the FSBC without hospital admitting privileges all had written backup arrangements with obstetricians.

For the home-birth mothers, arrangements for hospital backup were not so clear-cut. Twelve home-birth mothers (32 percent), irrespective of whether or not they had insurance, were assisted by lay midwives without hospital access. Most mothers made private arrangements with doctors to assist them in the event of complications or intended to use hospital emergency facilities. Frequently, these arrangements were less than desirable. As one mother stated when asked whether she had medical backup for her home birth:

Well, I had asked the last doctor I had seen and he was very, very nasty. He said, well, if you come to the hospital and you're dying, I'm not going to turn you away, so that was my medical backup. He was really awful about the whole thing. He said, I don't like to be a fireman after the fire, after the house has burned down.

Outcomes of Out-of-Hospital Deliveries
Medical Outcome

Sixty-seven of the seventy-six births (88 percent) had a positive medical outcome at the intended delivery site. However, nine problematic cases (12 percent) required hospitalization for either the mother or baby.

Of the women intending to deliver at the FSBC, a total of five mothers were transferred to the hospital. Three mothers transferred intrapartum for meconium staining, indicating possible fetal distress, and two transferred after birth, one for a retained placenta and one for postpartum hemorrhage. Two neonates were also transferred to the hospital, one for infection, the other for transient tachypnia. The second baby was hospitalized in the neonatal intensive care unit for three days.

For the home-birth mothers, two transferred to the hospital intrapartum, both for prolonged labor. One of these transfers involved a woman who had had the flu for several days before delivery and was suffering from extraordinary pain and weakness.

In all cases, the outcome was good, with hospital stays ranging from two hours to three days. Fortunately, in all cases in which hospitalization was required, excellent medical backup systems had been arranged in advance, and in all cases transfer was rapid and efficient. All of the mothers transferred to the hospital were attended by licensed physicians and midwives who either had hospital admitting privileges or whose partner or sponsoring physician had hospital admitting privileges.

Satisfaction with the Birth

When asked how she felt about her labor and delivery overall, Laverne Campbell had this to say:

In general, I felt it was the most high, exciting, wonderful time of my life. I was part of the creation of a new being.

It's a miracle.... There was excitement, I don't know, being absolutely, totally alive, every part of you is alive, keenly. It was so intense. I was happy, I was joyous. I was crying at different parts. It was just awe. I felt wonderful. I felt totally alive and wonderful.

Other mothers, delivering at home and in the FSBC, made similar statements:

Immediately following the birth, I would say I felt ecstasy.... I felt as if I had been through the most incredible experience and that I would probably never feel that good again.

After her shoulders were born.... I was just getting extremely eager and happy, getting elated with a sense of euphoria, and [the midwife] said I could reach down and take her under her arms and pull her out and that was just—I can't explain it! I can't put a good enough word on it! I was so joyful.

It was a peak experience. I felt a real sense of things being right, a lot of energy, a lot of love, a lot of joy ... on top of the world ... a feeling of accomplishment.... All was right with the world.

It was pow-er-ful. My labor was powerful. The delivery was—ecstatic. It was the kind of ecstasy that comes from knowing that you have something to do with it—but yet you don't.... I was awestruck.

[I felt] power. Is that an emotion?

The great majority of mothers experiencing out-of-hospital deliveries emerged from the birth experience exalted. They were awed by the work their bodies had done, and they experienced a surge of self-confidence and a "newfound respect for all mothers." The women took their ability to control the situation for granted, which freed them to become totally involved in giving birth. The result was a sense of mastery, a sense of satisfaction, and the discovery of inner strengths.

In total, 87 percent of the FSBC mothers and 95 percent of the home-birth mothers felt "positive" or "extremely positive" about their births (see Table 9.5).

Dissatisfaction with the Birth

Not all the women had wholly positive experiences, though. Two birth center mothers (5 percent of the FSBC sample) experienced highly mixed emotions, reacting both extremely positively and extremely negatively. The first woman was discouraged during labor as a result of intense pain, but after the birth she felt "happy, excited, and relieved." The second woman transferred to the hospital because of a retained placenta, and, though she was "elated" about the birth, she felt "impotent" when her baby was put under bilirubin lights for jaundice.

One home-birth mother emerged with negative feelings about her birth, and two FSBC mothers felt extremely negative about theirs. Thus, three of the women (4 percent) had an overall negative experience. Why?

The woman giving birth at home had experienced a sporadic forty-eight-hour labor in which she dilated slowly and felt lonely and frightened. When her baby was finally born, he refused to nurse for three days. Further, it was three days before she could find a pediatrician who would examine him because of the "fireman after the fire" syndrome noted earlier— the generally negative response to the fact that the baby had been born at home.

TABLE 9.5. Psychological Outcome

	Birth Center Mothers		Home-Birth Mothers		Total	
Reactions	No.	%*	No.	%*	No.	%*
Extremely positive	22	58	30	79	52	68
Positive	11	29	6	16	17	22
Neutral	1	3	1	3	2	3
Mixed reaction	2	5	0	—	2	3
Negative	0	—	1	3	1	1
Extremely negative	2	5	0	—	2	3

*Percents are rounded independently and may not add to 100 percent.

An FSBC mother described her birth as "the pits." She felt her first contraction eighteen hours after her membranes ruptured, and eight hours after that, her baby was born. Two hours later, the baby was transferred to the neonatal intensive care unit with an infection that she felt might have been prevented by a timely Cesarean section.

The other birth center mother who had a negative experience described herself as "a very self-controlling person." She felt embarrassed because she "lost control" ("made a lot of noise") in front of her husband and her daughter, which caused her to feel disappointment in herself and thus ruined her experience.

Impetus for Out-of-Hospital Birth and Medical Outcome in California

A 1977 analysis of data from the state of California (Birth Cohort File, State of California Department of Health Statistics)—the most recent year for which data have been analyzed—showed that the greatest number of out-of-hospital births occurred with "White non-Spanish Surname"[4] mothers (hereafter referred to as white), with just less than 2 percent of the total number of white births occurring outside a hospital. The only exception to this rule was in the age category fifteen to nineteen, in which Native Americans had the highest ratio of births outside hospitals. In general, Native Americans followed whites closely, with the second-highest proportion of out-of-hospital births. Among other prevalent ethnic groups in California, "White Spanish Surname" (hereafter Hispanic), Black, Japanese, and Chinese women had low out-of-hospital birth rates, all less than 1 percent of the total number of births for each respective population (see Table 9.6).

How does ethnicity relate to medical outcome? First, let us look at birth weight, the single most important indicator of a baby's health status. In 1977 for all minority groups, infants

---

[4]Ethnic identification is based on the ethnic group of the child. In this section of the chapter, "white mother" actually identifies the mother of a white baby, irrespective of the mother's ethnicity. In addition, the labels of "White non-Spanish Surname" and "White Spanish Surname" are the official categories of the state of California, which I have taken the liberty of shortening to "white" and "Hispanic" in order to avoid confusion.

TABLE 9.6. California Births according to Ethnic Group of Child, 1977

Ethnic Group	In-Hospital Births	Out-of-Hospital Births	
		No.	%
White	186,507	3,616	1.9
Hispanic	102,460	887	.09
Black	35,800	291	.8
Filipino	6,895	25	.4
Chinese	4,074	26	.6
Japanese	3,000	23	.8
Native American	2,574	46	1.8
Other	6,120	61	1.0
Total	(N = 347,426)	(N = 4,975)	1.4

Source: State of California Department of Health Services, Birth Cohort File, Sacramento.

born out of the hospital had lower birth weights than those born in the hospital. For example, the percentage of low-birth-weight infants—2,500 grams or less—was more than half again as high for Hispanic babies born out of the hospital as for those born in the hospital. For the black babies, it was almost a third higher. For white babies, exactly the opposite held true. The average birth weight of white infants born outside the hospital was higher than for those born in the hospital (see Table 9.7).

Although the death rate for out-of-hospital births was higher than the in-hospital death rate for all groups, the increased risk of neonatal death for Hispanic infants was more than twice as high as in the hospital: 15.8/1,000 out of hospital compared with 7.4/1,000 in hospital. For whites, the risk of neonatal mortality in out-of-hospital birth was only slightly higher than in the hospital: 8.3/1,000 out of hospital compared with 6.9/1,000 in hospital (see Figure 9.1).

What factors can account for these discrepancies between ethnic groups? As we know, a positive outcome results from good prenatal care and nutrition, low parity, adequate spacing between children, bearing children between certain ages, and, in general, good health. It is a telling fact, for example, that

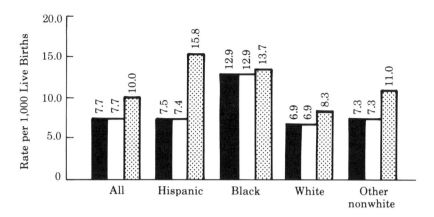

FIGURE 9.1. Neonatal Death Rate according to Ethnic Group of Child and
Place of Delivery, California, 1977

Key: Black Bar = Total Deaths; White Bar = In-hospital; Dotted Bar = Out-of-Hospital.
Source: State of California Department of Health Services, Birth Cohort File, Sacramento.

almost two-thirds of the white mothers delivering out of the
hospital in California (the lowest mortality group) began their
prenatal care in the first trimester of pregnancy, whereas
substantially fewer than half the Hispanic mothers (the
highest mortality group) started their care at that time. At the
other end of the spectrum, only 13 percent of the whites had
late or no prenatal care, while *almost a third* of Hispanic
mothers had late or no prenatal care (see Table 9.8).
    The California data show that the out-of-hospital birth rate
is highest among 1) those with low-birth-weight babies and a
high mortality rate (obviously, low-income groups) and 2)
those with high-birth-weight babies and a relatively low mortality rate. On the basis of this data, we can surmise that most
of the white out-of-hospital births may be by choice and
planned with adequate attendance and medical backup, while
most of the minority out-of-hospital births may result from
impoverished financial circumstances and the inability to
gain access to the hospital system. This supports the idea that

TABLE 9.7. Birth Weight and Ethnic Groups: In-Hospital and Out-of-Hospital Births, California, 1977

Place of Delivery and Ethnic Group	Total No.	%	Total Under 2,500	Under 2,500 Under 1,500	Under 2,500 1,501- 2,000	Under 2,500 2,001- 2,500	2,501 and Over
Total	340,888	100.0	5.3	0.8	1.0	3.5	94.7
White	183,023	100.0	4.5	0.6	0.8	3.1	95.5
Hispanic	100,672	100.0	4.6	0.7	0.9	3.1	95.4
Black	34,884	100.0	10.7	1.9	2.0	6.9	89.3
Other nonwhite	22,309	100.0	5.6	0.7	0.8	4.0	94.4
In-Hospital	335,963	100.0	5.3	0.8	1.0	3.5	94.7
White	179,436	100.0	4.6	0.6	0.9	3.1	95.4
Hispanic	99,802	100.0	4.6	0.7	0.8	3.1	95.4
Black	34,595	100.0	10.7	1.9	2.0	6.9	89.3
Other nonwhite	22,130	100.0	5.6	0.7	0.8	4.0	94.4
Out-of-Hospital	4,925	100.0	4.5	0.7	0.8	3.0	95.5
White	3,587	100.0	3.0	0.3	0.5	2.2	97.0
Hispanic	870	100.0	7.3	1.5	1.2	4.6	92.7
Black	289	100.0	14.1	2.8	3.2	8.1	85.9
Other nonwhite	179	100.0	6.7	1.7	2.8	2.2	93.3

*Percent calculations exclude birth weight not reported; 534 for total single live births, 451 for in-hospital single live births, and 83 for out-of-hospital single live births.

Percents are rounded independently and may not add to totals.

Source: State of California Department of Health Services, Birth Cohort File, Sacramento.

there are, in general, two categories of women having out-of-hospital deliveries: those who are driven to it out of economic necessity and those who could have hospital births but choose to give birth outside the hospital.

A study of 287 home births in Santa Cruz County in California showed that the complications of home delivery were not higher than those for a general hospital population, and that neonatal mortality and morbidity may actually be lower for an unanesthetized "natural childbirth population" than for the population as a whole (Mehl et al, 1975). Eighty-one percent of these births, which represented the practice of a lay midwifery group, had "unremarkable" outcomes at home. Of fifty-six women with complications (19 percent of the sample), forty-five (16 percent of the total sample, 80 percent of the group with complications) were transferred to a hospital during labor. The complications of those transported to the hospital were associated with one case of meconium aspiration, one case of toxemia of pregnancy, six cases of respiratory distress, and two cases of cervical lacerations. There was one stillbirth in the population. Others were transported primarily for prolonged or arrested labor. Overall, the complications were comparable with those for the general hospital population. This sample, however, represents a skewed situation of highly educated women with good prenatal care and, in general, an optimal situation for home birth. It is interesting that, with few exceptions, the mothers in this study were white and from middle-class backgrounds.

These results parallel those for the birth center sample I examined, particularly regarding both the impetus for giving birth outside the hospital and the medical outcomes. Thus, I would hypothesize that while philosophical incentives play a major role among some populations choosing to deliver out of

TABLE 9.8. Out-of-Hospital Births According to Ethnic Group of Child and When Prenatal Care Began

			When Prenatal Care Began			
Ethnic Group	Total Births	Total Reported*	First Trimester	Second Trimester	Third Trimester	No Prenatal Care
White						
No.	3,615	3,477	2,159	876	175	267
%			62.1	25.2	5.0	7.7
Hispanic						
No.	887	854	372	230	82	170
%			43.6	26.9	9.6	19.9
Black						
No.	291	272	147	75	12	38
%			54.0	27.6	4.4	14.0
Other nonwhite						
No.	181	168	82	46	17	23
%			48.8	27.4	10.1	13.7
	(N = 4,974)	(N = 4,771)	(N = 2,760)	(N = 1,227)	(N = 286)	(N = 498)

*Percents are rounded independently and may not add to 100 percent.
Source: State of California Department of Health Services, Birth Records, Sacramento.

the hospital, the increase in out-of-hospital deliveries may be attributable primarily to a tightening economic situation. As economic conditions improve, we will most likely see a decline in the total number of home births.

In the two-county area examined here, 76 percent of the home births occurred irrespective of financial considerations with a primarily white population. Nevertheless, even in this group, and in a relatively high-income area of the country, *nearly one-fourth of the women choosing home birth were effectively rejected by the medical system because of their inability to pay.*

Impetus for, and Outcome in, Home Birth

Reports on home birth in North Carolina, Washington state, Oregon, Alabama, and Arizona have appeared in the medical literature within the past few years. These reports, however, show contradictory conclusions and raise many questions about our ability to generalize from one population to another about the safety of home birth.

North Carolina

The North Carolina study of 1,296 home deliveries, which compared vital records of live births and neonatal deaths, showed that the home-birth population compared with the general population, was disproportionately young (mothers less than twenty years of age on average), primarily black, and with fewer than twelve years of education—all variables associated with high levels of infant mortality (Burnett et al., 1980).

The home deliveries in this study were associated with a neonatal mortality rate of 30/1,000. However, when this rate was broken down by whether or not the home births were planned, it was found that in planned home deliveries, the neonatal mortality rate was only 6/1,000 compared with 120/1,000 for unplanned home deliveries. Thus, the relative risk of unplanned home births was twenty times that of planned home births.

A home delivery was considered to be planned when the mother was attended by a lay midwife who had received a

permit specifically to attend that birth. In order for a permit
to be granted, the mother had to be approved by a health
department as being at low risk for complications. In contrast,
deliveries of infants weighing 2,000 grams or less, of which
there were fifty-one cases, were considered to be precipitate
and therefore unplanned.

This study showed that medical outcomes varied according
to both the place and circumstances of delivery. The classifica-
tion of in-hospital versus out-of-hospital births did not adequately group births according to risk of neonatal mortality
since the low mortality rate for the planned home births was
comparable with the state's in-hospital neonatal mortality
rate of 7/1,000. Planning, prenatal screening, and adequate
training of birth attendants emerged as the most important
variables in differentiating the risk of neonatal mortality in
North Carolina (Burnett et al., 1980).

Oregon

The Oregon study of 6,398 out-of-hospital births between 1975
and 1979 classified deliveries according to birth attendant
(Clarke and Bennetts, 1982). It reached conclusions remarkably
similar to the North Carolina study, in that when the birth
attendant was classified as "No attendant" or "Other attendant," the neonatal death rate was four times greater than
those deliveries attended by a "licensed attendant" or "midwife." The high mortality group was also associated with poor
prenatal care and parents with fewer than twelve years of
education.

The major categories of cause of death in the "No attendant" and "Other attendant" groups were Sudden Infant
Death Syndrome and external causes (motor vehicle accidents, drowning, assault, undetermined), which accounted for
nearly two-thirds of the deaths in that group.

Clearly, we need to consider the entire social and health
care environment surrounding the perinatal period, especially
that of the population served by other than licensed attendants.

Arizona

Although little information is provided regarding maternal
background in a report on four years' experience with home

birth by licensed midwives in Arizona, outcome data for 1,449 births are available. Fourteen percent of the mothers seeking to give birth at home were transferred to the hospital during labor. Eighteen percent of the women giving birth at home were attended subsequently by a physician, and 15 percent of those women were admitted to a hospital postpartum. The postpartum maternal hospitalizations totaled less than 3 percent of all the women delivering at home (Sullivan and Beeman, 1983).

For infants, only 3 percent had an Apgar score of less than seven at five minutes. A normal Apgar would be considered seven or above. Two percent of the infants were hospitalized after birth, primarily for respiratory distress, Apgar of less than seven, or jaundice. There were two neonatal deaths and three fetal deaths resulting from a breech delivery, congenital heart and lung anomalies, or unknown causes. At least one death may have been preventable with proper medical management. Two midwives' licenses were revoked in relation to these deaths. In the case of the baby with the heart and lung anomalies, the midwife's license was suspended for violation of several rules and regulations. The other license was revoked in connection with a fetal death in which the midwife falsely reported a heartbeat in order to allow her client to deliver at home. Subsequent examination indicated that fetal death had occurred four to twenty-four hours before delivery.

As in the experience of North Carolina and Oregon, Arizona's experience demonstrates that home births can be safe for women classified as low risk if they are attended by an adequately trained practitioner.

Alabama

An assessment of home births in Alabama from 1940 to 1980, with an emphasis on the period from 1970 to 1980, showed a decline in home births from 25 percent to .5 percent of all births during this period, along with a twofold increase in neonatal mortality for home births (Goldenberg et al., 1983).

Women delivering at home tended to be nonwhite, thirty-five or older, multiparous, and with less than a high school education and little or no prenatal care. Nevertheless, white, single primiparas less than twenty years old with less than a high school education and little or no prenatal care were at greatest risk for neonatal death.

The authors of this study attribute the increase in mortality rates to "granny" midwives who had attended most of the home births. These women, the authors state, did not practice in accordance with the medical standard of care of the day.

Like the other studies, the Alabama study points to the importance of having adequately trained practitioners attending home births.

Washington

In Washington state, birth certificates linked with death certificates and log books from tertiary-care hospitals were used to investigate 1,614 home births and 1,247 FSBC deliveries between 1975 and 1977 (Shy et al., 1980).

Home births were associated with grand multiparity (women with several babies), a disproportionate number of births to old and very young mothers, multiple gestations (twins, triplets, etc.), and nonprofessionally attended births.

Significantly more birth center deliveries than home deliveries were professionally attended, and FSBC deliveries were associated with an earlier onset of prenatal care, more prenatal visits, and a lower infant mortality rate than the home deliveries.

Impetus for, and Outcome in, FSBCs

In contrast to the range of outcomes reported for home birth in Santa Cruz County, North Carolina, and Alabama, the reported outcome at FSBCs shows a more even outcome.

Across the country, women choosing to deliver at FSBCs tend to be well educated and well prepared for childbirth through childbirth education courses. They have more prenatal visits than the home-birth population, and when medical protocols are strictly followed they generally have a favorable medical outcome, one that is comparable with in-hospital outcome (Bean, 1975; Bennetts and Lubic, 1982; Cohen, 1982; Cooperative Birth Center Network News, 1983; DeJong et al., 1979; Eakins, 1984; Faison et al., 1979; Lubic, 1975; Norwood, 1978; Reinke, 1982; Shy et al., 1980).

Only 5 percent of the births at FSBCs result in complications (Bennetts and Lubic, 1982), and the infant mortality rate
is 4–6/1,000, compared with 13/1,000, the national figure for
the United States.

The medical outcomes at FSBCs, though they are still in the
experimental stages and still being studied,[5] appear to be
excellent (Eakins, 1984). This seems to be a consequence of
both the socioeconomic background of the clientele and the
relatively uniform standard of care provided by the centers.
Further, the steady rise in FSBC births appears to reflect not
a tightening economic situation but rather a challenge to
dominant medical ideology. Ironically, it may be the current
difficult economic situation that ensures the survival of
FSBCs, since their services are cost-effective and therefore
attractive to insurance companies.

Regardless of whether the impetus to pursue out-of-hospital
births was financial or philosophical, the degree of satisfaction in these births, whether at home or in an FSBC, was, for
the sample I studied, very high. One possible explanation
might be that when a parturient woman feels a sense of
control over the external environment, she may be more
capable of controlling herself physically and mentally during
labor and delivery. A heightened sense of mastery, which may
lead to increased self-esteem, can result. This finding echoes
the conclusions of other studies, which indicate that giving
birth can be viewed by mothers as an important achievement
for themselves and for all women (see Seiden, 1978). As Alana
Bernard, age 35 and giving birth to her first baby, commented:

I was in awe of the whole birth experience.... This is amaz-
ing to me, that the human body can do this. I felt tremendous pride in being a woman—in that I could give birth. I
felt like I was very fulfilled and complete after having had
this experience ... gutsy.

---

[5]At present, there are two major studies of FSBCs under way, one by the
National Association of Childbearing Centers in Perkiomenville, Pennsylvania, and one by the UCLA School of Public Health.

CONCLUSIONS

This chapter has demonstrated that there are two groups of women most likely to give birth outside of a hospital: those who conscientiously prefer not to be admitted to a hospital in labor and those for whom cost precludes a hospital delivery. Most mothers choosing the FSBC as their birth site belonged to the first group, whereas home-birth mothers were divided fairly equally between the two groups. As the economic situation improves, we can expect to see a drop in the home-birth rate, although the birth rate at FSBCs will probably continue to increase, reflecting a philosophical divergence from the hospital experience.

Although medical outcomes at FSBCs parallel those of hospitals, for home births the medical outcome varies considerably between different ethnic groups. From this, it is clear that the medical system is not meeting the needs of a vulnerable, potentially at-risk, population. Thus, holding mothers responsible for their infants' sickness or death as a result of giving birth at home ("[The doctor said] that what I had done [by having a home birth] was equivalent to child abuse") does not take into account the fact that those home-birth mothers who are most likely to experience complications have been effectively excluded by the medical system because they cannot afford a hospital delivery. New arrangements must be made to accommodate home-birth mothers if doctors do not wish to be "firemen after the fire."

Conversely, for both the home-birth and FSBC mothers in this study, the psychological outcome of out-of-hospital delivery was outstanding. The ability to control the birth situation gave these mothers a heightened sense of mastery that enhanced their perception of themselves and their collective gender. This outcome might be produced in a variety of settings if women can gain more control over the external environment.

Assessing motivation and outcome in out-of-hospital delivery is critically important. However, this kind of analysis is by nature extremely complex, as conditions and results vary within, and between, subgroups of the population. This fact must be considered when generalizations are drawn regarding out-of-hospital birth populations.

REFERENCES

Bean, M. "Birth Is a Family Affair." *American Journal of Nursing* 75(1975):1,689-1,692.

Bennetts, A. B., and Lubic, Ruth Watson. "The Free-Standing Birth Center." *The Lancet* 1(1982):378-380.

Birth Cohort File, State of California Department of Health Statistics, Sacramento.

Burnett, C. A.; Jones, J. A.; Rooks, J.; Chen, C. H.; Tyler, C. W.; and Miller, C. A. "Home Delivery and Neonatal Mortality in North Carolina." *Journal of the American Medical Association* 244(1980): 2,741-2,745.

Clarke, N., in consultation with Bennetts, A. B. "Appendix F, Vital Statistics and Nonhospital Births: A Mortality Study of Infants Born out of Hospitals in Oregon." *Research Issues in the Assessment of Birth Settings.* Washington, D.C.: Institute of Medicine and National Research Council, National Academy Press, 1982.

Clarke, N., and Bennetts, A. B. "Out-of-Hospital Births," Letter to the editor. *Obstetrics and Gynecology* 62(1983):397.

Cohen, Richard L. "A Comparative Study of Women Choosing Two Different Childbirth Alternatives." *Birth* 9, no. 1 (Spring 1982), 13-19.

Cooperative Birth Center Network News 1(1981):1.

———. 1(1983):4.

DeJong, R. N.; Shy, K.; and Clark, K. C. "An Out-of-Hospital Birth Center Using University Referral." *Obstetrics and Gynecology* 58(1979):703-707.

Eakins, Pamela S. "The Rise of the Free Standing Birth Center: Principles and Practice." *Women and Health* 9(1984)9,4:49-64.

Faison, J. B.; Pisani, B. J.; Douglas, R. G., et al. "The Childbearing Center: An Alternative Birth Setting." *Obstetrics and Gynecology* 54(1979):527-532.

Goldenberg, R. L.; Hale, C. H.; Houde, J.; Humphrey, J. L.; Wayne, J. B.; and Boyd, B. W. "Neonatal Deaths in Alabama." *American Journal of Obstetrics and Gynecology* 147(1983):687-693.

Lubic, Ruth Watson. "Developing Maternity Services Women Will Trust." *American Journal of Nursing* 75(1975):1,685-1,688.

———. "The Rise of the Birth Center Alternative." *The Nation's Health* (January 1982):7.

Mehl, L. E.; Peterson, G. H.; Shaw, N. S.; and Creevy, D. C. "Complications of Home Birth." *Birth and the Family Journal* 2(1975): 123-131.

Norwood, Christopher. "Birth Centers: A Humanizing Way to Have a Baby." *MS.* 6 no. 11 (May 1978).

Pearse, W. H. "Trends in Out-of-Hospital Births." *Obstetrics and Gynecology* 60(1982):267–270.

Reinke, C. "Outcomes of the First 527 Births at the Birthplace in Seattle." *Birth* 9(1982):231–241.

Seiden, Anne M. "The Sense of Mastery in the Childbirth Experience." *The Woman Patient: Medical and Psychological Interfaces.* Vol. 1: *Sexual and Reproductive Aspects of Women's Health Care.* Eds. Malkah T. Knotman and Carol C. Nadelson. New York and London: Plenum Press, 1978.

Shy, K. K.; Frost, F.; and Ullom, J. "Out-of-Hospital Delivery in Washington State, 1975–1977." *American Journal of Obstetrics and Gynecology* 137(1980):547–552.

Sullivan, D. H., and Beeman, R. "Four Years' Experience with Home Birth by Licensed Midwives in Arizona." *American Journal of Public Health* 73(1983):641–645.

10

Nurse and Lay Midwifery in Vermont

REGI L. TEASLEY

Although midwifery is an ancient art, both nurse midwifery and modern lay or independent midwifery are of very recent origin in the United States. Begun in the 1920s on the fringes of the medical system, nurse midwifery began to move into hospital practice in the 1960s and 1970s. Although lay midwives have attended births for centuries, the recent independent midwife movement is an outgrowth of the home-birth movement that emerged in the 1970s.

The context in which modern lay and nurse midwifery have emerged is a product of the historical competition between traditional lay midwives and the allopathic (regular) medical profession in the United States. For most of the nineteenth century, the midwife was the typical birth attendant for the vast majority of women, as she had been for centuries. Even after the turn of the century, as physicians began to increase their competition for patients, midwives attended at least 50 percent of all births in the United States. By the late nineteenth century, however, the rise of allopathic medicine had begun in earnest, and by the time of the Flexner Report of 1910, the "man-midwives" (physicians) were edging out the lay midwives. This occurred first among the middle and upper classes and later (and less completely) among the working and poorer classes. Allopaths, especially obstetricians, eventually restricted or eliminated their female competitors (the midwives) state by state through legislation and licensure, coupled with public relations campaigns (Litoff, 1978:64–90). Midwives' numbers declined dramatically as their practices were legally restricted or outlawed. They were largely absent from the birthing scene by the 1930s, and hospital-based obstetric specialists employing forceps, anesthesia, and, not infrequently, surgery had defined childbirth as a medical event requiring the services of an obstetrician. Physicians had gained the bulk of the market for themselves and had become a dominant profession that regulated and restricted competitors with the assistance of the state.

At present, both lay midwives and nurse midwives are attempting to locate an occupational niche in an arena already monopolized by physicians. In order to do this, each group has developed a different strategy. Lay midwives have sought to locate an occupational niche outside, or on the perimeter of, the physician-dominated medical division of labor. Having grown out of the home-birth movement, independent midwives seek to attend deinstitutionalized births for a self-selected clientele that advocates the option of deprofessionalized maternity care.

In contrast, nurse midwives have taken up the strategy of professionalization in order to locate occupational turf in the medical division of labor. In the process, they have attempted to persuade the dominant profession to relinquish or delegate to nurse midwives specific tasks (e.g., the management of normal labors and deliveries in the hospital).

In the process of trying to locate an occupational niche, these emerging occupational collectives—lay and nurse midwives—have produced ideologies and tailored them to fit their social circumstances. World views specific to lay and nurse midwifery have grown out of training, clinical practice, and, of primary concern here, the struggle to obtain occupational turf. Taking a social movement perspective, this chapter examines how these unifying ideologies are produced, how they differ, and how lay and nurse midwives interrelate in Vermont in particular.

METHODS AND DATA

The information on which this analysis is based is drawn from a case study of northern and central Vermont (Teasley, 1983) and concerns the period from 1970 to 1980. Interviews conducted during 1980 and 1981 were the primary source of data. Twenty-five subjects were interviewed, including ten nurse midwives (all the certified nurse midwives practicing in the northern two-thirds of the state) and seven lay midwives (out of an estimated population of ten).

Other sources of information used include transcriptions from the hearings held by the Vermont House of Representatives subcommittee considering legislation to license lay midwifery. In addition, an independent midwife provided an extensive collection of clippings from state newspapers pertaining to home birth, birth reform, and lay midwifery.

Vermont is an attractive study site for examining the interoccupational relations in maternity care. Nurse midwives have worked in the state in various capacities since 1968, although their position in actual practice is still being negotiated. Legislation enabling the practice of nurse midwifery is of relatively recent origin (1974), and legislation concerning lay midwifery practice was discussed at some length in the state legislature in 1979 and 1980. Throughout the period examined in this study, the practice of lay midwifery was extralegal in Vermont (outside the legal system, neither prohibited nor sanctioned). The movement for home birth and lay midwifery was active in the state during the 1970s.

HOME BIRTH IN VERMONT

The home-birth movement in Vermont became active in the early 1970s, and both the numbers of home births and movement activism grew throughout the decade. The movement was successful in creating awareness of home birth and engaging the medical profession in public debate. However, it was less successful in achieving for midwives satisfactory working relations with obstetricians. Nonetheless, the movement was remarkably effective for its size, considering that at its peak the movement accounted for fewer than 2 percent of the births in the state (State of Vermont, 1975–79).

The movement was composed of a core membership drawn from the counterculture, back-to-the-land movement dating from the 1960s. The growing movement periphery consisted largely of more mainstream middle-class and professional couples whose expectations for birth had been raised by birth reform only to be quashed by traditional hospital practices.

The unifying theme of the movement was freedom from the medical profession's control of childbirth and its restriction of birthing options. It was a grassroots movement with no formal organization, whose goal was primarily the creation and maintenance of workable maternity care options that would meet the needs of its members. Thus, the movement advocated deinstitutionalization of childbirth and deprofessionalization of care giving as an option that could coexist with physician-attended hospital birth. However, as the movement encountered active efforts by the medical profession to eliminate it, it was increasingly forced to challenge the medical profession's authority, especially its claims to a monopoly on relevant expertise.

The central issues on which the ideology of the home-birth movement in Vermont was constructed were informed choice, personal autonomy, and individual responsibility. This is exemplified by one lay midwife's statement: "I do not *advocate* home birth." The reason given, as many respondents told me, is that "home birth is not for everyone." While many movement supporters suggested that ultimately up to 90 percent of all births could safely take place at home with properly trained attendants and adequate medical backup, most said that nowhere near that percentage of birthing families is currently prepared for such an undertaking. In this regard, movement participants use terms such as *prepared, responsible,* or *informed* home birth. Each of these terms emerged in part out of debates with the medical establishment. "Prepared home birth" distinguishes planned home births from births that occur at home but are accidental, unanticipated, or undesired. This distinction is necessary in part because organized obstetrics, in its efforts to delegitimate home birth, has included in its analysis of home birth data concerning accidental births, miscarriages, and unplanned home births (NAPSAC News, 1981:10).

"Responsible" or "informed" home birth are terms used to counter physicians' claims that home-birth parents are ignorant and cavalier about their choices. For example, a neonatologist at the university hospital in Vermont publicly charged that people who chose home births were "crazies who go off to caves and log cabins to deliver the newborn who has no say in the process"; he went on to say that home births were a "selfish fad" (Calta, 1977). From the point of view of the medical profession, the laity's choice not to consult it represents irresponsibility. Physicians make such charges (which they may sincerely believe) as a way of restating their claim to authority and a monopoly on appropriate expertise. In contrast, lay people's use of the terms *prepared, responsible,* and *informed* suggest that those who practice home birth have access to expertise, are reasonable and ethical, and both desire and deserve legitimacy. While some physicians charged that home-birth advocates were "antitechnology," or antimedicine, movement participants countered that technology and medical intervention were used when required. They readily acknowledged that hospitals and physicians were appropriate for abnormal pregnancies and births and for those who knowingly chose it. Thus, a key component of the concept "responsible home birth" was self-selection by participants augmented by midwives' screening.

A home-birth mother, writing in support of home birth in a local paper, emphasized these practices:

> No person will be attended at a home birth who hasn't been screened as thoroughly as possible for complications. Because of the risks involved in home births, the women are usually far better informed and prepared than those destined for the hospital. We, who are for home births or alternative birthing, feel ourselves not irresponsible but more responsible for our actions instead of putting ourselves in others' hands totally. If we had assumed any potential danger we would have used the available medical facilities (Brown, 1977).

Other supporters of home birth pointed out that screening and self-selection included consideration of psychological factors as well as geographic location and weather conditions. As one subject noted, "People who [successfully] do home births have to be super together.... [Some likely home-birth candidates choose to give birth in the hospital] because they're together enough to realize that [if they're] two miles up a dirt road in January . . . [it] is the better part of valor to come in."

While acknowledging the value of physician-attended hospital birth, movement participants criticize the medical profession and hospital practices. Obstetricians, in particular, are criticized for their colleague-centered, rather than client-centered practices. In addition, most physicians are charged with placing professional interests ahead of the provision of health care. For example, by withholding prenatal or backup care or delivering it in a punitive manner, physicians effectively restrict the availability of birthing alternatives. At the same time they make home birth more dangerous for those who choose it. (A few younger progressive physicians provide support for home births, and these physicians are highly valued and sought out.)

Professionals and an autonomous laity are, at least conceptually, at odds. Professionalizing occupations claim, among other things, a monopoly on relevant expertise (Larson, 1977:17), and freedom from lay intervention and evaluation is a hallmark of professional status (Friedson, 1970:24). At the same time, professions typically assert a conceptualization of the phenomena with which they work in a manner most consistent with their claimed capabilities. Professional conceptions of illness or disease and related cures may differ from those of the laity who, nevertheless, must be persuaded to consult the profession if the profession is to attain legitimacy (Friedson, 1970:21). Having achieved professional status and a monopoly on care giving, physicians have been remarkably successful at making both their claims and their definitions of the situation stick. The profession has encouraged the laity to acknowledge its ignorance and thus its dependence on physicians in order to most efficiently receive a cure and return to health (Parsons, 1964).

Illich (1976:42) claims that unchecked professional power results in the creation of a "radical monopoly" that not only inhibits access to competing services but also discourages the laity's choice to not consult by undermining self-care. In this way, the activities of professions may be viewed as strategies to disempower and de-educate the laity that then must become its clientele.

One response to such actual or potential professional

hegemony is a client revolt in which the laity seeks to counter the profession's monopoly on expertise by educating itself while simultaneously altering the professional-client relationship by "us[ing] the expert as consultant, not as authority figure" (Haug and Susman, 1969:158). In a more radical move, such as is manifested in the home-birth movement, the laity may also assert its right to choose not to consult the profession, relying instead on self-care or alternative care givers.

THE EMERGENCE OF LAY MIDWIFERY

While home-birth parents emphasize their own responsibility for birth, in Vermont they also typically support and promote lay midwifery. Thus, out of this anarchistic movement arose various birth attendants and midwives who are incipient leaders and the foci of the movement. While many of the home births in Vermont were planned and carried out by the families involved, the vast majority included prenatal consultations and birth attendance by lay midwives.

Becoming a Lay Midwife

For many of the midwives, attending the home birth of a friend as an observer or support person marked a turning point for them. They typically referred to this experience as transforming. For others, planning and having their own birth at home was crucial in their decision to become a midwife. Most of the midwives had had at least one home birth. Finally, some women came to midwifery through a larger concern for health care, often women's health care in particular. Here the influence of the feminist movement is more clearly felt and mentioned by respondents. While their stories are varied and intertwined, it is worth noting that there are several related routes into midwifery. The midwives perceive themselves as filling a need in the community. They all stressed that they do not seek out home-birth clients; rather, they are sought out. Apparently, the information that they are willing to attend home births spreads rapidly by word-of-mouth through friendship networks and some parent-oriented structures such as day care centers. Not surprisingly, many midwives refer to their choice as a kind of calling. Certainly they emerge as the key risk takers in terms of the movement as a whole, and they generally indicate a strong commitment to both their home-birth clientele and the viability of home birth as an option.

Once the self-selected birth attendants embark on the calling of midwifery, their path is far from clear. For example, one respondent recalled confiding to a friend her desire to be a midwife, but admitted knowing neither what it actually was nor how to go about becoming one. Because there were virtually no structured avenues to midwifery training and socialization, the midwives gathered information where they could and improvised as they went along. As one lay midwife explained, "lay midwives got responsibility and then scrambled [to learn adequate skills]." After the virtual obliteration of midwifery by the rising medical profession early in the twentieth century, there is little known tradition on which to build the work of midwifery. Thus, midwives find themselves reinventing what is probably the oldest form of health care. In Vermont, however, there were some variations on this theme. Midwives were aided in acquiring training by a physician who broke ranks with the medical establishment.

Most beginning midwives referred to themselves as birth attendants, emphasizing the centrality of parents' responsibility for birth. Given both movement ideology and their level of skill, they were both unwilling and unable to take responsibility for the birth. Instead, they noted that they came to assist the parents in carrying out a home birth.

The point at which the birth attendants began to call themselves midwives was problematic. One birth attendant explained that when people typically called her asking for a midwife, she responded with the caveat, "well, I have assisted at a number of births but I am not a professional midwife." Becoming a midwife suggested to respondents a higher level of skill and thus, perhaps, a somewhat altered relationship with the birthing parents. A woman who considered herself a midwife described the point at which she made the transformation:

Other people started calling me a midwife long before I was calling myself a midwife. [Meanwhile] the more births I attended, the more comfortable I felt. I was doing an enormous amount of self-studying and going to conferences.

Then one day it sort of fell into place. They'd say, "Are you a midwife?" and I'd say, "Yes." Instead of saying, "Well, no . . ." and going into a long explanation of what a midwife was . . . it got to be a hassle. I was competent at attending births. I did know what I was doing. . . . It was a couple of years before I felt comfortable. About forty births.

Most "birth attendants" charged little or no money for their services, while "midwives," often working in pairs, charged up to $450 for prenatal and postnatal care and attendance throughout labor and birth. The calling to service was thus transformed into an occupation.

While the process of becoming a midwife is not clearly marked, neither is the label used to indicate having completed that training. The medical establishment, and often the public, refers to midwives as lay midwives, emphasizing that they are not professionals. However, midwives themselves rarely use that term. As one explained to a newspaper reporter, "We prefer the term *independent* to *lay* because lay means unskilled, and we're not" (Reilly, 1977).

They also refer to themselves as "empirical midwives," indicating that while they have not chosen a scientific medical education, they may nevertheless have extensive training and practical experience.

The Role of the Lay Midwife

The position of the midwife in the home-birth movement is complex. She differentiates herself from her clientele as a skilled, independent practitioner, but at the same time she is, at least ideologically, firmly client centered. The midwives characterize their role as that of helper: providing information on birthing options and responsible birth (in any setting) and making viable the option of prepared/responsible home birth. But there is tension between midwifery's role as helper to an autonomous clientele and its development of expertise and skills. Two issues, screening for home births and taking responsibility for birth, will help illustrate this point.

The issue of screening out people who are at risk is problematic. Since most midwives view individual decision making as virtually sacrosanct, most are disinclined to deny care to women who might otherwise be categorically characterized as at risk. One midwife pointed out that independent midwives, nurse midwives, and physicians could agree on risk factors but would probably not agree on how to deal with them—that is, how to practice. She assumed that nursing and medical personnel would be more inclined to function according to medical standards of practice. Their categorical treatment of patients would occur in part because it is within the model and structure of medical practice that the data and prescribed practice for risk factors have been developed. In contrast, the midwives emphasized that because every pregnancy and labor is different, they resist categorical treatment.

Constructing a hypothetical situation of a woman "at risk" (multigravida, over thirty-five) but determined to have a home birth, a midwife explained:

> I, as an independent midwife, am committed to that woman out of my own ethics. I can explain to her why I think that she is "at risk" but I cannot refuse to give her care. I think a lot of midwives feel that really strongly. Because it's her decision. You share your knowledge but you don't make decisions for people. If you start making decisions for people, you're professional; you're turning people away, you're medical. Because the medical profession has turned away home birth people, all the time; that's partly why lay midwives started.

However, some evidence suggests that midwives may take a more active role in screening and management of labor and delivery than this statement would indicate. At least some midwives reported that they do actively screen and are unwilling to take on clients who smoke, for example.

Several of the midwives noted that their role in labor support and birth attendance was sometimes problematic. For example, a few birthing parents, whom the midwives had helped inform and train through prenatal classes, relinquished responsibility during the birth. A former birth attendant described this phenomenon as proof of the need for skilled midwifery as opposed to amateur birth attendance:

> Even though we made it really clear to all of our couples that the birth was their responsibility, we were just there to aid them. . . . There was still that. . . . It's just ingrained in

you that there's somebody else who's going to have the power to make everything OK. And when a woman's in labor, no matter what she has said prior to that about taking full responsibility, it changes. It's "please help me," "I need some assistance," whatever.... What I felt was, I don't feel like I have the skills to be handling this. I don't want this responsibility.

The inability of the client to maintain full autonomy during the birth required that the midwives be willing to share responsibility. And the transition from birth attendant to midwife included increasing acceptance of this role. However, midwives uniformly disliked situations in which clients fully relinquished responsibility during the birth since it forced them to assume a physician-like decision-making role. The more skilled midwives were able to cope with that role, though some considered it a risk factor indicating hospital care.

Practitioners attending home births were equally concerned, however, with clients who were extremely reluctant to go to the hospital should the need arise and who would not acknowledge midwives' shared responsibility. Midwives were aware of the potential negative outcomes, including morbidity and mortality as well as indictment, and occasionally had to do some fast arguing to persuade the couple to go in; the independent midwife is not in a position to demand it. For example, an obstetrician described having been contacted by a midwife who requested aid in convincing birthing parents that a complication requiring hospital care had arisen.

A midwife described the dual elements of exhilaration and relentless demands that coexist in the practice of empirical midwifery. She also implicitly acknowledged the tension in midwives' experience created by the struggle to balance the movement ideology of personal responsibility and deprofessionalization of care with the occupation's developing expertise and its altered relationship—sharing responsibility—with its clientele:

There's a mystique about being a midwife, there's an awe about it. It really is an incredible thing to be doing and I love it.... At the same time, it's an enormous amount of work. It can be so draining. You're on call all the time. You can go crazy. People just don't know what a heavy deal it is to be somewhat responsible for someone's life and death.

Laying Claim to Occupational Turf

The emergence of the occupation of independent midwifery was enhanced by both midwife training and the development of a formal occupational collectivity.

The first collective interaction of birth attendants in Vermont occurred in Burlington in 1973 when a group supporting home birth developed out of a free clinic's lay staff. In 1974, after becoming a supporter of home birth, a family practitioner in central Vermont began an informal course to teach basic skills to home-birth parents and birth attendants. The collective interaction made possible by this and subsequent training sessions facilitated the creation, in 1976, of a statewide organization of midwives: the Independent Midwives of Vermont. The organization's purpose was to discuss common concerns, provide mutual support, and to exchange and share information.

Among the items discussed was legislation licensing the practice of independent midwifery. In part, this was considered as a defensive measure aimed at countering physician efforts to eliminate independent midwives. However, when such legislation was introduced, it was initiated instead by a concerned state legislator who had discovered the dilemma faced by home-birth parents seeking capable birth attendants. Apparently unaware of the midwives' association, he had consulted a Canadian-trained domiciliary midwife practicing in Vermont. (The absence of an American counterpart for her foreign credentials cast her lot with the independent midwives.)

The bill called for the creation of a midwifery board comprising an obstetrician, a pediatrician, a nurse midwife, a lay midwife, and a consumer. The board would administer a standard test, passage of which would enable a state resident over the age of eighteen to obtain a license to practice midwifery in the state.

The bill was introduced into committee in 1979, after which time public hearings were held. After hearing widely divergent views, the committee tabled the measure. Having altered the legislation somewhat, the legislator reintroduced it in

1980, but it was again tabled after the committee heard testimony from witnesses representing the viewpoints of the major interested parties. At the time of this writing, the legislation had not moved out of committee.

After discussing the initial bill in 1979, the midwives' organization decided to support it, and they and other home-birth supporters used the hearings as a forum to make their claims to occupational turf. Their fundamental argument centered on the ability of an informed laity to responsibly choose home birth. As home-birth parents spoke about their right to self-care and home birth, they laid the groundwork for the midwives' argument that the occupation was responding to a felt need, since medical personnel with limited exceptions shunned home birth. In this way, the independent midwives could embark on the strategy of placing the home-birth movement out front, pointing to the client revolt as the source of both the challenge to the physicians' monopoly on care and the creation of alternatives to it. (This had the added bonus of placing conservative physicians in the unenviable position of having to argue for a "radical monopoly," which some did with great fervor.) Independent midwives thus claimed home birth as their turf and responsible home-birth parents who sought them out as their clientele.

In addition, independent midwives called for a strife-free working relationship with physicians. They enumerated the problems for the provision of optimum care occasioned by physician harassment of patients receiving prenatal care as well as those requiring hospitalization after beginning a birth at home. They wanted to be able to consult with physicians and refer patients to them when necessary.

At the same time, the midwives typically were not seeking a niche in the physician-dominated obstetrical division of labor. Instead they sought a state-sanctioned formal status outside or on the perimeter of that division of labor. Thus, they called themselves independent midwives in part to differentiate themselves from nurse midwives, who, with only one exception in Vermont, worked in the hospital as part of a health care team. Writing in response to nurse midwives' statements about midwifery legislation, an independent midwife noted:

The nurse-midwives... write... that they are qualified to practice independent management of labor "within a health care system which provides for medical consultation, collaborative management or referral." Independent domiciliary midwives have the same responsibilities, only our practice is in the home which the medical profession has defined to be outside the system. We must challenge the health care system to provide consultation and collaborative management for homebirth couples (Nolfi, 1979).

An important component of the midwives' rationale for their existence rested on the presence of an occupational vacuum created when the overwhelming majority of physicians and nurse midwives refused to attend home births. Simultaneously, independent midwives countered statements by medical personnel that home-birth attendance was unsafe for any practitioner by pointing out that physicians and the vast majority of nurse midwives currently in practice are trained for hospital births, not home births. They argued that midwifery skills are different from medical skills, though they do overlap. This position asserts that physician fears about home birth derive from their training, which is the treatment of abnormal births in a high-technology setting; home births leave them stripped of skills and resources. Independent midwives, in contrast, are trained to attend normal births, and they have learned to pay close attention to prenatal care, screening, and preparation of birthing parents. They travel light and treat birth as a natural event. This represents an implicit claim to the development of a different cognitive base and an explicit claim to a different mode of practice that is congruent with their claimed turf.

NURSE MIDWIFERY AS A PROFESSIONALIZING OCCUPATION

Nurse midwives undertook the project of professionalization at the national level, and a brief history will help locate the occupation's goals in Vermont.

The nurse midwives' professional organization, the American College of Nurse Midwives (ACNM) was founded in 1955 and

worked to standardize and upgrade nurse midwifery education. Required education consisted of registered nursing training coupled with additional training in midwifery in either a
certificate or master's program. The ACNM subsequently
provided a national examination for graduates of accredited
schools who, upon successful completion, received national
certification. Legislation enabling nurse midwifery practice
was passed state by state until by 1977 certified nurse midwives (CNMs) were licensed to practice in all but three states
(Rooks, 1978:42).

During the 1960s, the developing "team concept" in medical
care provided a rationale for the inclusion of nurse midwives
into the care of private maternity patients in hospitals, while
fears of physician shortages and a new "baby boom" provided
the impetus.

The ACNM negotiated with the American College of
Obstetricians and Gynecologists (ACOG) and the Nurses' Association of the ACOG (NAACOG) regarding the meaning
and practical implementation of the team concept. Interoccupational relationships were thus formally, if somewhat
vaguely, delineated at the national level through the 1971
"Joint Statement on Maternity Care" endorsed by each of the
organizations. The statement specified obstetrician direction
and supervision of the team, a relationship clarified in 1975
to include the use of standing orders and supervision by
means of protocols (lists specifying, typically in detail, the
prescribed care-giving activities of subordinates).

While protocols enabled physicians to retain ultimate
responsibility, and thus ultimate control, the joint statement
did acknowledge nurse midwifery's claim to "assume responsibility for the complete care and management of uncomplicated maternity patients." ("Joint Statement on Maternity
Care," ACNM, 1971).

For its part, the ACNM laid claim to its turf and CNMs'
relationship to physicians in the following statement:

Nurse-midwifery is the independent management of care of
essentially normal newborns and women, antepartally, intrapartally and/or gynecologically, occurring within a
health care system which provides for medical consultation,
collaborative management, or referral....

The nurse-midwife provides care for the normal mother during pregnancy and stays with her during labor and delivery. She evaluates and provides immediate care for the normal newborn. She helps the mother to care for herself and for her infant, to adjust the home situation to the new child, and to lay a healthful foundation for future pregnancies through family planning and gynecological services. The nurse-midwife is prepared to teach, interpret, and provide support as an integral part of her services (*Journal of Nurse-Midwifery*, 1980:ii).

The statement specified neither the location in which care would be delivered nor the specific relationship with physicians. In this way, it recognized both the variety of work settings and work relationships in which nurse midwives practiced and left open the possibility of independent practice.

The Introduction of Nurse Midwifery into Vermont

Nurse midwives first entered the state to practice in 1968. Their presence was the result of initiatives taken by the head of obstetrics and gynecology at the University Hospital in Burlington. Responding to concerns about projected physician shortages and high costs, he proposed a modified obstetrical division of labor in which obstetricians would concentrate on the care of the abnormal while nurse midwives took on the more routine management of normal labors and deliveries. While there was no physician shortage at the University Hospital, he and the nurse midwifery educator who subsequently joined him attempted to create a demonstration project for export to rural areas in Vermont and elsewhere.

By 1974 several nurse midwives had come and gone and only the nurse midwifery educator remained, the demonstration project having been stalled because of the legal ambiguity of nurse midwifery practice in the state. The nurse midwife and the department chair, with the support of the department of obstetrics and gynecology and the assistance of the state nurses' association, sought enabling legislation. This was granted in an extension of the Nurse Practice Acts in 1974. The revision stated that with appropriate advanced training nurses were allowed to practice in expanded roles working under protocols and guidelines for practice under the auspices of licensed physicians. It did not specify that CNMs were restricted to working under the supervision of obstetricians nor did it delineate the particular setting in which CNMs could work.

Although the enabling legislation was in place, the occupation's future in the state was unclear until 1976, when a private foundation came forward with funding to develop the practice of nurse midwifery at the hospital. By 1978 four nurse midwives had been hired by the large group practice of obstetricians-gynecologists who taught and practiced at the University Hospital. By that time, two instructors at the nursing school were also certified as nurse midwives. By 1979 three other CNMs were practicing in small private practices, and one had set up an independent practice.

Throughout the period of study, all but one of the nurse midwives were the employees of physicians, worked under protocols, and were unable to receive third-party reimbursement for their services. CNMs were structurally subordinate to physicians, although the effect on practical autonomy varied according to the nature of the practice. The nurse midwives who worked for individual physicians functioned as partners, with considerable autonomy in practice. However, nurse midwives who tried to fit themselves into the highly articulated division of labor and the teaching priorities of the hospital found their autonomy more circumscribed.

Efforts to Locate Turf

With their turf already legally laid out for them, nurse midwives cautiously embarked on the process of securing it and translating it into practice. Their emerging location in the medical division of labor obliged them to direct their energy toward negotiating their interoccupational relationships with physicians and nurses. Only after these relationships were somewhat settled did they turn their attention to the issues of their emerging clientele, the home-birth movement, and lay midwifery. Nurse midwives in Vermont began to develop a collective sense late in the 1970s, and their collective ideology was often fragmented, indicating their separate concerns and mirroring larger divisions within the national organization.

The Vermont CNMs described their claims to turf in terms consistent with the statement by the ACNM, noting their ability to indepehdently manage the care of women pre-, post-, and intrapartally within medical guidelines and with medical consultation. But, as subordinates, they were extremely attentive to the boundaries of their claimed turf. They emphasized that their considerable education and practical training enabled them to identify abnormalities, the care of which they promptly referred to physicians.

However, nurse midwives were unsure about the viability of their turf, and they were split in their assessment of physicians' ultimate willingness to delegate to them the care of normal birthing women. Some CNMs felt that obstetricians would, after some initial reluctance, gladly relinquish normal routine care, which they found uninteresting; this seemed especially likely in practices such as that found at the University Hospital in which physicians were salaried, and the emphasis was on teaching and research. One nurse midwife explained:

I think [they will be willing to delegate this work]. Because they don't like it. The more sick you are, the more pathology you can demonstrate, the more interesting case you become. The whole medical model is pathology oriented. The physicians aren't interested in normal. . . . They aren't interested in [routine work]. . . . They don't like to do it and they are delighted to have nurse-practitioners and nurse-midwives involved. They're giving up or turning over something they don't want to do anyway. Plus we do it better, that's what we're trained to do.

In solo or small group practices in which incomes were tied to patient fees, financial incentives could encourage the delegation of tasks; the relatively autonomous CNM could both expand the practice and help the obstetrician concentrate on more lucrative work, such as surgery. As one respondent explained, "Ob is not real profitable. What it mainly does is bring in gyn practice. . . . Surgery is much more profitable than what [CNMs] do." (Clearly, this division of labor does not hold in a nurse midwife–family practitioner team in which neither is trained as an obstetric specialist. In such a structure, both practitioners would perform similar work.)

Physicians' attitudes toward nurse midwives and their philosophies of care were cited by CNMs as crucial factors determining the nature of nurse midwifery practice.

A lot of it seems to hinge on the personal philosophy of the doctor. If the physician seems to feel that someone other than a physician . . . can take on some of the skills and do some of the things that have normally been restricted to doctors; if they believe [it] in their guts and you can demonstrate to them that you're good and you're competent, that you know what you're doing, that you're going to blow the whistle when it needs to be blown [then] you're going to get along. You can do it and create your own sphere of autonomy. [But] if they don't believe that and it's kind of done grudgingly or done because it looks good or because consumers are demanding it, it doesn't work. Because that's when protocol sheets get drawn up. That's when somebody's practice gets curtailed to be "exactly this" or "exactly that," and there's not much leeway to play with.

Another nurse midwife suggested that "the ideal would be to have a small practice with a physician who is fairly liberal." Describing a practice in which she was basically satisfied, one CNM observed:

This is a job where I can almost write my own ticket, as far as I am compatible with this physician. If either of us were different persons, it would be a different story. [But] like a marriage, as long as we're reasonably compatible in terms of philosophy [it works].

However, other nurse midwives worried that physicians might ultimately refuse to relinquish the mainstay of their practice, perhaps by so restricting the concept of normality as to "define us out of existence," as one CNM put it. Consensual delineation of occupational boundaries with nursing was equally problematic.

As nurse midwives attempted to locate turf somewhere between those tasks monopolized by physicians and those monopolized by nurses, each of the other occupations experienced some incursion. However, while physicians have structural power and may choose whether or not to delegate tasks, nurses have few legitimate means of resistance.

The Nurse-Nurse Midwife Relationship

Within the national nurse midwifery organization, ACNM, debates arose about the continued relationship with other nursing organizations and the necessity for RN training before advanced training in midwifery. Further, as nurse midwifery became more visible as a profession, more women who had commitments to feminism or midwifery but not necessarily to nursing entered the occupation.

The population of nurse midwives in Vermont mirrored this trend. While many CNMs considered themselves primarily nurses and had strong ties to nursing, others felt less affinity with the occupation of nursing. Nonetheless, all had had some difficulties with nurses, and all described these with regret. For some, encounters with nursing created a "no-win" situation:

> [My work relationship with nursing] has been kind of mixed. Overall, it has been very positive. There was some confusion about, for example, how much nursing care am I going to give? Am I going to usurp their bedside care? Some people would say, "You're a nurse, if you are going to be with a patient, why aren't you doing the vital signs?" and so forth. Why should I have to do that? There are some people you can't please. If I come in and do nursing care, they're mad because I'm usurping their job. If I don't do nursing care, they think I'm lazy.

For some nurse midwives, particularly those who did not feel an affinity with nursing, their day-to-day work with nurses could be problematic and frustrating:

> It's very tough to get along with nurses because of their passive-aggressive behavior, especially if you're trying to raise people's consciousness or work *with* women and here you have women fighting each other. Nursing is very jealous of the power that they don't have and they take it out in all kinds of devious ways. In some ways [the nurses] see us as a greater threat than [female physicians] because we're nurses; we're "super-nurses."

Behavior patterns such as this are typical of subordinates whose fortunes rest with the pleasure or displeasure of their superordinates in other structures as well. Nurses accurately judge the power of nurse midwives to be subordinate to that of physicians and understand that acting out displeasure at their competition may produce less direct consequences than similar behaviors directed toward physicians. By withholding their willingness to work supportively, nurses could make daily work for nurse midwives extremely uncomfortable.

Sometimes nurse midwives were discouraged about the emergence of a successful division of labor within nursing. Not only were they wary of the potential defensiveness of nurses, but more than one nurse midwife wondered whether with the presence of a reform-oriented nursing staff, much of their work (e.g., labor support) was not redundant.

On the whole, the nurse midwives were deeply concerned about their working relationship with nurses and sought to avoid competition and, ultimately, establish rapport with them. In part, the establishment of a cooperative working relationship was a pragmatic necessity. But there were several other reasons why CNMs avoided conflict with nurses. Some felt a strong sense of colleagueship with nurses; for others, feminist concerns made them unwilling to engage in power struggles with other women. Several CNMs recognized that it was physicians who were calling the tune to which they all danced.

For most nurse midwives, effective ties with the nursing staff were actively sought and maintained. As a nurse midwife noted:

It just took time [to defuse this mistrust]. It just took them getting used to seeing us there. Getting them to realize that we weren't trying to boss them around or take over their role. They still had a role there. We had a role, but we could work together.

The Nurse Midwives' Relationship with Clientele

CNMs typically placed their claims of a special contribution to care giving in the context of standard obstetrical practices. Thus, they emphasized that they brought the philosophy of normality to their care of patients who were experiencing pregnancy, birth, and the postpartum period. One CNM noted, "We have a commitment to keeping the birth normal," while another described it comparatively: "We're more patient than physicians. . . . We don't intervene as fast."

Nurse midwives described the care they gave their patients in terms suggesting that they are client centered, or at least far more client centered than physicians. They noted that they spent much more time with patients than did physicians and they considered patient education to be part of their contribution to care. Emphasizing their responsiveness to consumer desires and attentiveness to individual needs, they described their care giving as "personalized." However, their responsiveness was limited to the turf spelled out in the protocols.

Both nationally and in Vermont, CNMs aligned themselves with hospital birth reform and "prepared" or "natural" childbirth practices. Many of the nurse midwives interviewed considered themselves the embodiment of in-hospital birth reform, describing efforts to reform the institution as part of their work. They provided ongoing support for birthing alternatives for normal births in part through patient advocacy. In this context, their commitment to "keeping the birth normal" takes on new meaning, including at least some resistance to medical intervention when feasible.

A nurse midwife in practice at the University Hospital gave an example:

The residents, a lot of times, want to get their hands in there whether things are normal or not. It's wanting experience. Also, they're responsible. I have a problem with the number of people present at a delivery. People come to us because they don't want a cast of thousands.... [But] what happens depends on who's on [duty]. I can't just tell the resident to leave. I quite often do say, "Would you like to help?" or "Things are all right. I can handle it on my own." And it's up to the resident at that point if they want to be there.

This aspect of their contribution to care provided them with their clientele: patients who desired reformed hospital births and who were not convinced that physicians would provide it. While CNMs in small practices with physicians shouldered part of the work load and promptly made themselves relatively indispensible, the nurse midwives' turf at University Hospital was more fragile and the emergence of a clientele more essential, as one explained: "We're here because the patients want us. They want to have somebody they know there. They want to have a trusting relationship with somebody who's going to deliver their baby. They (correctly) believe we are their advocate." Several CNMs observed that both nationally and locally, growing consumer demand for their services was their critical resource in establishing their turf in the obstetrical division of labor. Their role as patient advocate helped win them their clientele, but the CNMs walked a thin line, as one explained: "We have to be careful not to appear antiphysician."

The birth reform orientation of nurse midwifery is consistent with the historical role of the occupation and is an outgrowth of its noninterventionist orientation to care giving. At the same time, birth reform is a vehicle for CNMs to attempt to redefine the turf in the care of pregnant and birthing women. Informed and active consumers with raised expectations for birth are likely to seek out nurse midwives for their hospital births. Consequently, CNMs may be able to utilize rising consumer demand as a way to expand their scope of practice, resisting physician incursion on their developing task boundaries and establishing a firmer foothold in the medical division of labor. This strategy has been used to advantage by other professionalizing occupations (Kronus, 1976).

CNMs and the Issues of Home Birth and Lay Midwifery

Home birth and lay midwifery were the most volatile issues for nurse midwives, and, not surprisingly, they found it difficult to develop a unified position. However, the emergence of the debate surrounding the legislation to license the practice of lay midwifery drew a response from them, in part because the legislation indicated that a person could be licensed to practice midwifery in the state after either completing the requirements for lay midwives (passing an exam) or holding certification in nurse midwifery. In addition, the legislation called for the board of midwifery to include a nurse midwife. While their primary collective strategy was to withhold public comment on the debate, the nurse midwives did make two public statements, one a statement to the House subcommittee considering the legislation and the other a letter to a Burlington newspaper.

In these statements, the nurse midwives formally distinguished themselves from lay midwives and the legislation, emphasizing that they were already licensed to practice under the Nurse Practice Acts. Seeking to increase the social distance between themselves and their "unprofessional competitors" (Larson, 1977:75), they emphasized their professional training, the ready medical backup that supported them, and the in-hospital birthing alternatives they provided. They disapproved of the legislation, indicating that it did not require adequate training.

In interviews, some CNMs stressed the value of their professional training as a guarantor of their ability that was visible to medical professionals and clients alike. A few CNMs avoided the term *midwife*, choosing instead to systematically distinguish lay from nurse midwifery. And regarding nurse midwifery's efforts to professionalize and seek legitimacy, one CNM complained that "lay midwives muddle the scene." Another echoed her, noting, "One of the problems now is that you can't differentiate who the lay people are, who the professional people are, and what the nurse midwife is."

While lay midwives actively distinguished their philosophy from that of medical workers (including nurse midwives), CNMs, when asked, suggested that their philosophies of care giving were probably not much different from lay midwives'. Instead, they pointed to differences in attitudes toward physicians and hospitals and, more important, to differences in skills. A nurse midwife observed, "Lay midwives feel like they've got the whole market on sensitivity and awareness and psychological responsiveness. I don't think that technical and theoretical training in nurse midwifery school precludes sensitivity."

While each of the nurse midwives interviewed regarded the informal and nonstandardized training of lay midwives a problem, their assessment of the value of lay midwifery varied widely. While one stated that "home is the most dangerous place to have a birth and you've got the least able people out there doing them," another observed, "What lay midwives need from us is training—what we need from them is role models. There is a lot lay midwives can teach nurse midwives about keeping hands off, staying out."

Paralleling this diversity, CNMs spoke with varying levels of ambivalence about home birth. More than one nurse midwife had had a home birth and several considered attending them, though only the CNM in independent practice openly attended home births. Interestingly, when she was faced with the loss of her hospital privileges as a result of physician resistance to her home-birth practice, other nurse midwives quietly supported her, noting that she was practicing legally (she did work under the nominal supervision of a progressive physician who provided her with backup).

Several nurse midwives agreed that there were valid social reasons for desiring home births, but their opinions varied significantly about the safety and viability of home birth in Vermont.

CONCLUSIONS

Seeking both turf and a clientele, emerging occupational collectivities have developed and asserted claims to special contributions to care giving. They have done this to distinguish themselves first from the laity and then from their competitors by asserting the value of their unique expertise and capabilities (Larson, 1977).

The populations to which these claims are directed may vary somewhat with the particular circumstances in which the occupation finds itself. However, occupations typically direct their claims simultaneously to their prospective clientele and legitimate authorities.

The independent midwives, who espoused an ideology of deprofessionalization, were increasingly emerging as a distinctive occupational group with a collective sense, emerging standards of practice, and claims to occupational turf.

Independent midwives narrowed their potential claims in order to fit the practice of lay midwifery into the social and interoccupational context of Vermont. To the public and the state legislature, they pointed to the client revolt as their raison d'être, taking the more defensible position of advocating "freedom of choice among viable options" in childbirth. The distinguishing label "independent midwife" itself suggested a congruence with a Vermont ethic of independence. To the medical establishment, they presented themselves as an uncompetitive occupation serving a preexisting market already outside that monopolized by physicians. Their critique of physicians and hospital practices was muted, and their primary concern was with ending physician harassment and developing working relationships. But even as the lay midwives narrowed their claims about home birth, the physician strategy to eliminate them required that they take the more radical step of challenging physicians' claims to a monopoly on relevant expertise.

The nurse midwives' strategy was professionalization and the creation and maintenance of working relationships with physicians to whom they were legally and structurally subordinate. Most of the physicians, especially those at University Hospital, strongly opposed both home birth and the lay midwifery legislation. However, in contrast with conservative physicians' statements, CNMs did not openly oppose lay midwifery; instead, they called for higher standards of training, leading one disgruntled lay midwife to complain that nurse midwives wanted lay midwives to become CNMs.

In the face of claims made by lay midwives, nurse midwives asserted their own claims to a special contribution to the care of pregnant and birthing women and their families. They claimed that they treated these processes as normal events and actively supported in-hospital birthing alternatives. While a few CNMs worried about physician incursions into their task boundaries (and thus the "naturalness" of their patients' births), they nonetheless regarded themselves as patient advocates and the actors who realized many hospital birth reforms.

Nurse midwives, with the exception of the CNM in independent practice, claimed reformed hospital births as their turf, and when their claims were disputed by physicians, they attempted to function as patient advocates. Their emerging clientele consisted of patients seeking in-hospital birthing alternatives. Nurse midwives attempted to guarantee them these alternatives while simultaneously avoiding alienating the physicians from whom they sought delegated task bundles. On the whole, their strategies were cautious and conservative. As one CNM explained, "Nurse midwives should stand our ground as much as we can; on the other hand, if you make big stands and burn bridges, you'll be on the outside looking in. There are no quick solutions."

In this way, a careful balance was struck between the two occupations who, at least during this period, implicitly honored one another's claims to occupational turf, recognizing that the medical profession, the legislature, and the laity were the likely arbiters of their respective fates.

REFERENCES

Brown, Mrs. Jeffrey L. "Letter to the Editor." *Burlington Free Press,* December 17, 1977.

Calta, Marialisa. "Expert Blasts Home Birth by 'Crazies.'" *The Times Argus,* Barre-Montpelier, Vt., December 9, 1970.

Freidson, Eliot. *The Profession of Medicine.* New York: Harper & Row, 1970.

Haug, Marie, and Susman, Marvin B. "Professional Autonomy and the Revolt of the Client." *Social Problems* 17(1969):153-161.

Illich, Ivan. *Medical Nemesis.* New York: Pantheon/Random House, 1976.

"Joint Statement on Maternity Care." American College of Nurse-Midwives, Washington, D.C., 1971.

Journal of Nurse Midwifery 25(1980):ii.

Kronus, Carol L. "The Evolution of Occupational Power." *Sociology of Work and Occupations* 3(1976):3-37.

Larson, Magali Sarfatti. *The Rise of Professionalism.* Berkeley: University of California Press, 1977.

Litoff, Judy Barrett. *American Midwives: 1860 to the Present.* Westport, Conn.: Greenwood Press, 1978.

NAPSAC News 6(1981):10.

Nolfi, Barbara, "Letter to the Editor." *Vanguard Press,* Burlington, Vt., October 23, 1979.

Parsons, Talcott. "Definitions of Health and Illness in the Light of American Values and Social Structure," in *Social Structure and Personality.* New York: Free Press, 1964, 258-291.

Reilly, John. "Midwives Charge Doctors Uncooperative." *Burlington Free Press,* December 11, 1977.

Rooks, Judith. *Nurse-Midwifery in the United States, 1976-77.* Washington, D.C.: American College of Nurse-Midwives, 1978.

State of Vermont Department of Health, Annual Reports of Vital Statistics, 1975-1979.

Teasley, Regi L. "Birth and the Division of Labor." PhD diss., Michigan State University, 1983.

11

African American Midwives in the South

LINDA JANET HOLMES

Southern African American lay midwives have been responsible for sustaining tradition and cultural continuity within the childbirth experience. Similar to traditional birth attendants worldwide, these midwives have functioned within community values that historically have reinforced culturally prescribed behaviors during labor, birth, and the postpartum period. While only vestiges of these traditions now remain in the United States, midwifery practices have provided the basis for the survival of these traditions since slavery.

Health department officials, medical men, and others responsible for regulating midwifery practice frequently categorize Southern lay midwives as "grannies." The term also has prevailed in the literature. Usually defined as middle-aged or older black women, these midwives acquired most of their skills through apprenticeships and personal childbirth experiences. In addition, most of these midwives also participated in short-term local health department training programs. Although sharing in support for natural childbirth, the Southern lay midwife should be distinguished from the more recently emerging nurse midwife in terms of educational background and ability to obtain practice privileges within medical settings.[1]

As recently as the 1970s, many southern black women continued to maintain a degree of freedom in their practices; even when requirements for obtaining midwife permits mandated that they officially abandon traditional practices, the midwife's empirical wisdom endured. In fact, as long as rural women continued to assist neighbors and relatives at the time of birth, direct opportunities were available to observe and reinforce traditional approaches to labor and birth. Resistance to health department efforts to destroy traditional midwifery was further strengthened by the fact that so many women were familiar with traditional roles and practices. One late nineteenth-century health department official who had the task of registering midwives wrote: "Every other Negro woman was a midwife" (Pierce, 1889). Another health department official commented, "There are as many midwives as there are grains of sand" (Bailey, 1887).

From its beginning, the Medical Association of Alabama, which has functioned as the state board of health since 1875, has tended to recognize the value of the black lay midwife only in circumstances in which medical services are not available. Quite simply, the "granny" midwife was seen as a "necessary evil." This view was reflected in the following statement written by an Alabama physician in a 1912 Alabama Medical Association publication:

> The existence of the midwife, as to numbers, locality and duration, automatically regulates itself. She will ply her art so long as people are too poor to pay a physician such fees as he is willing to take for his work, and so long as people live too far from doctors to obtain them with reasonable certainty for the hour of emergency. In proportion as these factors cease to operate, in measurably the same proportion will the midwife disappear from the scene of action (Cason, 1912:208).

[1]For a historical discussion of the nurse midwife, see Judy B. Litoff, *American Midwives: 1860 to the Present* (Westport, Conn.: Greenwood Press, 1978), 122-134.

THE ALABAMA STUDY

The state of Alabama was particularly appropriate for collecting information on traditional midwives because as recently as 1977, the Alabama Health Department's listing of registered lay midwives included approximately 200 women, an unusually large figure compared to other southern states that eliminated African American midwifery practices in previous decades. Meanwhile, Alabama legislation passed that year prohibited the issuance of new lay midwife permits and provided the impetus for dramatically phasing out remaining lay midwife practices. By 1981 most midwives had been displaced. Medicaid reimbursement to physicians also contributed to the further eradication of midwives by providing an incentive for increased hospital use.

While all the midwives interviewed in the Alabama study had acquired lay midwife permits, they varied substantially in experience. Some women were, indeed, senior midwives who were highly specialized from having attended more than 2,000 births over decades of practice; others had only occasionally assisted neighbors or family members. The project also included a small number of interviews with mothers who had never acted officially as midwives, but who sometimes supported family members and friends at birth.

This chapter will present aspects of the practices and philosophy of Southern African American midwives from a midwifery point of view. I will refer here only briefly to medical assessments of midwifery practices, statistical outcomes, and overall health care policies governing lay midwives. The primary focus will be the opinions of the midwives themselves as expressed in tape-recorded interviews conducted in Alabama in 1981. While scholarly documentation of Southern lay midwife practices are scarce, the Alabama midwife experience generally appears to reflect the historical role and practices of lay African American midwives in other southern states (Robinson, 1982; Mongeau, 1973; Mongeau et al., 1961; Dougherty, 1978 and 1982).

SPIRITUAL DEPTH

All the midwives I interviewed in Alabama believed in the power of divine intervention in the birth process and regularly incorporated various activities in their midwife work to maintain communication with spiritual forces. This spiritual dimension of midwifery is in harmony with a traditional cosmological view that does not fragment the secular and the religious. Many midwives believed that God's presence permeated their lives, but they felt particularly close to Him during a birth. One midwife explained that she had never witnessed a birth without pausing to say, "Thank you, Jesus," when she heard the first cries of a newborn.

Because spiritual depth is highly valued in many African American communities, it is not surprising that individuals who were unrelenting in their recognition of almighty powers occupied multiple leadership positions in their communities. Several midwives were in their church's most recognized position of spiritual wisdom, Mother of the Church. In addition, midwives assumed various leadership positions in missionary organizations, burial societies, and church auxiliaries.

Giving God the credit for successful outcomes in complicated situations and emergencies was common among the midwives. In several instances, when a midwife encountered a complication for the first time, she found strength through prayer. In fact, many of the midwives considered their ability to make rapid and appropriate judgments as much a spiritual experience as it was a synthesis of past technical knowledge. The midwives' specific examples of complications that required the inner confidence of prayer included delivering triplets, managing breech presentations, and delivering a retained placenta.

One midwife, Mrs. Rosie Smith, eighty-four years old, recalled how she relied on spiritual sensibilities in a situation that required her to operate outside the usual limitations of her practice. Although Mrs. Smith's opportunities for formal education were limited, she frequently referred to the value of fireside learning gained from her grandmother, an ex-slave. Having worked many years as a tenant farmer and still living in predominantly black Lowndes County, Mrs. Smith said that her ingenuity came from the Lord:

If they got where they couldn't deliver the afterbirth, then we just had to have a doctor to get it cause we wasn't allowed. Now I did it one time, but I knew it was against the law. I got one one time from a lady. We were a long way.

It was on a Saturday. All the men people were out of place. We didn't have a doctor nearer than Benton. We didn't have nobody to go get the doctor. So the girl laid there but t'wasn't nothing we could do. We put her over the slop jar and it wouldn't come. So finally, I just decided. I said, now I know this is against the law. I hope this don't come against me now. I said, I know this is against the law, but it is against the law for you to lay there in this condition too long. I said, it just won't come. The afterbirth dropped off of the cord and that made it drop back in her abdomen. . . . I had to put my hand inside. I greased my hand and put it inside and lifted up. When I did that, it come right on. Oh, they used to give me all the praises. I just near about knew what to do for a lady. I don't know. The Lord must have put in into me . . . you know, what to do for a lady when she was sick.

Although not a formal prerequisite for midwifery practice, the ability to summon the Holy Ghost for support, guidance, and "miracle working," as the case might require, became apparent in many of the midwives' practices. Even before leaving their homes, these midwives frequently assumed the meditative state of prayer in preparation for attending a birth.

Mrs. Louvenia Taylor Benjamin, eighty-six years old, was another retired midwife who offered personal testimony regarding the power of prayer. Beginning her midwife work in the early 1920s, Mrs. Benjamin also devoted many years to her work as a school principal and teacher in Baldwin County, where she lived. Specifically, Mrs. Benjamin recalled how her personal relationship with God had helped her overcome her nervousness when delivering triplets:

Oh Lord, I always prayed. Oh, yes ma'am, I always prayed. I'd get on my knees and tell the Lord what to do to help me. Anytime, anytime I'd have a case, I would always tell the Lord before I went and then I'd thank Him afterwards, after I delivered. Sometimes I'd do it right there, get on my knees and pray. When I had them three, that's when I talked to the Lord more—I think the Lord got tired of me that night because I was nervous about those three. I just says, Lord, now you come here because I can't do this by myself. I would talk to Him like I was talking to another man. Yes sir. And, I don't care when any of them would come and tell me that they were in labor, I'd get on my knees and tell the Lord about it. I'd say, now Lord, I'd got to go out and get this baby. I can't get him by myself. You have to help me to get him. Everything usually comes out all right. Oh yeah, I prayed. I pray yet. I pray.

Another example of spiritual preparation for the birth event was reflected in the remarks of Mrs. Georgia Richardson, forty-eight years old, who indicated that she attended her first birth nearly thirty years ago. While no longer an active lay midwife, Mrs. Richardson continues to work as a nurse's assistant in a major urban hospital. She recalled that she sometimes asked her husband, a deacon in the church, to pray with her:

I asked God to give me His guidance and understanding and not let anything come that I couldn't handle. I always want Him to be there. And, if it is any complications, I want Him to straighten it. It always worked. And, if I kind of feel myself a little down, I always go to my husband and when he prays I just get things over with. And, I have my Bible. I take my Bible with me and I always read it.

The influence that these women exerted in the birthplace is also directly related to the communitywide respect for individuals who openly expressed their personal relationships with God. Many midwives viewed themselves as providing comfort throughout labor and birth as instruments of the Lord; the power they exercised was primarily God's power. Since midwives often lived in the communities that they served, direct opportunities existed for community members to observe these midwives in acts of propitiation and devotion as witnessed in prayerful responses, heartful moaning, and singing. As a result, some midwives were respected as spiritual forces even by individuals who may have never called on them for their midwifery services.

A prominent minister who headed one of Montgomery's major black Baptist churches recalled the status that his grandmother, a midwife, occupied in the rural community where he grew up. The minister explained, "Her hands looked like the gift of God. When a woman was having a baby, just seeing her there somehow let them know that everything was all right" (Carver, 1981). This particular midwife's preparation for birth included reading the Bible and drenching her hands in olive oil, which was then rubbed on the mother's stomach while asking for the Lord's blessings.

In fact, actual entry into midwife practice was often initiated by supernatural calls in the forms of visions or dreams. These kinds of spiritual calls received special consideration from senior midwives when they determined the readiness of younger women for midwifery apprenticeships. Several midwives also spoke of having spiritually inherited midwifery practices from living and dead family members.

Mrs. Lizzie Major, fifty-nine, who practiced as a midwife only briefly, explained how it was revealed to her at the age of thirty-eight that she was to work assisting the sick in her small rural community. Mrs. Major told of the significance of her heeding the call to do midwife work:

> I prayed. I asked the Lord to give me a job or something to do and that's what He showed me to do and I didn't do that at the time He showed me what to do. After I didn't do that at the time He showed me, I got down sick, but didn't no where hurt me. So I told Him, if that what He had for me to do, I would do it. I got just as healthy as if I were a child. I sure did the whole time I was in that field I never did feel bad. I never did get sick no more.

The fact that many midwives viewed themselves as being chosen for midwifery was also supported by what they considered to be unusual childhood interests in caring for the sick. This concern for the sick in the community was also expressed in their adult lives. An ability to heal through the laying on of hands is a specific example of the kinds of activities that sometimes preceded midwifery.

Mrs. Mattie Hereford, eighty-one years old, was another woman with a long-term interest in care for the sick. As a midwife, Mrs. Hereford attended more than 900 births and served as president of the Lay Midwives Organization of Madison County until her death in 1982. While she lived for many years in a middle-income community in Huntsville with her husband and other members of her family, Mrs. Hereford possessed vivid memories of tenant farm life:

Well, anytime anybody—there were about eighteen families on that farm—anytime anyone got sick and went to the bossman and told him that they wanted a doctor for so and so and they were going to the hospital, he'd tell 'em, well, go tell Matt. I'll go get Matt and let Matt stay with 'em until the doctor gets there. Well, now I did that for eight to ten years before I came to be a midwife. Didn't care what was the matter, night or day, people would come and get me.

The fact that midwifery abilities were sometimes viewed as a spiritual gift created some ambivalence among midwives regarding payment.[2] Although midwifery has not always been defined as a form of employment, most midwives expected a fee for their services. Health department rules also frequently fixed midwife fees. When beginning their practices, many midwives recalled charging two or three dollars per delivery, as well as frequently receiving payments in kind. Several midwives, however, also acknowledged that the opportunity that midwifery work provided for independent moneymaking was a motivating factor. Yet nearly all midwives provided care in several instances when no payment was expected. Midwife Smith expressed both a characteristic disappointment in lack of payment and an acceptance of the intangible rewards that comes from providing charitable acts:

I had a Christian heart about that. If they didn't have nothing, I didn't worry 'em for nothing. I figured if they had the right kind of heart, when they got something, they would give me something. Some of them—some of the poorest ones—I went in and they would have my money under their pillows somewhere where they could give it to me. Now you take some of these call themselves living well, I ain't got their money now. I'll have it Saturday. I ain't never seen them no more. Some children in the world grown and I don't know them and I don't know their parents neither and I ain't never got a dime from them. That was real disencouragement. I was so patient with people and I was so nice to people and then I would come out so bad sometimes. My husband used to tell me a lot of times, they used to laugh

---

[2]For another discussion of midwife attitudes regarding payment, see Marie Campbell, *Folks Do Get Born* (New York: Rinehart Company, 1946), 44-48.

at me. They thought I ought to compel people to the money, but you know a person got a job—don't nobody know like you. My husband used to tell me somtimes, he said, when Rosie come in the gate, I can tell when she ain't got paid. Sometimes she come in the gate, she got a smile on her. She looked happy. If she looked dry and pitiful, I know she ain't got nothing.

Appropriate models of midwifery behavior were also generally outlined in terms of Christian virtues. Along with spirituality, good morals, patience, kindness, and temperance often were cited as midwifery attributes. While not all midwives were regular churchgoers, community members generally expected a midwife to be kindhearted and to have good moral character.

Mrs. Thelma Shamburger, now retired and living in the highly industrialized section of Plateau in Mobile, began her midwife work forty-one years ago. Having attended an estimated 3,000 babies both in rural Wilcox County and in Mobile County, Mrs. Shamburger served as president of the Mobile County Midwife Association for nearly thirty years. Unlike the overwhelming majority of the midwives, Mrs. Shamburger never married or had children. She explained the kind of behavior that she believed midwifery required:

You dedicate yourself. I don't think I missed two cases in my whole time. No use to being a midwife being over yonder dancing. No use to being a midwife being over yonder on the party, they got to look for you. If you got patients, due three in the month, stick around and wait for them.

POSTPARTUM TRADITIONS

Midwives have acted as significant tradition bearers in maintaining various customs and rituals, particularly in the postpartum period. Some of these traditions have African origins. There are similarities, for example, between African American descriptions of the postpartum seclusion period and the description of rituals among the Akamba and the Gikuyu (Mbiti, 1969:148-149). Similar to the cultural patterns that remain in other aspects of African American life, the fact that this tapestry of childbirth practices has withstood tendencies by the dominant society to eliminate them is testimony to their strength. Of course, long-term contact with Native Americans and local whites has modified many of these practices. The collective adherence to tradition by many senior women in the community, however, has provided an effective base for midwives to maintain many aspects of these practices.

The midwife was responsible for instructing the mother in the performance of prescribed precautionary measures during the particularly vulnerable postpartum period and overseeing rites to celebrate and protect the newborn. Since the acceptance of a range of living spirits, good and evil, is not unusual, the community valued the midwives' roles in providing instructions on how to mitigate such forces during the postpartum period. While only a limited number of senior midwives in the Alabama study could recall their personal roles in presiding over these once-essential practices, most midwives could recall the responsibilities of senior midwives who waited on them in childbirth.

One of the functions that the midwife performed with care and sometimes with ceremony was preparing for the burying of the afterbirth. Although the disposal of the afterbirth was an obvious public health concern, the meticulous care provided for it also reflected the pervasive view that the afterbirth was an extension of the human body, a part of life. The specific procedure for its burial often included sprinkling it with a handful of salt, making certain that it was buried deeply in the ground, at least three to four feet under the earth, selecting a spot that was near the house and highly visible, and sometimes covering it with a rock or turned over tub with a rock on top. The belief that animal or human tampering with the afterbirth would adversely affect the mother's health was another reason for ensuring that the afterbirth was properly buried.

Tradition also dictated special treatment of the fire that was burning at the time of birth. This special fire has been identified as a ceremonial birth fire (Goldsmith, 1984:85). There are specific African practices that have survived in the United States forbidding removal of fire from the ceremonial birth fire that was maintained continually throughout the initial postpartum period. Custom also dictated that the ashes from the birth fire be safeguarded for a prescribed period of time. Nathefenia Davis, who lives in rural Dallas County and is still in her childbearing years, explained: "It would be a month before they threw the ashes away. If you smoked a cigarette in there, you couldn't take fire out of the fireplace where they burned the afterbirth."

Another one of the midwife's important duties in the postpartum period was to officiate in "taking the mother up." This ritual, which provides for a reintegration of the mother into her everyday role, involved taking the mother outdoors for the first time. In some instances, this ceremony also included smoking the mother's undergarments and/or outer clothing with the bran sifted from cornmeal as a method of purification.[3] The "taking up" ceremony occurred anywhere from three days to a month after the birth. Women recalled midwives permitting them to walk around the perimeter of the house on the ninth or tenth day after childbirth, while other midwives required a month-long period of seclusion. Other variations in the taking-up ceremony included differences in whether it was customary to pray, sing, call in the baby's spirit when returning to the house, or carry a thimble of water that was to be swallowed after returning indoors. In any case, there was a certain dramatic element in this ceremony that is reflected in Mrs. Richardson's following description of the practice:

The old midwife would be there. They would take 'em around the house—them and the baby around the house. And a heap of them never get out. Used to hear my grandmother saying that when they see the light, they will faint and that's why they be there to get 'em back in the bed. Then the next time they would get 'em and take 'em around the house and they would carry a chair, take a chair with them. And if they would get tired or feel like they're going to faint again, you have the chair and let them sit in it until they go all the way around the house. They take 'em all the way around the house—the mother. Then the old midwife would take the baby and go all the away around the house.

[3]For another description of "smoking" practices, see Ruby A. Tart, "Carry Dykes—Midwife," in *From Hell to Breakfast*, ed. Mody C. Boatright and Donald Day (Dallas: Southern Methodist University Press, 1944).

Mrs. Hannah Williams, ninety-seven years old, attached particular significance to performing this ritual. In rural Butler County where Mrs. Williams assisted many women in childbirth, this retired midwife said she often recited the Lord's prayer or sang a hymn as she carried the infant around the house. Mrs. Williams also recalled the influence a midwife could exert on a growing child: "If you are a good woman, doing good work, when you take the baby around the house you say, don't be like your mother. Don't be like your father. Be like your sister or your granny who brought you in this world."

In a custom reminiscent of African naming ceremonies, midwives sometimes named babies after walking around the house with the infant. Generally speaking, the midwife's association with these postpartum practices strengthened her position in the community as long as such traditions were valued.

PHILOSOPHICAL VIEW

Most of the midwives defined birth as a healthy and normal event requiring little or no technological intervention in most cases. Regardless of educational background and experience, the midwives emphasized that their extended supportive roles in being with women during labor and birth provided a qualitatively different birth experience from orthodox medical management.

The ability to view birth as a natural phenomenon was strengthened by the many opportunities southern black women had to observe births and by their own birth experiences. In the past, countless women either chose or were forced to give birth without a birth attendant of any kind. Even when relatives were nearby, some women selected to accept responsibility for their own care. Mrs. Richardson recalled her own birth experience before becoming a midwife:

I didn't even let them know that I was in labor. I got up. I fixed my bed. I got my clothes out and everything. Those pains were eating me up and I got up and I took my left hand and I lifted up my stomach. I walked all the way around the bed. Sometime that pain hit me so hard I had to take both of my hands and hold my stomach. I didn't grunt. I wouldn't let my mother know nothing about it. And my brother heard that I was being sick. He knew I was sick because I didn't have no business being up that time of night. It was around two o'clock. So I walked around there and I was beginning to get where I couldn't walk. I just couldn't hardly walk. I got down at the foot of the bed. I couldn't get back to the other end of the bed. One mind said, now you just get in that bed and push your baby on out. So I just got in that bed and I reached down and I grabbed these here feet, and I was waiting on the next pain. When the next pain came, I pushed that baby on out and I called and say, hey, mama. The baby said, whaaa. She said, that baby's being born.

In many situations, Alabama women expressed matter-of-fact attitudes about past birth experiences and simply refused to view birth as a complicated situation. For them, birth was a natural, spontaneous event. Nevertheless, there were instances in which women sought assistance at the time of birth but were denied medical care; however, it should be understood that remaining active throughout labor and simply catching one's own baby with minimal assistance from other women had been both the traditional way and the chosen way for many childbearing women (Anderson and Anderson, 1982:183–184).

Mrs. Smith commented:

I never hardly had no trouble with my pains. Most of the times, I be done birthed my babies when the midwife got there and if I didn't be done birthing them, they wouldn't have much trouble before my babies would come out. I delivered all my babies pretty good. Well, I would walk around long as I felt good enough to walk around. Some of 'em I found in the bed. And some of them, I found them on the floor. I just put a little pallet on the floor and get down on my knees.

Although there were instances in which women described being alone at childbirth, most recalled birth experiences that included social interaction. For example, Mrs. Thelma Caver, forty-six, never practiced as a midwife but often attended births in her rural community. She explained that with the majority of families living in two-room houses—a bedroom and a kitchen—everyone would naturally surround the mother at the time of birth. Mrs. Caver, who began her childbearing years when she married at the age of fifteen, described the kind of supportive roles that women shared:

When I was younger and I had good nerve, I was with a lot of people that had babies. In fact, I was with one woman by myself one time. I was kind of scared cause I was pregnant myself. They always told me, the old saying say, if you are pregnant, you shouldn't be around another woman having a baby. So I was kind of scared to be around that woman, but I didn't have no other choice. We lived real close together and her husband left to get the midwife. At that particular time, there weren't any cars. They walked to get the midwife. It was just a thing when a woman got ready to have her baby, all the women would go and try to help out.

So entrenched were many midwives in community-based experiences and values that midwives continued to support a variety of practices that lacked official medical sanction. The use of various labor stimulants such as castor oil, ginger tea, black pepper tea, and May Apple root is one example. The refusal to forgo traditional birth positions is another. Many Alabama midwives were adamant in their support of alternative birth positions, such as getting down on one's knees, using a chair for a head-down-on-chair position, and sitting halfway down against a turned over chair. Recently, interest in natural childbirth has led to greater scientific investigation and documentation of the worth of a variety of practices that minimize technological intervention (Cadeyro-Barcia, 1985:22–26; Thacker and Banta, 1983; Flynn, et al., 1978). From time immemorial, however, midwives have asserted that providing a supportive birth environment, remaining ambulant during labor, and using upright birth positions are all helpful during birth.

Mrs. Margaret Smith, a seventy-five-year-old midwife, described how she accepted and encouraged various birth positions. Having worked for more than thirty years in predominantly rural and low-income Greene County, Mrs.

Smith continues to maintain her basic attitudes regarding the appropriate approach to childbirth, even though she no longer practices:

But you know we were told not to let them deliver on the floor. But when you in misery, if there is any way you can ease that misery, you gonna ease it. You are not going to try to make nobody worse than what they are feeling. And, if they want to throw a quilt down on that floor and they get down on their knees, I let them do it and catch it behind them and let them get back in the bed. That's just the way I have done it several times.

CURRENT DILEMMAS

Despite the burgeoning interest in childbirth alternatives, the decline of traditional midwifery within southern black communities continues for several reasons. Although as recently as the 1950s, significant numbers of black women were attended by midwives, traditional practices were sacrificed in most instances when women could obtain obstetrical care. Similar to Third World women who adopted bottle-feeding because they associated this feeding practice with upper-income groups, southern blacks sometimes abandoned the midwife because hospital birth symbolized social and economic status. In fact, the failure of the certified nurse midwife to elicit significant interest and support in middle-income black communities may reflect lingering associations of the "granny" midwife with second-class health care and poverty (Robinson, 1984:250).

Midwives now face a formidable medical superstructure in efforts to reclaim their position in the field of birth. Southern black lay midwives in particular have lacked the organization and political leverage needed to counter the medical profession's high-powered antimidwife campaigns. Although the medical profession has been prone to link the high maternal and infant mortality rates that have plagued the South with the presence of lay midwives, economics factors (including a large rural, poor, and black population) remain the most salient ones affecting birth outcomes. Specific maternal and child health concerns among Southern black women continue to be the effects of nutritional deficiencies, parity, spacing of children, general environmental conditions, access to prenatal care, and the availability of emergency medical support. In a recent anti–lay midwife medical study of neonatal outcomes over an eleven-year period in Alabama, in only three years did neonatal mortality differ significantly for nonwhite high-risk mothers having their babies at home. The study did find significant increases in neonatal mortality for the few remaining white out-of-hospital deliveries. Birth weights for home births, however, did not differ significantly from those of in-hospital births for both blacks and whites (Goldenberg et al., 1983:689).

While many Alabama local health departments have reported excellent outcomes overall for the experienced midwives practicing in their districts, the truth remains hidden. These mostly middle-aged and older low-income black women have had little opportunity for formal education and historically have been denied access to mechanisms for influencing policies and regulations that govern midwifery practices and training programs. In short, they lack political power.

The most recent manifestation of this lack of political power has been the ability of local health department officials to phase out currently licensed and practicing midwives with little or no notification. A poignant example of official attitudes toward current midwife practices is reflected in a letter from the Autauga County Health Department addressed to Autauga midwives, dated April 14, 1978, which reads:

> Because of the "lay" or "granny" midwife law passed last year by Alabama State Legislature, there are many changes in the law. You must have an Autauga County physician (member of Autauga County Medical Society) that you could call in "case of emergency or complications of labor, delivery of infant." Since none of Autauga County physicians deliver babies you will have no one to call. Also, your permit must be signed by the Chairman of the Board of Health (a Prattville physician) and they will no longer do this. Therefore, as of this date, April 15, you are *not* to deliver any babies. To do so is against the law and could lead to prosecution.

Women living in Autauga County must now use major hospitals in neighboring counties for maternity care because there are currently no in-hospital obstetrical units in Autauga County.

In 1983, the governor of Alabama, George Wallace, reiterated the state's opposition to lay midwifery. In a letter addressed to the members of a small rural community in Autauga County, who had written the governor in support of lay midwives, Wallace expressed direct opposition to home birth. "I support the concept of providing a hospital birth for all pregnant women in our State," the Governor said (Wallace, 1983). While endorsing programs to train nurse midwives, Wallace cited the lack of basic skills such as checking blood pressures and monitoring fetal heartbeats as reasons for eliminating the lay midwife. Even when lay midwives do possess such skills, however, specific health department policies have tended to prohibit them from rendering care that is considered to be within the realm of nursing. For the most part, midwives who have expressed interest in officially expanding their roles in the birthplace have not been offered opportunities or support for effectively expanding their knowledge base.

Despite dominant medicine's long-term efforts to limit the midwife's roles, traditional midwives have always been much more than birth assistants. Most recently, they have acted as advocates for women in clinics and hospital settings; historically, they have been family counselors, herbologists, household assistants, and general care providers for various members of the community. In fact, many midwives continue to occupy positions of esteem even though they may no longer practice as midwives. Indeed, celebration of the common traits that successful midwives tend to possess—independence, spirituality, straightforwardness, and nerve—is ongoing.

While the ubiquitous presence of traditional birth attendants worldwide has demanded varying degrees of public and community support, the United States historically has offered little legal protection for the traditional African American Midwife (Owens, 1983:445–447). There is beginning, however, to be some increased recognition of the benefits of selected aspects of traditional birth practices. Nevertheless, the women, as practitioners, continue to be denigrated. Certainly, those midwives who have demonstrated their skills and have provided culturally sensitive care to women in their communities for generations are worthy of the broad-based political support needed to guarantee the survival of their occupation.

REFERENCES

Anderson, Helen K., and Anderson, Richard N. "Traditional Onitsha Ibo Maternity Beliefs." In *Anthropology of Human Birth*, edited by Margarita Kay. Philadelphia: F. A. Davis, 1982.

Bailey, [?], Talladega County. Letter to Jerome Cochran, State Health Officer, December 28, 1887. State Health Department Records, Alabama Department of Archives and History, Montgomery.

Cadeyro-Barcia, R. "Position of the Mother During Labor and Birth." Paper discussed at Interregional Conference on Appropriate Technology for Birth, World Health Organization, Fortaleza, Brazil, April 1985, 22–26.

Carver, George Washington, minister. Interview, Montgomery, Alabama, November 24, 1981.

Cason, Eugene P. "Obstetrical Work in Alabama." *Transactions of the Medical Association of the State of Alabama*, meeting of 1912, 207–211.

Dougherty, Molly C. "Southern Lay Midwives as Ritual Specialists." In *Women in Ritual and Symbolic Roles*, edited by Judith Hoch-Smith and Anita Spring. New York: Plenum Press, 1978.

———. "Southern Midwifery and Organized Health Care: Systems in Conflict." *Medical Anthropology* 6(1982):113–126.

Flynn, A. M.; Kelly, J.; Hollins, G.; and Lynch, P. F. "Ambulation in Labor." *British Medical Journal* 2(August 1978):591–593.

Goldenberg, Robert L.; Hale, Christiane B.; Houde, John; Humphrey, Joan L.; Wayne, John B.; and Boyd, Beverly W. "Neonatal Deaths in Alabama: III. Out-of-hospital Births, 1940–1980," *American Journal of Obstetrics and Gynecology* 147(November 1983).

Goldsmith, Judith. *Childbirth Wisdom*. New York: Congdon & Weed, 1984.

Mbiti, John S. "Birth and Childhood," in *African Religions and Philosophy*. New York: Doubleday, 1969.

Mongeau, Beatrice. "The 'Granny' Midwives: A Study of a Folk Institution in the Process of Social Disintegration." PhD diss., University of North Carolina, 1973.

Mongeau, Beatrice; Smith, Harvey L.; and Maney, Ann C. "The 'Granny' Midwife: Changing Roles and Functions of a Folk Practitioner." *American Journal of Sociology* 66(1960):497–505.

Owens, Margaret. "Laws and Policies Affecting the Training and Practice of Traditional Birth Attendants." *International Digest of Health Legislation* 23(1983):441–473.

Pierce, Thomas W., Greene County. Letter to Jerome Cochran, State Health Officer, April 28, 1889. State Health Department Records, Alabama Department of Archives and History, Montgomery.

Robinson, Beverly J. *Aunt (ant) Phyllis.* Los Angeles: Women's Graphic Center, 1982.

Robinson, Sharon. "A Historical Development of Midwifery in the Black Community, 1600-1940." *Journal of Nurse Midwifery* 29(July/August 1984):247-254.

Thacker, Stephen B., and Banta, David H. "Benefits and Risks of Episiotomy: An Interpretive Review of the English Language Literature, 1860-1980." *Obstetrical and Gynecological Review* 38(June 1983):322-338.

Wallace, Governor George C. Letter to the Jones Community, November 16, 1983, in response to community correspondence expressing support for the renewal of lay midwife permits for Mrs. Lula Moten and other midwives in Autauga County, Alabama.

12

Unionizing Midwifery in California

DEBORAH LEVEEN

The readmission of midwives[1] into the established medical system can be viewed as a major victory by feminists, childbirth advocates, and others seeking transformation of the health care system. For feminists, midwives represent a challenge to the male-dominated, technologically invasive medical system. For childbirth advocates, midwifery represents a return to a more humane, family-centered experience of birth. For those seeking more general kinds of health care transformation, midwifery represents the demedicalization of American society, the democratization of the health profession, and the rationalization of the health care system through an emphasis on cost-effective preventive care. And to all of these groups, the reacceptance of midwifery represents

[1] Although the focus of this paper is on nurse midwives—midwives who are registered nurses and who have had formal midwifery training—the term *midwives* will generally be used throughout the paper. Neither the midwives nor most of the other people I spoke with use the more formal terminology, and there may be substantive reasons as well as convenience in using the shorter term: the term *midwives* emphasizes their continuity with a broader historical tradition of midwifery.

292

the possibility of significant change through grassroots, self-help kinds of efforts—indeed, transforming the system quite literally "with our own hands."[2]

At the same time, the process of institutionalizing midwifery care—that is, gaining permanent acceptance of and support for midwifery care from the dominant institutions of the health care system—is problematic at best. First of all, simply gaining access to the system remains difficult. Training, licensing, definition of scope of practice, and access to other conditions necessary to practice—such as physician supervision, malpractice insurance, third-party reimbursement, and hospital privileges—are dominated by the established medical profession. In most states, only certified nurse midwives are allowed to practice—midwives who have been trained and licensed as registered nurses and who have in addition had one or two years of midwifery training and have been certified by the American College of Nurse Midwives (ACNM). Lay midwives—midwives whose training is more eclectic and who are not ACNM certified—are for the most part limited to home births. And given the continuing threat posed by midwives to established obstetricians—the threat of economic competition, which is growing steadily as the number of obstetricians increases disproportionately to the birth rate, and the threat of professional competition, as midwives offer a direct challenge to the established medical model of childbirth—many physicians still refuse to provide the support needed to allow nurse midwives to practice.

Furthermore, even those midwives who have found opportunities to practice face significant pressures against their efforts to offer midwifery care, both economic (pressures to spend less time, to see more patients in order to generate more

[2] The resurgence of midwifery has been acclaimed by many writers. For the essential feminist perspective, Rich (1976) is one of the best sources. Most advocates of midwifery as a means of reclaiming childbirth are also feminists: Arms (1975), Corea (1977), Rothman (1982). At the same time, some childbirth reformers advocate midwifery from a more traditional perspective, as Rothman makes clear. Edwards and Waldorf (1984) provide a comprehensive account of the entire childbirth reform movement. As far as the role of midwives in helping to create broader transformations of the health care system, certainly they illustrate the need for demedicalization advocated by Illich (1976) and the kind of democratization, humanization, and rationalization advocated by Victor and Ruth Sidel (1983).

revenue) and professional (pressures to use more intervention and to use them sooner than the midwifery model would prescribe). And there are additional pressures stemming simply from the nature of the hospital context that make it difficult to offer midwifery care.

Indeed, there is some question whether midwifery care can really be offered by nurse midwives in hospital settings (Arms, 1975:197-206; Rothman, 1982:71-77, 245-274). And if midwifery cannot be practiced within a hospital context, the readmission of midwives may represent not significant institutional change but rather another instance of cooptation, in which those seeking change are absorbed into the established institutions as a means of gaining control over them and reducing the pressure for change (DeClerq, 1983:167; Ruzek, 1980:336).

Certainly there are elements of cooptation in the readmission of nurse midwives: nurse midwives are much more acceptable to the health care establishment than are lay midwives attending home births. And certainly there are serious limits on the practice of midwifery in hospital settings, as well as powerful pressures to modify the substance of midwifery to accommodate those limits.

Nevertheless, it would be premature to conclude that the readmission of midwives offers no hope for a broader transformation of the health care system. Cooptation may be one of the motives for those who have offered nurse midwives the chance to practice. But unless those midwives abandon their commitment to midwifery and adopt the values as well as the practices of the dominant institutions, they have not been coopted. Indeed, some would argue that adopting the appearance of cooptation is a major strategy for change, allowing those seeking change "to get a foot in the door" and thereby establish the basis for more extensive institutional change.

This raises significant questions about the prospects for institutionalizing midwifery care and the most effective strategies for enhancing those prospects. This chapter will address these questions by examining the experience of nurse midwives in seven county hospitals in California and then focusing on the efforts of the Highland General Hospital midwife service, which adopted an unusually militant strategy in its efforts to institutionalize midwifery care.

I will begin by reviewing the conditions under which midwives have been readmitted into the health care system and the conflicts between those conditions and the conditions necessary to the provision of effective midwifery care, for it is those conflicts that impede the institutionalization of midwifery care. Then I will examine some of the ways in which midwives have responded to these conflicts, along with the strategies that have been adopted to increase the prospects of institutionalization.

METHODS

Most of the field research for this paper was conducted during a sabbatical leave in 1982. I visited various midwife services and interviewed (in person and/or over the phone) midwives, doctors, and administrators. In addition, I worked with the Highland General Hospital midwives during their contract negotiations; I served as a recorder during the bargaining sessions and helped prepare analyses to be used in the negotiations. This allowed me to spend a great deal of time with them in a wide variety of settings and thus repeatedly to hear and observe their central concerns. I have continued to work with the Highland midwives; I have also maintained contact with most of the others whom I interviewed in 1982, allowing me to update my analysis of their situations. In describing the experience of midwife services in general, I have drawn upon the cumulative research, quoting occasionally but not identifying particular sites or sources. All of the quotations are from my field notes. The seven county midwife services that are described in this chapter are Fresno, Highland, Humboldt, Los Angeles, San Diego, San Francisco, and San Luis Obispo.

THE READMISSION OF MIDWIVES INTO THE MEDICAL SYSTEM

Three major reasons for the readmission of nurse midwives into the established medical system are generally recognized: 1) consumer pressure, 2) concern with health staffing shortages in medically underserved areas, and 3) the professional interests of obstetricians. Consumer pressure has been expressed through both the home-birth movement and the pressure for more humanized hospital birth. The women's health movement more generally, along with a stable or falling birth rate, has helped intensify this pressure (Ruzek, 1980:348). This pressure has resulted in institutional changes such as the creation of alternative birthing centers within hospitals, the passage of legislation allowing the certification of nurse midwives, and, to a more limited extent, the hiring of nurse midwives.

The concern with health staffing shortages has been expressed by public health officials concerned with the needs of low-income populations (Germano, 1979:6–7). Nurse midwives have been seen as a cost-effective means of providing care in areas shunned by the dominant medical establishment because of its preference for more lucrative and congenial practice sites. Thus while not entirely absent, medical opposition to practice by nurse midwives in medically underserved areas has been weaker than its opposition elsewhere, and it has been possible to establish nurse midwifery programs in such areas.

The third, more recent reason for the increased acceptance of nurse midwives is the professional interests of obstetricians. As articulated in a 1981 presidential address by J. Robert Willson to an annual meeting of obstetricians and gynecologists, obstetricians are grossly overtrained for the routine tasks that occupy much of their practice and consequently "may do them reluctantly and less well than do nonphysician associates prepared specifically for that purpose" (Willson, 1981:860). He recommended that most "primary care" be delegated to nurse practitioners and nurse midwives, freeing obstetricians for more specialized work. And although Willson did not mention this in his address, the more specialized work is also the more lucrative work and hence is a better use of the physician's time in terms of financial as well as professional interest.

The California Situation: Support for Nurse Midwives

Support for midwives in the seven California counties reflects all three of these general factors. Consumer pressure for midwifery has been extremely strong in the state, as has competition for maternity patients. California achieved national renown for its home-birth movement, and the fact that the number of in-hospital alternative birth centers (ABCs) in-creased from three to seventy between 1975 and 1978 is strong evidence of the effectiveness of more conventional consumer pressure (DeVries, 1980:50).

And consumer pressure, along with the competition for maternity patients, has affected county hospitals. In the rural counties, the desire to limit home births was an important factor in the establishment of midwife services. In the urban counties, it was a need to reverse the dramatic decline in county hospital use, in large part the result of the MediCal (California's version of Medicaid) program, which allowed women to go to any physician and hospital that accepted MediCal (Blake and Bodenheimer, 1974:335), that increased the hospitals' willingness to try new ways of attracting patients. This was particularly important in teaching hospi-tals, which are associated with four of the seven county mid-wife services. As the chief resident at one of them said, "Eight years ago patients were precious, and so we had to be creative, use gimmicks, to find new patient material for the medical school."

Public health concern with medically underserved areas has also been important. The state's Department of Health Ser-vices has a long-standing tradition of supporting the use of nurse midwives in medically underserved areas, dating back to the Madera County demonstration project in 1960 and continuing through various initiatives during the 1970s (Kouyoumdjian, 1983:4–18). California public health officials see midwives as providing cost-effective prenatal care, helping to reduce the costs of caring for preventable infant morbidity. All but one of the county hospitals had a state grant to help start and in some cases maintain their midwife services. Federal support was also important: three of the county hospi-tals had federal grants for nurse midwife educational pro-grams as well.

Professional physician interest in using midwives has also been present; several of the doctors I interviewed cited the Willson address. They prefer the more specialized work not only because it is more professionally challenging but also because it is much more lucrative than routine care and has a more predictable schedule. Most private physicians also expect midwives to be cost-effective. That is, through a com-bination of referrals generated for more specialized and lucrative work for the doctors and revenues for midwives' own work, to generate more than enough revenue to cover their costs to their employers.

In sum, then, midwives have benefited in their efforts to reenter the medical system from the strong support of certain members of the system. Indeed, for whatever combination of reasons, midwives in most of the county sites have had strong "institutional patrons"—doctors or public health officials willing to use their influence to help establish and maintain the midwife service. At the same time, however, nurse midwives have been readmitted because they meet certain specific needs and interests of those who control access to the system. Those interests essentially define the terms under which midwives can practice, and they do not always coincide with the midwives' orientation to their work or with the conditions necessary to providing effective midwifery care.

Conflict between the Terms of Midwifery Practice and the Needs of Midwifery Care

The key source of conflict between the terms of midwifery practice and the needs of midwifery care revolves around the issue of time and the costs of supporting time-intensive care. Good midwifery care requires much more time than standard or even high-quality obstetric care. Midwifery requires the time needed to develop a personal relationship with a woman, to educate her in the importance of prenatal health, to ensure that she receives whatever additional services (nutritional, psychosocial, and so on) she might require, and, finally, to stay with her during labor (labor sitting) and to provide support in order to maximize her sense of control in the birthing process and minimize the need for drugs or other interventions. Midwives are known for spending about a half-hour per routine prenatal visit (Dempkowski, 1982:11) while some doctors estimate three to five minutes as sufficient. Midwives are committed to being with women through active labor; most doctors are present only for periodic checks, if necessary, and at the final moments of delivery.

This kind of time-intensive care is extremely costly, requiring more staff time per patient, hence more costs per unit of service, and more costs relative to the revenues generated, which are based on units of service rather than units of time.

The problem is compounded by the fact already noted that routine obstetrics is less well reimbursed than more specialized obstetrics or gynecological surgery; indeed, most obstetricians try to limit the amount of their practice devoted to routine obstetrics and often regard the more lucrative work as subsidizing the lower-paying care. As already noted, this is one of the main reasons why doctors have been willing to cede normal obstetrical practice to midwives: if midwives cost less than doctors, and they can both generate referrals and free doctors for more lucrative tasks, they may be quite attractive from the perspective of cost-effectiveness. However, the physicians' desire for cost-effectiveness conflicts sharply with the midwives' desire to provide more time-intensive care.

The problem of cost-effectiveness is particularly acute in county hospitals in which public-sector reimbursements for obstetrical care are much lower—by a half to two-thirds—than private-sector reimbursements. Here there is even greater pressure to maximize the number of patients seen and thus reduce the time spent with them; yet there is also a greater need for midwifery care—for the extra support and support services—because of the high concentration of medical and socioeconomic risk factors among low-income women.

The conflict over time and cost-effectiveness may reflect an underlying philosophical difference between doctors and midwives. Doctors try to minimize the time they spend in routine obstetrical care not simply because of financial considerations but also because of professional interest in more specialized care. But this may entail more than the sense of being overtrained for routine obstetrics; it suggests that they find routine obstetrics "boring," as one put it; or, as another doctor who was extremely supportive of midwives said, he didn't want to do "all that shit" that midwives do. Thus, to doctors, the kind of caring for pregnant women that midwives offer is not as interesting and perhaps not even as important as nonroutine care.

Needless to say, this view of the inherent interest and importance of extensive caring for pregnant women conflicts dramatically with that held by midwives. Supporting a woman, ultimately empowering her—giving her not simply a better understanding or her health needs but the sense that she did it, she birthed her baby—this is what excites midwives.

The contrast between their view of pregnancy and birth and that of doctors is a fundamental source of conflict between obstetricians and midwives, surfacing continually in the doctors' failure to appreciate or support the time commitment that midwives want to make.

The county hospital context creates additional pressures against midwifery care. As Rothman (1982:245–274) has argued, the hospital setting itself, with its rigid scheduling of scarce resources, mitigates against the midwives' individualistic and time-intensive approach to labor and delivery; in county hospitals, where resources are even scarcer, these pressures may be still greater. County hospitals are notorious for their staffing and management problems. Understaffing translates into higher work loads for midwives, hence less time for midwifery care. Management problems make it difficult to obtain the coordinated support services that are often critical to the patients served by county hospitals. Finally, the time pressures created by high caseloads and low levels of staffing, along with professional pressures if the hospital is a teaching facility, may force midwives to resort to medical interventions more frequently and earlier than they otherwise would choose.

Lastly, midwives for the most part have a relatively strong sense of independence: if they began as RNs, a major reason for choosing to become midwives was to increase their professional autonomy; if they began as lay midwives attending home births, they were essentially in charge of the birth process and furthermore were quite consciously offering a kind of care that was very different from that offered in institutional settings. Working in a county hospital setting, under the supervision of a group of doctors, produces many obstacles to the kind of autonomous decision making that midwives value both in itself and as a necessary means to the provision of what they regard as quality midwifery care.

Thus, midwives have been readmitted to the health care system but on terms not wholly compatible with the needs of midwifery care. Midwives were hired as a means of attracting patients back into the system and as a cheaper means of providing routine obstetrical care, particularly to underserved populations. Although some members of the medical profession genuinely support midwives, even these may not fully support the midwives' style of practice, particularly when the costs are recognized. This paradox creates a serious dilemma for those seeking to institutionalize both midwives and midwifery care.

Strategies of Response

How have midwives responded to this dilemma? Is there any way to maintain support for midwives while at the same time increasing the prospects for institutionalizing midwifery care?

The predominant strategy has been for midwives to try to meet the needs for which they were hired as effectively as possible with the hope of thereby developing leverage—through their increased value to their employers—to use in bargaining for more adequate institutional support. However, this strategy requires either an avocational approach—providing the necessary care regardless of institutional support (e.g., adequate pay for the hours worked)—or some adaptation of the midwifery model.

An avocational approach is generally necessary in the early stages of any social change effort, and midwives have recognized the need for personal sacrifice in order to "get a foot in the door," leading some of their patrons in the establishment to note their willingness to "work their buns off." However, this kind of effort seldom can be continued indefinitely; as one midwife put it, "You have to be able to prove yourself without killing yourself." Perhaps even more important, the institutional context may make it practically impossible to provide such care regardless of the midwife's commitment. For example, scheduling a midwife to see thirty prenatal patients a day or to handle four to six women in labor and delivery makes it physically impossible for her to spend the time needed to provide midwifery care.

Thus, some modifications of the model become necessary. Prenatal visits must focus on medical rather than educational and psychosocial issues. Continuity of care is abandoned, and the role of the midwife is redefined; from being a kind of "saint," establishing an intense one-to-one relationship with her clients, the midwife becomes more of a facilitator and coordinator, trying to ensure that the woman receives adequate care from an integrated team of support services. Labor sitting is reduced, perhaps delegated to other nursing staff or labor coaches, perhaps replaced by machinery (e.g., fetal monitors).

This strategy has been relatively effective as a means of institutionalizing the acceptance of nurse midwives; when the midwife service has expanded not only in terms of numbers but also in terms of the functions served by midwives in the system, the institutional position of midwives seems to have become more secure. But what about increasing support for midwifery care? Do these modifications of the model suggest that midwives are being coopted? Or are they simply making rational adaptations to the profound limits on the provision of midwifery care?

On the one hand, one could argue, as one midwife did, that "the midwifery model isn't marketable; it rips you off." Indeed, she held that real cooptation was trying to follow the midwifery model in the absence of institutional support. On the other hand, this kind of adaptation led one of the midwives' staunchest institutional patrons to claim that "midwives are practicing more and more like doctors. They don't think so, but I do." Yet numerous midwives as well as doctors have argued that the accommodation was to some extent mutual: that is, doctors were adopting some of the midwives' techniques, and midwives were being used in the instruction of medical students. And, as one midwife said, "If you want to make these kinds of changes, you can't make the doctors the enemy." And certainly all of the midwives I spoke with would argue that despite the compromises they have had to make in their practice, their care is still qualitatively different—more personal, more humane, more fundamentally supportive of pregnant and laboring women—than that of doctors.

These questions of adaptation and cooptation are extremely complex, and I do not propose to try to answer them here. What I do want to do is examine an alternative strategy, one in which the midwives did, to a certain extent, make the doctors the enemy. The Highland Midwife Service in Oakland chose to challenge its employers directly by unionizing and trying to use the process of collective bargaining to gain what they had failed to gain through a more cooperative approach. An analysis of their experience will help us address the broader question of the prospects and strategies for institutionalizing both nurse midwives and midwifery care as well.

THE HIGHLAND MIDWIFE SERVICE

During the 1970s, Highland General Hospital was increasingly troubled. Like other county hospitals, its birth census had declined; and since 1974 its obstetrical service had consisted of a group of private physicians who maintained significant private practices and had little commitment to the hospital.

Then in 1978, infant mortality suddenly became an intense local political issue. The county had released statistics showing that infant mortality in certain areas of East Oakland was twice the state average and six or seven times the average in more affluent areas of the city, and the Coalition to Fight Infant Mortality (CFIM) was formed to lobby for more effective perinatal health care.[3] During a campaign visit to East Oakland, then-Governor Jerry Brown promised to fund a special program to address the problem of infant mortality. The Oakland Perinatal Health Project—OPHP—was the result. It provided funding for innovative efforts to reduce infant mortality.

The Highland Midwife Service (HMS) was created as part of OPHP. (See Appendix A for a summary chronology of the Highland Midwife Service.) Its origins can probably be traced to a labor and delivery nurse (who later became an HMS midwife) who suggested to the hospital's chief obstetrician that Highland establish a midwife service and seek OPHP funding. The doctor agreed, in part because none of the existing doctors was using the two new ABCs that the hospital, in an effort to attract more patients, had just opened. In January 1979, the first Highland midwife was hired. She succeeded in getting OPHP funding for the Highland Midwife Service, which began in July 1979 with three certified nurse midwife (CNM) positions.

In the meantime, community concern with infant mortality had focused on Highland's Obstetrical service. In September 1979, demonstrations were held at the county board of super-

---

[3] Data on infant mortality rates in Alameda County can be found in the Alameda Contra Costa Health Systems Agency 1980 Plan. At a time when the infant mortality rate in California and for Alameda County as a whole was 13.2/1,000, it was 3.6/1,000 for the affluent white North Oakland Hills/Piedmont Health Planning Area and 26.3/1,000 for the low-income black East Oakland Health Planning Area.

visors, who agreed to request a grand jury investigation; at the same time, the CFIM undertook its own study of county perinatal health needs. That winter, three out of the four staff obstetricians resigned, and an acting chief was appointed. The midwife service continued to grow, and by July 1980 there were four full-time midwife positions.

That summer, the grand jury and the CFIM reports were released; both had high praise for the midwife service but demanded a new obstetrical service with a full-time commitment to the hospital and to serving a community-based perinatal program.

The group chosen for the new service was Gynecology and Obstetrics of Highland (GOH), and it was regarded by the larger community as well as by the midwives as a progressive and committed group of physicians. The midwife service, which by then included six midwives (two full-time, four part-time), would become part of GOH, and the midwives and the doctors held planning meetings during the months preceding July 1981, when GOH officially began operation. During those meetings, problems began to surface.

Institutional Weakness of HMS

Despite exceptionally strong community support, overall institutional support for the midwives at Highland was weaker than at other county sites.

First of all, Highland was not a teaching hospital, and thus lacked both the need for "teaching material" and the institutional resources associated with a teaching hospital. And although community support for the midwife service was unusually strong, the pressure generated by community mobilization tends to be more ephemeral and weaker than pressure stemming from the needs of a well-established academic institution.

Second, the state subsidy was also ephemeral: as a result of the hospital's failure to comply with the requirements of the state grant, the state refused to fund the midwife service for its third year—1981–1982.

However, the most important problem was the fact that GOH was a for-profit partnership. Its revenues—apart from a few small county subsidies—were limited to what could be generated from patient charges, and it had to use those revenues to provide all of the services (including the midwife service) required by the county contract. Thus, any costs for the midwife service beyond the reimbursements received for the midwives' work would have to come out of the doctors' earnings. And this fact heavily influenced their view of midwifery care.

Finally, the HMS lacked the kind of institutional patron present in most of the other services. Although the doctors in GOH were very supportive of midwives, they did not feel the same interest in having midwives as did doctors at other sites. Thus, although births at Highland had increased dramatically since the creation of the HMS, the doctors, unlike the rest of the community, did not recognize the role of the midwives in "turning Highland around" (See Appendix B for birth trends at Highland General Hospital). And they questioned the midwives' cost-effectiveness, often suggesting that a team of physicians and nurse practitioners could see more patients in less time than the midwives could. (One of the doctors claimed that he was at his best when he was delivering eight women at once.) Neither the doctors nor any county health officials had actively worked to create the midwife service; rather, they had essentially acquiesced. Indeed, the patron relationship was to some extent reversed for the Highland midwives: they predated GOH, they worked to help bring GOH to Highland, and they believed that they could help GOH establish itself successfully at the hospital.

Thus, although the HMS did benefit from community support and a state subsidy, and although the GOH doctors were supportive of midwives, the overall institutional support for midwives was weaker than at other sites. The state subsidy was short-lived; support from the doctors was limited by the fact that they were a for-profit group. And the indirect subsidies—residents and attending faculty to provide consultations and backup for the midwives, leverage in negotiating with the hospital and county health care system—that a teaching hospital would have provided were absent. The relative weakness of the institutional support for the midwives intensified the problems they faced in trying to provide midwifery care.

"Cadillac Care when Chevy Would Do"

The most fundamental conflict between the midwives and the doctors concerned the issue of cost-effectiveness and its implications for quality care and work load. This was exacerbated by their different perceptions of the political and administrative exigencies of the situation.

Because of their financial structure, the doctors were extremely concerned with cost-effectiveness, defined simply in the narrow sense of costs relative to revenues generated. The original state grant for the midwife service had projected financial self-sufficiency for the midwives, and the doctors initially expected them to cover their costs through revenues generated by their own work. However, as already noted, routine obstetrics is not generally cost-effective in this sense of the term, much less routine obstetrics reimbursed at Medi-Cal rates; and even with the midwives' relatively lower salaries, the doctors believed that the midwives were not meeting their costs. Although the extent of the deficit was not clear—the midwives' revenues were not precisely calculated, and their estimated costs varied, depending on how much they were charged for overhead and physician backup—the doctors pressured the midwives to be more efficient: to see more patients in less time in order to generate more revenue.

The midwives, however, were intensely committed to providing "first class care," particularly to patients who traditionally had received inferior care and to those, like black women, who had a tendency to regard midwives as second-class care. Furthermore, as a group, the midwives were unusually political: they shared a feminist and class analysis of the health care system and the need for institutional change; most of them had had prior political experience and had been involved in the mobilization of community pressure to bring better obstetrical care to Highland Hospital. They believed that they had a community mandate to provide first-class care and were not about to compromise their commitment in order to meet what they perceived as the doctors' misinformed and, more important, misguided concerns with cost-effectiveness.

At the same time, the midwives were not willing to continue providing that care on an avocational basis. Four of the six midwives were already half-time because they could not sustain the full-time load; however, the nature of the job combined with their avocational orientation meant that the half-time midwives were working thirty-five to forty hours a week for half-time pay, while full-time midwives were logging fifty-five to sixty hours a week. With a salary range of $24,000 to $28,000, the midwives estimated that the part-timers were earning six dollars an hour, and the full-timers were earning nine to ten dollars an hour.

The midwives thus were determined to make the doctors recognize the necessity both of limiting their work loads and of ensuring that the necessary care would be provided. And they argued that clinical as well as political factors necessitated their time-intensive work load.

First of all, prenatal care for many women was provided at community-based satellite clinics, where midwives had the major clinical as well as administrative responsibility. In addition to the extra care required by a low-income Third World population, the midwives' clinical work was complicated by various other factors: waiting for translators or for consultations with doctors back at the hospital; ordering tests and then ensuring that test results made their way from Highland to the patients' charts in the clinics; providing adequate charting to ensure that whoever delivered a woman would have all of the necessary information (e.g., whether syphilis had been treated, or whether a patient had a communicable disease); ensuring that patients' charts were at the hospital when they delivered. Furthermore, the midwives usually received less clerical and nursing assistance than the doctors did. Finally, the midwives had various general administrative responsibilities at the clinics.

As far as labor and delivery were concerned, the midwives likewise argued that labor sitting was not an optional feature of the midwifery model but a clinical necessity: the hospital suffered from chronic understaffing, which was borne most heavily by the midwives because the nursing staff gave priority to the doctors and often did not work in the alternative birth rooms, where many midwife patients chose to deliver.

The midwives held weekly meetings to review cases. All the patients whose due dates were approaching were discussed, and the midwife providing prenatal care briefed the other midwives on the particular needs of her patients. This was necessary to provide continuity of care, since patients were delivered by whichever midwife was on call when the patient came in. The midwives also undertook several outreach projects, such as providing regular tours of the ABCs in a variety of languages, holding predelivery parties, and developing a slide show about the Highland obstetrical service.

The midwives had hoped that the doctors would not only recognize the importance of providing first-class care but also support the midwives in their efforts to provide that care. The doctors, however, not only failed to provide adequate help; they also refused to recognize the necessity of all of the work that the midwives were doing. They did not share the midwives' political analysis, nor did they see the clinical need for all the extra time and work. The most sympathetic believed that the midwives were inefficient; the least sympathetic referred to them as "mothering and smothering" their patients, "mollycoddling" them, "providing Cadillac care when Chevy would do."

The Decision to Unionize

This kind of conflict is present, in varying degrees, in many midwife services. However, it was more intense at Highland because of its particular institutional and political context and the midwives' refusal to either modify their concept of necessary care or continue to provide it on a voluntary basis. The midwives held a series of meetings with the doctors to try to win their support, but they were unsuccessful. Agreements would be made and then rescinded or forgotten, and the midwives became increasingly frustrated by their powerlessness in relation to the doctors. Increasingly, it became clear that the "big happy family" approach taken initially by both the midwives and the doctors was not going to work. Rather, the midwives were going to have to develop a separate basis of power from which to force the doctors to take their concerns seriously.

The first need, the midwives decided, was for a written contract, and for legal assistance in contract writing, which led to the decision that the best source of help would be a union. Deciding to join the union, however, was not an easy or automatic decision, as it entailed shifting from a "professional" to a "worker" conception of their job, from defining the work load in terms of *what was needed* to defining it in terms of hours and pay. However, the midwives felt that they were not paid well enough to maintain the professional concept of work load; indeed, that was seen as an ideology that served only to rationalize their continuing exploitation. A union would give them not only legal and technical assistance but also bargaining power with the doctors.

And so in the fall of 1981 the midwives approached SEIU 616 (Service Employees International Union, AFL-CIO), the union that represented RNs at the hospital. The midwives were a tiny bargaining unit because they were private-sector employees (the doctors were a private partnership). However, the union agreed to represent them both because of the union's involvement in the infant mortality struggle and its recognition of the importance of the midwife service in this struggle, and because the union was concerned about the growing county practice of contracting out to the private sector and saw this as an opportunity to challenge the antiunion implications of that practice.

Joining the union not only committed the midwives inexorably to a confrontation strategy with their employers, but it also immediately intensified the conflict. The doctors were hurt and outraged; to them, the union represented the destruction of the GOH family and a serious threat to the collegiality they expected in their professional relationship.

Collective Bargaining
Writing a Contract Proposal
The central goals of the midwives were to use the collective bargaining process to force the doctors to recognize the necessity of midwifery work and at the same time to develop some means of limiting their work load. And the most important institutional mechanisms by which these goals were to be achieved were a finite workweek and a job description that included all of the necessary components of good midwifery care. The midwives also sought to maintain the maximum amount of autonomy for the midwife service. Pay itself was not so much an issue as pay relative to hours worked; however, benefits were extremely important, as GOH had

refused to continue the health plan coverage that the midwives had finally won from the previous group of doctors.

The first task was to translate the work load issues into contract language. The midwives' initial "bottom line" in terms of hours was forty-five to fifty for full-time and thirty-five to forty for part-time, with part-time increased from one-half to three-quarter time; the professional model was still with them. The union suggested a different approach: first, to clearly distinguish the work that had to done by midwives and the work that could be reduced or eliminated either through the use of ancillary personnel or through more efficient administrative support and second, to propose a forty-hour workweek with overtime and night differentials.

This became the core of the first union proposal. Other key work load and autonomy provisions included a long and detailed job description, a description of the midwife service that specified a separate midwife caseload, seniority based on date of hire with the HMS, representation of GOH decision-making committees, veto power in midwife hiring, and responsibility for scheduling and outreach. The salary range for the basic forty-hour workweek was modest: $26,412 to 30,576; it would have been increased substantially by overtime and the nighttime differential. Other important demands included leaves—and particularly the right to use sick leave for appointments and dependents—and demands specific to the union, such as dues checkoff, the automatic deduction of union dues from paychecks.

The doctors, having initially threatened to challenge the unionization election, finally agreed to negotiate; however, they sought to minimize their own involvement in the process. They hired a firm called Human Resources Management (HRM) to draw up a contract and do the negotiating for them. For HRM as well as the union, it was the first time they had dealt with a midwife contract; however, the problem was made even more difficult for HRM by the relative inaccessibility of the doctors. Thus HRM's initial contract proposal, drawn largely from a nursing contract and referring throughout to nurses, was irrelevant to the actual situation on the critical issue of work load: it proposed an indefinite workweek (essentially as much work as was necessary to provide the necessary services) yet referred to an hourly basis of pay.

Negotiations

Negotiations began in March 1982. The doctors categorically opposed the idea of a forty-hour workweek, believing that it would be economically disastrous. They proposed to continue the current work load and to raise the salary only to the level proposed by the midwives for a forty-hour week. They also refused to provide full health coverage. The midwives were appalled.

Nonetheless, because of the custom in contract negotiations of beginning with the supposedly easier noneconomic issues, the questions of pay and benefits were deferred while other issues were discussed. But in the midwives' case, these issues were not necessarily easier: while agreements were reached relatively quickly on minor or uncontroversial issues, such as the union bulletin board or including sexual preference and family status in the nondiscrimination clause, the midwives' proposals regarding job description and service autonomy were extremely controversial.

To some extent the collective bargaining process itself compounded the problems. The legally binding character of the contract made the doctors extremely hesitant to yield any further to the midwives than absolutely necessary, even though in practice they actually preferred to allow the midwives considerable autonomy, as it reduced their own administrative burden. Furthermore, HRM had its own interest in writing as strong a contract as possible in order to enhance its reputation, and because of the doctors' inexperience, they tended to defer to HRM even when they themselves might not have felt so strongly about an issue.

Thus, the GOH "management rights" clause was practically all-inclusive and furthermore reserved for the doctors all rights not specifically granted to the midwives. The midwives, in their struggle for service autonomy, had to negotiate for a decision-making role with regard to each specific issue—such as preparing the work schedule, scheduling vacation leaves—and resisted signing off on the management rights section until near the end of the negotiations. And HRM regarded including a job description in the contract as a major breach of management rights; here, however, the doctors were opposed for their own reasons—namely, the extensiveness of the proposed job description.

Thus not only was there no progress on the economic issues, but progress on the noneconomic issues was also problematic, and impatience mounted on both sides. In early May, the midwives sent a letter to the doctors accusing them of bad faith for failing to attend the negotiating sessions, and the doctors, who were paying the HRM on an hourly basis, began to pressure the firm to move more quickly. On May 13, the HRM representative made his first reference to the possible need for a mediator.

Finally on May 18, GOH put forth a proposal to limit the midwives' work load: caseload guidelines that used births as a measure of work load and established a formula linking number of births to midwife position time thereby ensuring staffing increases proportionate to work load increases. The birth ratio proposed was eight to ten births per month for each fulltime midwife position. Thus, additional hiring would take place when births exceeded the ratio and layoffs would occur when they dropped below. The proposal also sought to reduce the use of part-time midwives by requiring that staffing increases be implemented first by increasing existing part-time midwives to full-time; the doctors claimed that having part-time midwives was more costly in terms of benefits and administration.

The midwives reacted negatively to both parts of the proposal: the birth ratios were too high, and the opportunity to work part-time was essential. However, they did finally decide that they would get nowhere with a contract proposal based on hours and furthermore that they needed to demonstrate their own willingness to negotiate.

Thus on May 20 the midwives submitted their own alternative to a forty-hour workweek as a means of limiting their work load; the proposal consisted of three components. First, they accepted the concept of caseload guidelines, which are used at least informally in various other midwife services, but proposed a lower ration: the maximum births per full-time midwife per month would be eight. Second, they developed a two-part job description, with the first part describing those tasks that were required as part of the midwife job and the second part describing those tasks that were optional and that would be done either for extra compensation, if GOH approved, or on a strictly volunteer basis. Third, they proposed to increase all part-time positions from half-time to three-quarter time. This would essentially recognize the amount of work that the part-timers were already doing and compensate them accordingly.

In the game of collective bargaining, "the move off hours" (i.e., abandoning the demand for a forty-hour week) was a major concession, one that required the doctors, in turn, to make some significant new offers. Accordingly, though they found the birth ratios proposed by the midwives too low and the increase in part-time hours too expensive, they did make concessions in other areas that were regarded as extremely significant. A job description would be included in the contract, and although the doctors retained ultimate control in the case of disagreement, its content would be developed jointly by the midwives and the doctors. Joint decision making was to be allowed on various other issues. And, in what HRM described as "a giant step for womankind," seniority for noneconomic purposes (e.g., priority in resolving conflicting vacation requests) was to be based not on date of hire with GOH (and alphabetically for those hired on the same date—namely six of the seven midwives who were part of the HMS before the establishment of GOH) but on date of hire with the HMS. In addition, the caseload guidelines were dropped from eight to ten to seven to nine. Furthermore, the doctors began to send a representative to the negotiating sessions.

The midwives, too, made some additional moves; most important, "in the interest of reaching agreement," they signed off on management rights. However, they were becoming increasingly impatient: the GOH concessions were still far from the midwives' demands, and, there had been no movement on other major issues. In early June, they notified the state conciliation service that they might want a mediator. At the same time, they began to explore ways of increasing pressure on the doctors; their first step was to solicit letters of support from some of the community clinics.

On June 15, perhaps in response to the fear thus created that an impasse was imminent, GOH offered another major compromise: immediately following settlement, staffing for the midwife service would be increased to 5.5 full-time positions. This was justifiable in terms of the caseload guidelines proposed by GOH because the births averaged more than seven per month per full-time midwife at that point, and in earlier meetings HRM had deliberately emphasized that the guidelines would permit additional hiring when the birth ratio was anywhere between seven and nine. It was a conditional increase, however, limited to four months, during which time the midwives would have to increase their births to the nine per full-time midwife per month required to maintain the 5.5 positions. But it did provide temporary relief, and furthermore it established the principle of flexible position time; the midwives could distribute the additional position however they chose. (And one fulltime position would allow the midwives to increase the five existing part-time midwives from .5. to .7 position time per midwife, bringing each from half-time to almost three-quarter time, which was much closer to their actual work time.)

The midwives, however, remained adamant: six to eight was the maximum birth ratio they could accept. Furthermore, various other demands were still outstanding (health benefits, seniority for salary purposes, the union issues). At last an impasse was declared; the union called the mediator, while the midwives sought to further increase community pressure by circulating a leaflet describing their struggle with the doctors.

Settlement

The mediator came the following week and spent a day hearing both sides' positions and trying to identify possibilities for movement. The next session, on July 9, 1982, was a marathon session, starting at eight in the morning and ending at about 9:30 that night. The doctors offered some new concessions: full health plan coverage for the first year, but without a maintenance-of-benefits clause (i.e., without any obligation to cover cost increases in subsequent years), and the use of sick leave for appointments and dependents. And agreement was reached on a few other items. But there was still no movement on the other key issues, and again an impasse developed.

In her final caucus with the midwives, the mediator offered her assessment of the situation and gave them some advice. She emphasized the gap between what would be acceptable in practice and what could go into a formal contract, particularly a first contract, when management was especially nervous about its potential implications. And she described what she called "the control issues"—the job description, the caseload guidelines—as "brick wall issues," issues on which the doctors were unlikely to move regardless of pressure because they had to protect their ultimate rights as management to define the job. However, she thought that if the midwives focused on one issue, such as pay, they might be able to get it. They had to decide where they might be able to move. She suggested that they consider filing a ten-day notice of a work action—such as a slowdown; they might not have to do anything, for the notice alone might create sufficient pressure to bring the doctors back to the negotiating table. Furthermore, it would allow the mediator to schedule another meeting, and perhaps help set an endpoint to the negotiations. In the meantime, she would explore the possibility of progress on wages; she thought that might be possible if they took everything else off the table. However, she concluded, "it's your judgment. If you're going to take a beef, it might be better to take it over principle—it's sometimes more persuasive."

The following week, after lengthy consideration, the midwives agreed to file notice of a work action; however, although the decision was unanimous, it was not uniformly supported. Some felt that pressure was the only way to get any further movement from the doctors; others believed that the doctors would negotiate if the midwives expressed a willingness to compromise and feared that further pressure would be counterproductive.

Two weeks later, the midwives reversed their decision and decided that they were ready to settle. Several factors influenced their decision. First of all, they were increasingly aware of the dilemmas they faced in trying to create pressure. Anything in the nature of a work slowdown, aimed at pressuring the doctors, would hurt their patients and might, as a consequence, reduce their community support. Efforts to mobilize further community pressure—such as a demonstration at the hospital—seemed extremely difficult given the nature of the clientele: largely low-income women and Third World women, who had too many problems maintaining their own survival to be easily mobilized to demonstrate. Moreover, it appeared that the midwives' efforts to generate pressure were becoming counterproductive: increasing the doctors' intransigence without increasing their need to negotiate. Finally, the midwives were exhausted, and as their own resources were steadily depleted, the prospects of an immediate pay raise, particularly for the part-timers, became increasingly attractive.

In addition, there was a growing awareness of some of the larger problems facing GOH as a service. GOH's first-year community evaluation had raised some critical questions; MediCal cuts had just been passed by the state legislature; and the midwives were concerned about the potentional vulnerability of GOH in relation to this larger context.

And so the midwives informed the doctors that they were willing to settle in return for a pay increase. The doctors, however, were divided: although some were willing to talk, one had threatened to quit if there were any further negotiations with the midwives; and so the doctors refused to meet.

The stalemate was finally broken through an informal meeting between one of the more moderate midwives and the most intransigent doctor; the two were close personally, and they were on call together the night before the final meeting scheduled by the mediator. The midwife managed to persuade the doctor that the future cooperation that was necessary to their clinical effectiveness required the doctors to recognize the midwives' willingness to settle. The doctor finally agreed but only on the condition that the midwives would address only the issue of a $1,000 salary increase.

The rest of the midwives were polled, as well as some of the other doctors, and when the mediator arrived the next day, the basis for settlement had been established. In addition to the $1,000 pay raise, the doctors agreed to establish seniority for purposes of salary through a separate letter of agreement that essentially recognized the seniority accrued through HMS.

Thus, the bargaining was over: after five months of time-consuming meetings and intense bargaining, the midwives had a contract. Did they also have more protection and support for their desire to provide midwifery care? Did they have more power in their relations with the doctors? How effectively did unionization help them meet their needs and objectives as midwives?

Contract Gains and Losses
The midwives initally felt a sense of defeat. They had won a settlement, but only by abandoning their position on some key

issues: caseload guidelines, the job descriptions, dues checkoff. However, most of these concessions were mitigated by other gains, and with the perspective of time and experience with the new contract, the balance sheet on the contract began to look more positive.

The higher caseload guidelines were softened immediately by the staffing increase of one full position as well as by the right to distribute the extra position in any way they chose; this increased the resources for the service as a whole, increased the recognition of and compensation for the contribution of the part-timers in particular, and preserved the midwives' right to work part-time. And although it was on a trial basis only, contingent on increasing the number of births to meet the 9:1 ratio, achieving an increase was no problem—the service caseload has increased steadily since its inception—and the 9:1 ratio turned out to be workable. Equally important, the caseload guidelines ensured that staffing levels were maintained and increased as soon as warranted, a contract guarantee that became increasingly important as GOH felt increasing financial pressure and sought to make cutbacks wherever possible.

The job description was much narrower than the midwives wanted, and, as they expected, the doctors were not willing to pay for many of the tasks in the extra-pay category. Nevertheless, there were some compensating factors. The first responsibility listed on the job description was to maintain a caseload of clients choosing a nurse midwife delivery: the separate caseload was preserved. And the director's job included responsibility for scheduling, assigning midwives to various tasks/clinics, and coordinating with the hospital and the clinics. This autonomy in scheduling, combined with the staffing increase, which was not rigidly linked to increased clinical responsibilities, allowed the service to provide at least limited support for extra administrative and political tasks by reducing the clinical duties of midwives who took on additional work. And the midwives also gained voting representation on such joint decision-making committees as were needed.

As far as pay, although the salary range increased only $1,000 above the original GOH proposal and was considerably below what the midwives had demanded, it was $2,000 to $5,000 higher than the 1981 salary range and was particularly dramatic for the part-timers, with their increase from .5 to .7

position time. And there were various other important gains—seniority, health plan coverage, the right to use sick leave for dependents and appointments.

Thus the process of collective bargaining did allow the midwives to win some additional institutional supports for their efforts to provide midwifery care. However, for a more thorough assessment of its effectiveness, we need to look at the broader impact on the process of institutionalizing midwifery care.

CONCLUSIONS

Midwives universally must confront the dilemma caused by the fact that their employers tend to be supportive of midwives for reasons that conflict with the provision of midwifery care. Thus in seeking long-term institutional security, midwives must strike a balance between winning support for themselves as midwives, by meeting the needs for which they have been hired, and winning support for midwifery care, which may force them to challenge some of the reasons for which they were hired. Most midwives, as we have seen, have placed primary emphasis on increasing support for midwives and thus have adopted a more cooperative strategy than the Highland midwives. And while this may win them greater support from, and even increased leverage with, their employers, the danger is that they will not gain sufficient support or leverage to allow more extensive provision of midwifery care and thus will continue to have to choose between compromising their practice of midwifery and/or providing it on an avocational basis.

The Highland midwives refused to either modify their concept of midwifery care or provide it on an avocational basis, and when efforts to win support from their employers failed, they abandoned that effort and chose instead a strategy aimed at generating sufficient leverage to force the doctors to support midwifery care. The strategy did succeed in winning some additional institutional support for midwifery care, but the danger of that approach is that it will not generate sufficient leverage to counteract the reduction in support that it is likely to cause, thus threatening the prospects for the institutionalization of both midwives and midwifery care. What does the Highland experience suggest?

Certainly unionization increased the midwives' leverage with the doctors; indeed, some would regard this as its most important result. The contract allowed the midwives to *claim* rather than simply be *allowed* certain gains; it freed them, on those issues that were enshrined in the contract, from dependence on the doctors' good will and protected them from changes in that good will. On those issues, the midwives won real power in relation to the doctors. Thus, when the doctors sought to impose cutbacks on the midwife service, the contract prevented it. The midwives also felt empowered by having won a contract: the process as well as the product increased their sense of independence.

However, although the contract increased the midwives' power in relation to the doctors, it by no means eliminated the need for cooperation. The fundamental asymmetry in their relationship remained: the doctors still had ultimate control over most of the necessary conditions of practice. The doctors held the contract with the county that included a midwife service; the doctors decided whether or not they were willing to provide physician supervision for the midwives; and of course the doctors exercised the medical authority entailed by that supervision. Furthermore, to the extent that both the doctors and the midwives shared a commitment to improving perinatal care in the county, a cooperative effort to pursue that commitment would have helped; unfortunately, their different assessments of what was necessary was one of the issues that led to unionization.

But this leads to the next question, namely the value of unionization in relation to the broader constraints on the provision of quality care—indeed of adequate care—to low-income people. The political economy of health care in the United States makes it extremely difficult to provide first-class care to low-income people. Health care is considered a commodity and provided on the basis of profit; doctors, along with other members of the medical-industrial complex, expect and can command a high rate of return; and the general antipathy to the welfare state severely limits the resources available for the provision of care to those who cannot pay enough to make it profitable. At the same time, those who are least able to pay tend to have the greatest need.

These structural factors took their toll on GOH. After the

first year, in which the doctors grossed what some in the county regarded as excessive profits, GOH suffered the next two years from a combination of reduced county support and cuts in the levels of state MediCal reimbursement. Their profits disappeared, and they were forced to lower their incomes below what they considered acceptable and to reduce the services that they could offer.

And as their problems worsened, some of the doctors came to resent what they saw as their subsidy of the midwife service: though never precisely calculated, estimates ranged up to $100,000 per year for the costs of providing medical supervision to the midwives. This perceived subsidy, further aggravated by the fact that fees to HRM for the union negotiations were $28,000, led some of the doctors to seek ways to eliminate or at least cut back the midwife service. And while the union contract prevented them from reducing the midwife staffing below the caseload guidelines, it did not prevent them from trying to reduce the midwives' caseload through such means as lowering the threshold of risk at which a patient had to be transferred from the midwives to the doctors.

Even more important, the union contract could not prevent the doctors from abandoning their practice at Highland altogether. And when their financial problems became too severe, and the county refused to renegotiate their fee structure to allow them to increase their revenues—and maintain the level of services, personnel, and income that they believed were necessary—that is what they did. On October 31, 1984, after giving the required six-month notice, GOH disbanded. With its disbanding, the midwives' hard-won union contract and all of its protections vanished, leaving the midwives vulnerable to whatever pressures arose in the aftermath of the GOH departure.

And those pressures have been substantial. Despite the six-month notice, the county was unable to find another obstetrics group to replace GOH—a fact that further indicates the genuine difficulties of providing good·obstetric care at Highland Hospital. The interim solution—lasting supposedly only until July 1985—was to make independent contracts with a chief of obstetrics, one additional full-time physician, and a string of fourteen to sixteen part-time physicians. With this kind of fragmented system of care, reduction in quality was inevitable. Not only was there no continuity of care for the patients, but in addition, the midwives, who rely heavily upon physician consultation and supervision in a high-risk population such as the Highland clientele, found it extremely difficult to establish and maintain the kinds of working relationships with the physicians needed to provide effective care.

The midwives were also hired as independent contractors: although all but one of the Highland midwives signed contracts—albeit not without substantial reservations about the implications of the new arrangement—the midwifery service itself no longer exists. All of the mechanisms for autonomy written into the union contract—the midwifery caseload, the director's responsibility for coordination, the joint participation in decisions affecting the midwifery service—are gone. The chief value of the union contract was in establishing a baseline for subsequent pay and benefits that was certainly higher than it would otherwise have been.

Thus, with the exception of pay, the institutional supports for midwifery care that were won through unionization were almost all eliminated. Furthermore, there was evidence of increased opposition from various members of the health care establishment. The hospital administration was not happy with all of the trouble caused by the midwives' unionization. The new chief of obstetrics, although a long-time midwife supporter, was apprehensive about working with a tight-knit group of outspoken midwives and reportedly regarded their desire for a midwifery caseload as a desire to provide "elite care" to a select group of patients. The county began conducting productivity studies to determine how many midwife positions were really necessary, and there were reports of county officials blaming the midwives for creating such a "political cauldron" in obstetric services that it was impossible for the county to recruit qualified physicians.

All of these pressures slowly eroded the midwives' willingness to continue to fight. By June 1985, five of the seven midwives working until the GOH dissolution had resigned. Some felt they could not provide the quality of care that was necessary; others were simply exhausted after the years of struggle. Those remaining became more cautious about speaking out about conditions at Highland for fear of losing their jobs.

However, the Coalition to Fight Infant Mortality (CFIM) did not have those constraints. They blamed the hospital administration for the departure of GOH, which they saw as a major tragedy for the East Oakland community. The extraordinarily fragmented system of physician care, combined with the longstanding problem of serious nursing shortages, were expected to seriously reduce the quality of care, and the CFIM monitored the situation closely. As evidence of deterioration began to accumulate, the CFIM provided a steady stream of letters documenting problems and making recommendations to the hospital administration. When the administration, predictably, failed to respond, the CFIM turned to the state and in June 1985 requested a complete investigation of perinatal services at Highland.

The resulting state investigation confirmed all of the concerns of the CFIM and the midwives: the problems were serious enough to threaten the hospital's accreditation. At last the board of supervisors began to take seriously the community's demands. Additional funding and additional nursing positions were provided, and the top administration of the hospital, which had long been regarded as a major barrier to change, was finally removed. The part-time obstetricians were slowly replaced by full-time physicians.

So what does all of this suggest about strategies for institutionalizing the presence of midwives and the practice of midwifery care in the established medical system? The confrontation strategy adopted by the Highland midwives was reasonably effective for the duration of the union contract and regarding the issues covered by that contract. Unionization provided a vehicle for effective collective action and enabled the midwives to press for and win increased institutional support for midwifery care. However, it could not address the larger structural problems that ultimately led to the termination of the contract. And with the loss of protection offered by the contract, the midwives became more vulnerable than ever to opposition from other members of the medical system, opposition that had intensified because of the midwives' unionization. Thus, as the system of care continued to deteriorate, the midwives felt both increasingly concerned about the quality of care and increasingly powerless to deal with the situation. For many of them, resignation seemed the only option.

And herein lies the real danger of a confrontation strategy: that it will generate increased opposition without being able to generate and maintain sufficient leverage to counteract this increased opposition and to continue pressing for change. This danger was compounded in the Highland situation by the fact that the problems that had led the midwives to choose a confrontation strategy were actually worsening.

But what was the alternative? The confrontation strategy was motived first and foremost by concerns for quality of care that the established system regarded as "cadillac" or "elite," but that the midwives believed was required for all women and particularly for the high-risk women served by Highland Hospital. Indeed, even GOH eventually came to realize that some degree of confrontation would be necessary if they were to provide an adequate level of care, and they too antagonized the hospital administration. Certainly the state investigation provides dramatic evidence of need for improvements in the system of care. Cooperation in that situation meant accepting a status quo that desperately needed to be challenged.

Furthermore, while the more cooperative strategy taken by other midwife services may seem to have brought them more security, we cannot be too sure. Their more cooperative approach in part reflected greater institutional support to begin with, and that support is now beginning to erode. Indeed, many of these services are beginning to face serious institutional problems—the retirement of the only physician willing to provide backup for the midwives; the termination of the educational grant that supports half of the midwife positions. Others are reaching the limits of their avocational commitment and are beginning a more direct struggle to challenge what they see as exploitative arrangements. On a broader scale, reduced funding for health care services and training programs, combined with the growing physician surplus and the malpractice crisis in obstetrics, threaten to undermine what support for midwives there is within the medical establishment. Midwives universally will need much more active support if they are to retain their position within the medical system.

In the final analysis, we cannot underestimate the extent to which the provision of midwifery care challenges the existing health care system. Ironically, this challenge is nowhere greater than in that segment of the system in which midwives have found the greatest acceptance, namely the low-income segment served by county hospitals, where midwives have been hired to provide less expensive care and find themselves unable to provide midwifery care because it is too expensive. The Highland midwives' experience demonstrates the potential effectiveness of a direct conflict strategy. It also reveals the critical importance of our willingness as consumers, and as the larger community, to join the struggle to make the system change.

REFERENCES

Alameda Contra Costa Health Systems Agency. 1980 PLAN. Oakland, Calif.: Alameda Contra Costa Health Systems Agency, 1980.

Arms, Suzanne. *Immaculate Deception: A New Look at Women and Childbirth*. New York: Bantam, 1975.

Corea, Gena. *The Hidden Malpractice: How American Medicine Treats Women as Patients and Professionals*. New York: William Morrow, 1977.

Declerq, Eugene R. "The Politics of Cooptation: Strategies for Childbirth Educators." *Birth* 10(Fall 1983):167-172.

Dempkowski, Alfreda. "Future Prospects of Nurse-Midwifery in the United States." *Journal of Nurse Midwifery* 27(March/April 1982):9-15.

DeVries, Raymond G. "The Alternative Birth Center: Option or Cooptation?" *Women and Health* 5(Fall 1980):47-60.

Edwards, Margot, and Waldorf, Mary. *Reclaiming Birth: History and Heroines of American Childbirth Reform*. Trumansburg, N.Y.: The Crossing Press, 1984.

Germano, Elaine. "Obstetricians vs. Midwives: The Effect of the Professionalization of the Practice of Obstetrics on the Practice of Midwifery in the United States." Unpublished manuscript, Fall 1979.

Illich, Ivan. *Medical Nemesis*. New York: Bantam, 1976.

Kouyoumdjiam, Hrant E. *A Legislative and Political Analysis of AB 1592: The 1981 California Nurse Midwifery Scope of Practice Bill*, unpublished manuscript, 1983.

Rich, Adrienne. *Of Woman Born*. New York: W. W. Norton, 1976.

Rothman, Barbara Katz. *In Labor: Women and Power in the Birthplace*. New York: W. W. Norton, 1982.

_____. "Medical Response to Women's Health Activities: Conflict, Accommodation and Cooptation." *Research in the Sociology of Health Care* 1(1980):335-354.

Sidel, Victor W., and Sidel, Ruth. *A Healthy State: An International Perspective on the Crisis on United States Medical Care,* rev. Ed. New York: Pantheon, 1983.

Willson, J. Robert. "Obstetrics-Gynecology: A Time for Change." Presidential Address to the Second Combined Annual Meeting of the American Gynecological Society and American Association of Obstetricians and Gynecologists, Montreal, May 20-23, 1981. *American Journal of Obstetrics and Gynecology* 14(December 15, 1981):853-863.

APPENDIXES

APPENDIX A. Chronology of the Highland Midwife Service

1978	Politicization of infant mortality in East Oakland
	Formation of CFIM (Coalition to Fight Infant Mortality)
	Creation of OPHP (Oakland Perinatal Health Project) by Governor Brown
1979	
January	First midwife hired at Highland General Hospital (HGH)
June	Highland Midwife Service (HMS) funded through OPHP (three full-time positions)
September	Demonstrations at board of supervisors call for investigation of obstetric (OB) services at HGH
October	Board requests grand jury investigations of OB at HGH
	CFIM undertakes concurrent study
1980	
Winter	Three of four staff obstetricians at HGH resign
Summer	HMS increases to four full-time positions; new director hired
	Grand Jury and CFIM reports released: both praise HMS; both call for new OB service at HGH
1981	
Spring	GOH (Gynecology and Obstetrics at Highland) selected
	Preliminary meetings with HMS
	HMS redistributes full-time positions and hires two new CNMS: total now six CNMs, two full-time, four part-time
July	GOH officially begins
	Meetings continue with HMS
Fall	HMS joins SEIU Local 616
1982	
January	GOH agrees to recognize the union
March	HMS adds seventh CNM, part-time; total full-time positions, 4.5
	Union negotiations begin
June	Impasse declared; mediator called in
July	Second impasse reached; HMS gives notice of work action

August	Settlement reached
	HMS up to 5.5 full-time
1983	GOH experiences increasing financial problems and frustration in contract negotiations with HGH administration
1984	
April	GOH gives six months notice of intent to terminate contract
November	GOH dissolves
	Obstetric services provided by independent contractors
	HMS terminated; midwives become independent contractors
1985	
Spring	CFIM submits complaint to state's Department of Health Services
	Four midwives resign
July	State investigation finds serious deficiencies in obstetric services at HGH
Fall	County board of supervisors provides additional resources for HGH, removes top administration of HGH

APPENDIX B. Birth Trends at Highland General Hospital and in the Highland Midwife Service

Highland General Hospital, Total and as Percent of County Births, 1972-1982

	1972	*1974*	*1976*	*1978*	*1979*	*1980*	*1981*	*1982*
HGH Births	676	506	568	560	746	767	867	1,087
County Births	—	14,009	14,276	15,458	16,637	16,744	17,936	18,160
Percent of County Births	—	3.6	3.9	3.6	4.5	4.6	4.8	6.0

Sources: Highland General Hospital (HGH), 1972-77: Williams, Ronald L., *Vital Record Data for Use in the Planning of Perinatal Health Services,* April 1980. 1978-79: State of California, OSHPD, *Annual Report of Hospitals,* 1978, 1979, Sacramento. 1980-82: Alameda County Health Care Services Agency, Systems Management and Analysis, phone interview, July 1984. Alameda County, 1972-82: Alameda County Health Care Services Agency, Systems Management and Analysis, phone interview, July 1984.

Highland Midwife Service, 1979-1984, Fiscal Years

	(March-June) 1979	*1979-80*	*1980-81*	*1981-82*	*1982-83*	*1983-84*
HMS Births	17	153	251	377	512	869
Percent of HGH Births	7	20	29	43	54	64

Source: Highland Midwife Service, July 1984. Data taken from the labor and delivery birth logs and the birth logs of the HMS.

EPILOGUE

A Note on the Future of American Birth

DOROTHY C. WERTZ
PAMELA S. EAKINS

Parents want both safety and humanity in birth. The preceding chapters have described different scenarios for reconciling conflicts between these two desires: in-hospital birthing suites, free-standing birth centers, home births, certified nurse-midwives, lay midwives. For most parents, however, a possibly inevitable conflict will remain between desire for maximum safety and desire for a humanized, woman-centered birth. In today's world, few can have it both ways.

For today's parents, safety is seen primarily in terms of the child and the child's future mental development. Mothers may be willing to take risks for themselves, but few are willing to risk having a child who receives B's instead of A's in school on account of an accident at birth. People want children who are not only free from biological defects, but who are above average, ready to achieve in a competitive society. It is this desire for the "perfect" child, that, above all else, will keep most births in the hands of obstetricians, hospitals, and high technology.

As Nancy Schrom Dye documents, Americans have long placed their faith in science. This meant the abandonment of midwives, who trusted in nature, in favor of physicians, who promised to improve upon a faulty nature through the use of medical art. When hospital birth became an option for most private patients in the 1920s, parents came to regard an expensive in-hospital birth as a "best buy," even though it could cost as much as a white-collar worker's annual salary. Families believed that a hospital birth, attended by an obstetrical specialist, surrounded by the latest technology, was the best insurance against having a damaged child.

Today, the desire for perfect children and the belief that increased technology will contribute to increased perfection are stronger than ever. Several recent social trends have coincided to make the birth of a less-than-perfect child a greater disaster than it was even fifty years ago. Families are smaller; parents now value each child as an object of intense emotional and monetary expenditure rather than a source of labor for the family (Zelizer, 1985:169-207); mothers now have jobs or career goals that will be curtailed if they must care for a less-than-perfect child; sources of social support, such as grandparents or extended families, are no longer as readily available. Furthermore, the availability of legal abortion has redefined "responsible parenthood" for many American families (Luker, 1984:158-191). Parenthood is now seen as a matter of choice. This has led to greater social and psychological pressure, for those who decide to become parents, to use every available technical option to ensure that the child is as nearly perfect as possible and will not be a burden to self, family, or society.

Within the next generation, early prenatal diagnosis within the first trimester of pregnancy will probably become routine, at least for private patients. This will keep most pregnancies and births firmly under medical control and will serve to reinforce most parents' trust in high technology. As Barbara Katz Rothman (1986:116-154) has shown, it will also fundamentally change the character or pregnancy by assigning sex and other discrete human characteristics to the fetus. Women who have had prenatal diagnosis become aware much earlier than others of the fetus as a distinct and separate being (Kolker and Burke, 1987:1). In the future, this awareness, together with technologies that permit the survival of ever smaller neonates, will lead to renewed social and ethical debates about how to balance the interests of the fetus with the autonomy of the mother, particularly in the last trimester. The attempts of some physicians to get court-ordered in-hospital births or Cesareans are only the beginning. In the future we will see court battles over whether society may confine pregnant women who do not follow accepted medical advice to control their use of drugs, alcohol, or diet in order to prevent damage to the fetus. Those who argue for such control will argue that the woman's right to choice ended with her choosing to carry the child to term. Once having made this choice, she is obligated to follow medical advice (as established by physicians) to make sure that the child has the optimal chance of being normal. The issues of women's autonomy, freedom of choice, and responsibility toward viable fetuses will be extremely difficult to resolve, and will only become more complex with the advent of new scientific discoveries.

New technologies not only raise new ethical debates about control over birth, but are rapidly making birth more expensive. In order to fulfill parents' desires for perfect children and to protect themselves from lawsuits, doctors are using more tests and procedures than ever before. The cost of "normal," vaginal birth is increasing so rapidly that any figures we provide will soon be out of date. The average in-hospital vaginal birth in 1986 cost approximately $3,500. Prenatal diagnosis, whether by amniocentesis or chorionic villus sampling, increased the cost by about $1,000. Cesarean birth costs roughly twice as much as vaginal birth, and the Cesarean rate now hovers around 18 percent (Placek et al., 1983:861–862). Within the near future, when the average vaginal birth costs $5,000, most parents will probably still consider this a "best buy." Doctors do not make money out of the extra procedures; most of the added costs go to hospitals, laboratories, or suppliers of equipment. In fact, the cost of birth has escalated out of the control of any one group, largely as a result of malpractice suits by parents whose children were less than perfect, even though (or sometimes because) they received maximum birth technology. Small wonder that "normal" birth is the medical procedure that tops the list, in terms of total dollars expended, for insurers of employees of some Fortune 500 companies. To control costs, one company has begun offering bonuses to women who volunteer to leave the hospital within two days after birth, but none has yet offered financial incentives to women who choose out-of-hospital birth (*Wall Street Journal*, November 16, 1983).

If in-hospital costs continue to increase, however, some employers may begin to encourage use of free-standing birth centers (FSBCs) in an attempt to keep their insurance premiums down. In 1982, for example, the average charge for hospital birth was $1,713, with a range from $550 to $3,750. FSBC charges in that year averaged only 47.7 percent of hospital charges for "comparable care,"meaning nonsurgical delivery (Cannoodt, 1982:4). Insurers have already begun to regard the FSBC as a financially attractive alternative. Of forty-nine birth centers surveyed, 69 percent reported reimbursement by one or more of forty-two commercial insurance companies; all reported payment by Blue Cross/Blue Shield, and 24 percent were reimbursed by Medicaid (*Cooperative Birth Center News*, 1983:4–8). It would be ironic of a movement begun for the purpose of creating a more natural and homelike environment for birth were to succeed primarily because it reduces companies' insurance premiums.

Today's parents say they want a humanized birth as well as a safe birth. For some, this means that the woman has total control over the entire process. Families who wish to retain this kind of control, or anything close to it, must usually choose to have births outside the hospital, preferably in their own homes. When confronted with the roles, rules, and rituals of the medical profession on its terms and on its turf, parturient women are forced to conform to the role of the sick patient. They surrender personal judgment to experts. Authority is transferred, symbolically and actually, as the consent form provided by the emergency room receptionist is signed.

For women who wish to retain control and whose worldview enables them to trust in nature even if something may go wrong, out-of-hospital birth is the logical alternative. In the future, home birth, nurse-midwifery, and lay midwifery will serve a small but increasing minority who believe that they can find both more humanity *and* greater safety (because drugs and other treatments and interventions that might harm the child are not given) in out-of-hospital birth. To do this, particularly with a home birth and lay midwife, requires courage and an unwavering determination to stand by one's own values.

Most families, however, will continue to use hospitals. As long as the husband or another person of the mother's choice is present, the mother is conscious, rooms are nicely decorated, and staff is pleasant, most women's requirements for a humanized birth will probably be satisfied. These requirements can be met even with continuous fetal monitoring or a "family-centered" Cesarean operation. The reorganization of many maternity wings into "birthing suites," where the woman labors and delivers in the same homelike room, has enabled hospitals to retain some clients who might otherwise have used free-standing birth centers. These women perceive that the reality of the American hospital, to whatever extent it denies the complexity of their experience in childbirth, cannot be wished away. Women in labor must, and do, relinquish control. Giving over control, however, makes childbirth less problematic in the sense that these parents are freed from responsibility for the outcome.

In the future, we will see several kinds of "turf battles" over birth. One will be in the area of professional control. Although obstetricians have long controlled birth, there is increasing consumer revolt and dissatisfaction. Furthermore, obstetricians' services have become too expensive for families who neither have insurance nor wish to use public clinics. As Light (1987) has shown for other professions, notably psychiatry versus lay therapy, wherever established, orthodox physicians have failed to satisfy large numbers of consumers or have priced themselves out of the market, new or fledgling professions have entered the field, captured a segment of the market, achieved legitimation either through licensure or court decisions, and eventually received third-party reimbursement, the final evidence of legitimation. If lay psychotherapists, chiropractors, and osteopaths have succeeded in their turf battles, lay midwives can do likewise. Lay midwives serve families who have found that in-hospital births or obstetrical services do not meet their needs. Lay midwives charge a fraction of obstetricians' charges and are almost never sued because their clients rarely blame them if something goes wrong. Nurse-midwives are in a more difficult situation because they tend to practice in medical settings and under physician control. They *are* sued (though the rate of suits is low compared to that of obstetricians) and recent increases in malpractice premiums have threatened the continued existence of the entire profession of nurse midwifery.

The second type of turf battle will be between different hospitals as they compete for private patients by advertising attractive frills, such as candlelit champagne dinners or personally monogrammed kimonos for the new parents. Hospitals now have too many maternity beds and too few private patients. The added frills serve to further polarize the two-class system of birth that divides private from clinic patients. The importance of this two-class system to the future of American birth cannot be overemphasized. The system means that, as Sandra K. Danziger and Margaret K. Nelson inform us, a woman's response to physicians is highly dependent on her location within the social structure. Her social position determines, in part, how much power she will have to effect change and how far-reaching that change will be. The two-class system also means that poor mothers are still more likely to have premature or low birthweight babies and have higher rates of maternal, neonatal, and infant mortality. Finally, this system means that poor women have fewer alternatives with regard to place of birth and provider. The freestanding birth center is most often, unfortunately, the province of the private or well-insured patient and not an alternative for the clinic patient.

For the present, we can expect the two mainstreams in American birth to continue. Childbirth will become increasingly technical. There will, concurrently, be a growing movement toward "humanization." What is needed to solve the incongruities in these apparently divergent trends is a new vision: a vision that combines excellent outcomes for the child with a truly woman-centered experience. To be successful, this new vision must overcome the unresolved disparities in the two-class system of care.

REFERENCES

Cannoodt, Luk J. "Alternatives to the Conventional In-Hospital Delivery: the Childbearing Center Experience." *Acta Hospitalia* 22(1982).

Cooperative Birth Center News 1(1983).

Kolker, Aliza, and Burke, B. Meredith. "Amniocentesis and the Social Construction of Pregnancy: Preliminary Findings." *Marriage and Family Review* 11(1987).

Light, Donald W. "Turf Battles Between Physicians and Competing Providers: Professional, Economic, and Organizational Interests," in Dorothy C. Wertz (ed.), *Research in the Sociology of Health Care* 7(1987). Westport, Ct.: JAI Press.

Luker, Kristin. *Abortion and the Politics of Motherhood.* Berkeley, Ca.: University of California Press, 1984.

Placek, Paul J.; Taffel, Selma; and Moren, Mary. "Cesarean Section Delivery Rates: United States, 1981." *American Journal of Public Health* 73 (1983).

Rothman, Barbara Katz. *The Tentative Pregnancy: Prenatal Diagnosis and the Future of Motherhood.* New York: Viking, 1986.

Zelizer, Viviana A. *Pricing the Priceless Child: The Changing Social Value of Children.* New York: Basic Books, 1985.

ABOUT THE CONTRIBUTORS
and
INDEX

About the Contributors

JANET CARLISLE BOGDAN has taught at Hobart and William Smith Colleges and at Syracuse University. She is currently completing her doctoral dissertation on "Childbirth in America."

SANDRA K. DANZIGER is a research associate at the Institute for Research on Poverty at the University of Wisconsin at Madison. She has published articles on childbirth in the *Journal of Human Resources*, the *American Journal of Public Health*, and *Social Science and Medicine*.

NANCY SCHROM DYE is an associate professor of history at the University of Kentucky. She has authored the book *As Equals and As Sisters: Feminism, the Labor Movement, and the Women's Trade Union League of New York* and published articles on childbirth, the history of women, and the American labor movement in *Feminist Studies*, the *Journal of American History*, the *Journal of Social History*, *Signs*, and the *Bulletin of the History of Medicine*.

PAMELA S. EAKINS is an adjunct scholar with the Center for Research on Women at Stanford University and a public policy analyst studying the free-standing birth center movement at the School of Public Health, University of California at Los Angeles. She is president and cofounder of the California Association of Free-Standing Birth Centers and consults on women's health and professional liability for California State legislators. She is also former

341

director of a free-standing birth center and author of *Mothers in Transition*.

MYRA GERSON GILFIX is an attorney in private practice in Palo Alto, California. She has authored several articles on informed consent, technology in childbirth, and medical malpractice that have appeared in *ICEA News*, the *American Journal of Law and Medicine*, and the *Brain Trauma Quarterly*.

LINDA JANET HOLMES is an assistant professor of nurse-midwifery at the University of Medicine and Dentistry of New Jersey. She has published several articles on women and health and is currently producing a film on traditional midwifery practices.

DEBORAH LEVEEN is an associate professor of urban studies and public administration at San Francisco State University. She has written on protest movements and social change and has recently served on the Alternative Birthing Methods Study Committee for the State of California.

MARGARET K. NELSON is an associate professor of sociology at Middlebury College in Vermont. She has published a number of articles on pregnancy and childbirth and is currently investigating the provision of family day care as an occupation for women.

ANN OAKLEY is deputy director of the Thomas Coram Research Unit of the University of London Institute of Education. She is the author of *Women Confined*, *Becoming a Mother*, *The Captured Womb*, and numerous other works on childbirth.

WENDA BREWSTER O'REILLY is executive director of The Birth Place Childbirth and Resource Centers in Menlo Park, California. She is also an adjunct scholar at Stanford University's Center for Research on Women. Dr. O'Reilly is the author of *The Beautiful Body Book*.

GARY A. RICHWALD is an assistant professor in the School of Public Health at the University of California at Los Angeles. He is the medical director at Los Angeles Childbirth Center and has written several articles on childbirth.

BARBARA KATZ ROTHMAN is an associate professor of sociology at Baruch College and at the Graduate Center of the City University of New York. She has authored *In Labor: Women and Power in the Birthplace* (entitled *Giving Birth* in paperback) and *The Tentative Pregnancy: Prenatal Diagnosis and the Future of Motherhood*.

DIANA SCULLY is an associate professor of sociology at Virginia Commonwealth University in Richmond. Dr. Scully is the author of *Men Who Control Women's Health*.

PAMELA S. SUMMEY is a Ph.D. candidate at the State University of New York at Stony Brook. She is completing her thesis on "Ideology and Obstetrical Care," and has published several articles on Cesarean delivery and the history of obstetrics.

REGI L. TEASLEY has taught at Hobart and William Smith Colleges. Her doctoral work concerned the structure of the practice of midwifery. Currently, she is working in applied sociology in health care in Ithaca, New York.

DOROTHY C. WERTZ is an associate research professor at the School of Public Health at Boston University. She has authored *Lying-In: A History of Childbirth in America* (with Richard Wertz) and numerous articles on childbirth and genetic counseling.

Index